The Medical Mandarins

The Medical Mandarins

The French Academy of Medicine in the Nineteenth and Early Twentieth Centuries

GEORGE WEISZ

McGill University

New York   Oxford
OXFORD UNIVERSITY PRESS
1995

Oxford University Press

Oxford   New York
Athens   Auckland   Bangkok   Bombay
Calcutta   Cape Town   Dar es Salaam   Delhi
Florence   Hong Kong   Istanbul   Karachi
Kuala Lumpur   Madras   Madrid   Melbourne
Mexico City   Nairobi   Paris   Singapore
Taipei   Tokyo   Toronto

and associated companies in
Berlin   Ibadan

Library of Congress Cataloging-in-Publication Data
Weisz, George.
The medical mandarins : the French Academy of Medicine in
the nineteenth and early twentieth centuries /
George Weisz.
p.   cm.   Includes bibliographical references and index.
ISBN 0-19-509037-3
1. Académie de médecine (France)—History—19th century.
2. Académie de médecine (France)—History—20th century.
3. Medicine—France—Societies, etc.—History—19th century.
4. Medicine—France—Societies, etc.—History—20th century.
I. Title.   [DNLM: 1. Académie de médecine (France)
2. Societies, Medical—history—France.
WB 1 GF7 P2A2W 1995]
R504.W45   1995   610'.6'044—dc20   DNLM/DLC   for Library of Congress   94-12531

1 3 5 7 9 8 6 4 2

Printed in the United States of America
on acid-free paper

For Zeeva

Acknowledgments

In the course of working on this book, I have accumulated many intellectual debts. First of all, I would like to thank Jack Ellis, Matthew Ramsey, and Charles Rosenberg for reading an earlier and much longer draft of the manuscript. Their thoughtful comments forced me to rethink some of my basic assumptions. In addition to providing me with an unusually congenial and stimulating intellectual environment within which to work, my colleagues in the Department of Social Studies of Medicine—Don Bates, Alberto Cambrosio, Margaret Lock, Faith Wallis, and Alan Young—read and discussed some of the papers and articles whose contents were incorporated in this book. Christophe Charle was generous with his knowledge of the fine points of prosopographical research in France; he and Nancy Davenport were also kind enough to share unpublished research materials with me.

Over the years, I have benefited from the work of outstanding research assistants. It is a particular pleasure to thank Donna Evleth, Don Fyson, and Elsbeth Heaman, all of whom have become fine historians in their own right. Sovita Chander and Harvey Blackman provided able editorial assistance.

The research for this book would not have been possible without the help of the staffs at several libraries. I especially wish to thank the librarians at the Académie de Médecine and at the Osler Library, Health Sciences Library, and Humanities and Social Sciences Library of McGill University.

It is a pleasure to acknowledge financial support for necessary research from the Social Sciences and Research Council of Canada, the Hannah Institute for the History of Medicine, and the Graduate Faculty of McGill University. A pleasant and stimulating semester spent as a fellow of the Camargo Institute in Cassis, France, resulted in rough drafts of two chapters in this book.

A number of chapters are based on previously published articles that have been extensively revised for this book. Permission to reproduce materials from these articles was granted by the *Bulletin for the History of Medicine*, *Medical History* (Copyright The Trustee, The Wellcome Trust), and John Libbey Eurotext.

My most heartfelt thanks go my family, who put up with the intense work necessary to research and write a book of this sort. Since I could not be coaxed away from my computer, my children, Talia and Jonathan, took to writing stories on their own computer, which was a few feet away from mine. I hope that their memories of these moments are as sweet as mine. To Zeeva, who has been my partner and companion for these many years, I dedicate this book.

Contents

Abbreviations

AGM	*Archives générales de médecine*
AM	Archives of the Academy of Medicine
AN	Archives Nationales
AP	Archives de Paris
BAM	*Bulletin de l'Académie de Médecine*
Bull. Soc. fr. hist. méd.	*Bulletin de la Société française d'histore de la médecine*
CRAS	*Comptes rendus de l'Académie des Sciences*
JGM	*Journal général de médecine*
MEM	*Mémoires de l'Académie de Médecine*

N.B.: All French sources listed in the notes were published in Paris unless indicated otherwise.

Between 1808 and 1914, 100 French francs were worth roughly 4 pounds sterling and 18.5 U.S. dollars.

Introduction

Throughout much of the Western world in the early eighteenth century, institutional medical power was vested in a multitude of regional corporate elites; by the end of the nineteenth century, it was wielded by national elites whose power derived from the control of key institutions—notably medical schools, hospitals, licensing bodies, public health agencies, and national academies or their equivalents. In England corporate elites adapted to new conditions and gradually transformed themselves into an elite of the modern type.[1] In France, however, this process occurred with remarkable rapidity and involved far greater discontinuity between old and new elites. Political intervention, moreover, consistently played a decisive role. In many ways it was the state, in the form of successive governments of markedly different political stripes, that created the medical elite and the modern profession of medicine in France.

It was the state that, during the decade of the French Revolution, set up a system of medical education that soon became the locus of elite medical power. In 1820 the government of Restoration France established the Royal Academy of Medicine as the primary instrument of its public health policy. This new institution brought together hitherto disparate medical specialties as well as the assorted institutional elites that had come into being since the French Revolution. It served as the major medical advisory body to the government on health-related matters, while at the same time functioning as the primary arbiter of new medical knowledge. It evaluated medical and scientific writings, awarded prizes in annual competitions, collected and examined epidemiological information, administered smallpox vaccinations, supervised secret remedies and mineral waters, and frequently provided the government with expert knowledge on health-related issues. The academy, it is true, in many ways failed to fulfill initial expectations. Nevertheless, it was by international standards a unique medical institution, enjoying a remarkable degree of responsibility and prestige.[2]

The institutional significance of the academy is not, however, the sole reason I have chosen to make the first century of its existence the subject of this book. The academy was implicated in virtually every aspect of French medical life in the nineteenth and early twentieth centuries. Little of significance occurred in the science, practice, or politics of medicine that was not in some way reflected in its activities, deliberations, or internal structures. Consequently, the academy provides a uniquely strategic location from which to observe the development of French medicine more generally.

The fact that the academy extended into so many areas of French medical and social life creates a unique set of problems for the historian. There is, on the one hand, a complex institutional history to recount. At the same time, nearly every form of academic activity raises broader issues fundamental to the history of French medicine. Although one cannot explore in detail all the subjects raised, one can certainly select a small number for extended discussion. Such issues constitute an integral part of the academy's history; they do not, however, fit neatly into the framework of conventional institutional narrative.

The need to reconcile these differing imperatives has dictated a less than conventional narrative structure for this book. Part I attempts to provide a history of the academy and its major activities from 1820 to 1939. The next two parts, while concerned with the academy's institutional history, also use the institution as a window to explore broader issues. Part II examines a number of rather different academic activities relating to medical science. Part III uses both qualitative and quantitative research methods to explore the nature of elitism and hierarchy in French medicine.

Chapter 1 examines the creation of the academy in 1820. The campaign to establish an academy is recounted in the context of efforts to either dominate or overturn the elite medical institutions created after the French Revolution. The academy that was finally fashioned brought together, for a time at least, the various conflicting elite factions, though it did little to mitigate the intense professional conflicts characteristic of French medical life. My account underscores the tensions generated by a system of centralized medical stratification conferring enormous status and power on a Parisian elite. It also emphasizes the will of successive governments to temper the ambitions of academicians and to limit the academy to a technical advisory role.

Chapters 2 through 5 focus on the institutional structures and activities of the academy. To better describe long-term developments, I have eschewed a chronological narrative in favor of a thematic treatment that describes the evolution of different structures and activities during the institution's first century. Chapter 2 examines the academy's administrative arrangements and physical setting. I emphasize, in particular, that during the course of the nineteenth century the academy evolved from a broadly based medical institution to a narrower academy of professors. This shift was, in part, a consequence of academicians' burning desire to raise their relatively low-status institution to a level closer to that of the more prestigious Academy of Sciences. Despite their desire to emulate scientists, a close look at the associate members of the Academy of Medicine suggests that the nonmedical scientific elite was gradually excluded from that institution as the worlds of elite medicine and elite science increasingly drifted apart.

Chapters 3 and 4 enlarge on the theme of the academy's gradual transformation by describing the evolution of its major functions. These functions can be divided into two overlapping categories: the presentation and evaluation of the results of medical science and the provision of public health expertise to state authorities. Each of the activities was associated with specific textual genres—reports, debates, oral

presentations, academic eulogies—and each went through its own specific development, whose natural history will be examined in detail. A common thread in my
narrative is the twentieth-century decline in the evaluative scientific functions of the
academy and the growing magnitude of its public health and professional interventions. Closely connected with this shift is the evolution of the academy from an
institution suffering from relatively low public status while still serving a pivotal intellectual role for the medical profession to one that had by the twentieth century
become a recognized part of the public "establishment" while losing its central intellectual position in French medicine.

Chapter 5 examines the role of the academy in representing the self-images and
historical memories of the Parisian academic elite. I first discuss the spatial disposition of works of art in the institution, suggesting that the effort to concretely embody
medical history within its walls was severely constrained by academicians' lack of
control over artistic elements that were donated in most instances. I next discuss the
variety of academic eulogies presented in that institution. Within these genres, the
functions of social representation and collective memory coexisted with elaborate
scientific evaluation. I argue that this unstable combination gradually fell apart as scientific evaluation came to predominate in the early twentieth century.

Part II returns to specific academic genres in order to more fully explore certain
aspects of clinical science. Underlying these studies is the notion that, rather than
being an "art" gradually transformed by laboratory science, clinical medicine in its
elite spheres involved continuous efforts to create a distinctive applied science of
medicine. It developed its own indigenous scientific practices, like clinical examination and postmortem dissection, and borrowed procedures liberally from other
scientific and, occasionally, administrative domains. The results were frequently un-
satisfactory because the problems dealt with were complex and the extent to which
borrowed procedures were valid for medical science had to be laboriously worked
out. Like other scientific domains, clinical medicine had areas and activities that were
deeply influenced by institutional, social, and professional realities and "interests,"
several of which are explored. But unless one also recognizes that the medical elite
was deeply committed to the development of medical science as a rigorous intellectual activity and not just as a rhetorical device to raise the status of the medical
profession, one will overlook an essential aspect of the academy's history.

Chapter 6 explores the academy's central role in the administration and scientific
study of spas and mineral waters in France. In so doing, it raises the issue of the
therapeutic specificity of French medicine in comparison with that of North America. I argue that the continuing popularity of water therapy in France can partly be
explained by the historical commitment of the Parisian medical elite. Until the 1920s,
the academy played a predominant role both in administering the system of spas and,
perhaps more important, in helping to formulate a science of hydrology that legiti-
mized water cures. Academic hydrology embodied many of the difficulties faced by
all "clinical" sciences, but it was distinguished by its close association with the administrative needs of the state and with the economic interests of a growing capitalist
industry. I also suggest that academic hydrology contributed to "medicalizing" the
water cure in France to a far greater degree than was the case elsewhere. The roles
of chemistry and, in the twentieth century, physiology in academic hydrology pro-

vide illuminating perspectives on the complex relationship between laboratory science and clinical medicine.

The interpretations offered in this chapter come close to "social constructionist" tendencies in the sociology and history of science. While such perspectives are indispensable for the analysis of certain subjects, they are not the only ones possible. I take a rather different approach to medical knowledge in Chapter 7, which examines a number of debates about therapeutic innovations that erupted in the academy during the middle decades of the nineteenth century, the golden age of academic debating. My goal here is to better understand both therapeutic reasoning and the way clinical "facts" were constructed during this critical period in the history of medicine, when traditional notions of disease as disequilibrium of bodily elements coexisted uneasily with newer doctrines of organic localism, as well as techniques of pathological anatomy, physiological and chemical experimentation, and clinical statistics. My discussion calls into question a number of common historical assumptions about Parisian medicine of this period relating to the supposed dominance of therapeutic nihilism, hostility to therapeutic innovation, and opposition to clinical statistics. More important, I document the problematical process of constructing "facts" in the messy arena of clinical medicine and scrutinize the various strategies that could be used to negotiate or impose a consensus. My discussion also points to the ways in which the academy was able to influence medical perceptions of innovation.

Academic judgment and evaluation could sometimes blend into another characteristic form of scientific activity, namely, the production of historical myth. Chapter 8 analyzes this process in detail by examining the posthumous reputation of René-Théophile-Hyacinthe Laënnec, inventor of mediate auscultation and perhaps the most famous representative of Parisian clinical medicine of the early nineteenth century. My account begins and ends in the academy, which played a central role in the construction of Laënnec's reputation, but it places academic judgments in a larger context by examining the many individuals and institutions that also contributed to Laënnec's emergence as an emblematic hero of medicine. I argue that during the half century following his death Laënnec evolved from the inventor of auscultation to the man who had associated pathological anatomy with clinical medicine, and finally to the founder of the Paris school of medicine and the greatest French physician of the nineteenth century. In the twentieth-century academy, I suggest, he came to represent and justify a tradition of clinical medicine linked to pathological anatomy that had been rendered somewhat old-fashioned by the experimental laboratory. My discussion thus touches on the way in which Laënnec's posthumous reputation in the twentieth century intersected with those of Claude Bernard and Louis Pasteur. I argue that the evolution of Laënnec's reputation occurred as various groups in search of precursors and emblematic heroes linked their own fortunes to that of the inventor of auscultation.

Part III examines the Parisian medical elite from a number of different perspectives. During the past two centuries no aspect of French medicine has generated more controversy than the career structures responsible for profound stratification and polarization within the profession. These structures have been attacked repeatedly for being inegalitarian and divisive and for seriously impairing the ability of French medicine to respond to the exigencies of medical science.[3] I do not attempt to evaluate such criticisms; rather, I seek to better understand the medical elite produced by these career patterns.

Chapter 9 describes how this elite looked from the inside in the early nineteenth century. It scrutinizes the academic eulogies of the academy's first permanent secretary, Etienne Pariset,[4] with a view to understanding the social imagery embedded in them. My discussion refers back to the eulogies of the eighteenth century in order to understand both traditional and innovative elements in Pariset's utilization of a rich array of images and metaphors; these images portrayed a medical elite that had only recently attained prominence and saw itself in some of the metaphorical terms characteristic of economic, political, and military life. I emphasize the theme of the academician as "self-made man," which stands out in high relief, alongside topoi of military and political courage. There is also a rich and complex vocabulary of medical virtue that Pariset manipulated adroitly.

Chapters 10 and 11 utilize prosopographical analysis of the membership of the academy to explore from the outside the meaning of elite medical status in Paris. Chapter 10 focuses on the evolving nature of elite careers represented in the academy. It documents the increasing career uniformity centering on the system of competitive examinations (*concours*) that came to predominate among academicians and elite doctors more generally. A study of the role of the Academy of Sciences in elite medical careers further develops the theme of the growing chasm between medical and scientific elites in Paris.

Chapter 11 attempts to situate elite medical status within the larger social world of the French bourgeoisie. Basing my argument on various data (social origins, marriage patterns, wealth, and place of residence) I suggest that the medical elite, which had been somewhat isolated socially in the early nineteenth century, ascended rapidly into the higher echelons of the French bourgeoisie in the last years of the century. In the early decades of the twentieth century there was a retreat into a more narrowly medical milieu, which I suggest reflected the intensely competitive and absorbing character of elite medical careers. But there is no indication that this affected the economic and social status of the by now well entrenched and quite wealthy medical elite.

It should be readily apparent that no grand theoretical design lies behind the various chapters of this book. I do not, for instance, present the academy in Foucauldian terms as a producer of "discourses" and "disciplines" which brought increasingly large sectors of social life under medical authority. Nor do I use the academy to illustrate the "professionalization" of French medicine or the way in which medical science is "socially constructed." Each of these approaches neglects most of what I regard as significant and illuminating about the academy's history. I have chosen instead to be guided by the rich source materials which the academy provides the historian. While my choice of sources and subjects undoubtedly reflects my specific intellectual preoccupations, I nonetheless see this book as an exercise in historical exploration rather than as an effort to elucidate a particular thesis.

The specific questions posed and the sources at the historian's disposal have dictated the methodologies used in the different chapters. Some chapters seek to piece together a coherent historical narrative from the fragmented archival record and published materials. Others use techniques of collective biography pioneered by social historians in France. A number of chapters have been deeply influenced by recent work in the sociology of science. And if I am profoundly irritated by much of the literary theorizing that is applied to historical analysis, throughout this work I have sought to treat my sources as complex textual productions in their own right and not just as raw materials to be mined selectively. The starting point of my research has been the assumption that a multifaceted institution like the academy can be grasped only through multiple perspectives and methodologies. Thus I have deliberately chosen to bring together social, cultural, and medical history.

For all my interest in the larger issues of medical history, the Academy of Medicine is very much *the* subject of this book. The fact that I have been able to roam relatively widely and can so easily envisage radically different narrative treatments reflects nothing so much as the variety and richness of this institution's history. I hope that I have conveyed at least some of this wealth and diversity in the pages that follow.

NOTES

1. This, at least, is the argument advanced by Jeanne Peterson in *The Medical Profession in Mid-Victorian London* (Berkeley, Calif., 1978).

2. Although there exists no good historical study of the academy, one can read with profit Paul Ganière, *L'Académie de Médecine: ses origines et son histoire* (1964) and the collective volume *Centenaire de l'Académie de Médecine, 1820–1920* (1921).

3. George Weisz, "Reform and Conflict in French Medical Education, 1870–1914," in *The Organization of Science and Technology in France, 1808–1914*, ed. Robert Fox and George Weisz (Cambridge, 1980).

4. Although the surname "Etienne" is now written with an accent over the first "E," usage was fluid in the early nineteenth century and Pariset himself consistently wrote it without the accent. I have followed his usage.

I

THE ACADEMIC INSTITUTION

1

Creating the French Royal Academy of Medicine

The creation of the Academy of Medicine in 1820 did more than bring yet another Parisian medical institution into existence. It was a major and perhaps the final step in a process begun during the French Revolution leading to the formation of a national medical elite in France. Like other stages in this lengthy process, the establishment of the academy was part of a struggle for power to define and control the medical domain.

The final four decades of the ancien régime were instrumental in setting the pattern for extensive state intervention in health care. Recent historical work has emphasized continuities between postrevolutionary medicine and that of the ancien régime.[1] Such continuities, however, should not obscure the massive institutional transformations that were set in motion after 1789. These unfolded in a gradual way over the course of the next half century. The years 1794–1803 saw the establishment of a state system of medical education and licensing. In 1820 the state's role in health care was further extended when the government of Restoration France established the Royal Academy of Medicine as the primary instrument of its public health policy. This new institution brought together hitherto separate medical specialties as well as the diverse institutional elites that had sprung up since the French Revolution.

The process leading to the creation of the academy reflected the growing determination of successive governments since the eighteenth century to expand and consolidate the role of the state in public health and medical care. Events also reflected the intense competition among medical groups, both old and new, for the right to represent and profit from this growing state authority. In the pages that follow I shall first analyze the system of professional and institutional power which emerged from the dislocation of revolution. I shall go on to describe the unsuccessful campaign from 1814 to 1817 that attempted to end the domination of the postrevolutionary elite by effecting a separation between medicine and surgery. This is

3

followed by an examination of the process which led to the establishment of the Royal Academy of Medicine in 1820; the process, I shall argue, was in large measure a continuation of the struggle for medical supremacy begun in 1814. Finally, we shall see the way the struggle was resolved or at least abandoned *within* the academy during the early years of that institution's existence. This resolution set the limits of the academy's future role.

The Medical Domain

As in so many other spheres, the Revolution of 1789 brought a new degree of centralization to the medical domain in France. Despite a general movement toward more centralized forms of authority, medical institutions of the eighteenth century had remained highly fragmented among conflicting corporate groups. Rather than referring to a single medical domain, one must speak of several, each with its own practices, cognitive foundations, and forms of authority.

Professional authority during the ancien régime was extremely dispersed, partly following traditional guild divisions and partly as a result of the government's penchant for creating institutions as new needs arose or as the performance of existing institutions was judged inadequate.[2] "Regular" medical practitioners were divided into three types of professional guilds—medicine, surgery, and pharmacy—each with its separate institutional structures. Medical jurisdiction was also fragmented along regional lines, with the authority of each institution confined to a limited geographical area. Both licensing powers and disciplinary authority over member practitioners were vested in these corporate institutions. The king, moreover, could authorize any practitioner, whatever his credentials, to practice in Paris by naming him to the court medical staff, which itself constituted a major source of institutional power in medicine.[3]

Physicians were licensed and more or less educated in nineteen faculties and fifteen colleges of medicine located throughout the kingdom. The former awarded diplomas, although fewer than half provided instruction on a regular basis. Colleges offered limited instruction but could not award degrees. It was ordinarily necessary to become an *agrégé* of either type of institution in order to practice within the area of its jurisdiction. Since the main function of both types of corporate guilds was to control professional privileges within a jurisdiction, corporate conflict over monopolies was widespread.

Apprenticeship of one sort or another remained the primary form of training for most surgeons and pharmacists; but they were increasingly being educated in programs of study organized in guildlike colleges of surgery or in the course of extended hospital service. In order to practice within a jurisdiction, they had to be admitted to one of four hundred surgical communities. The existence of relatively autonomous hospital training provoked further tensions. To complicate matters still more, lectures and instruction useful to future practitioners of medicine and surgery were available privately and in a wide variety of institutions including the Collège du Roi and Jardin du Roi.

Authority over the development of medical science was gradually being displaced from the Paris Faculty of Medicine (not without noisy protest) to state institutions of science that contained large numbers of doctors, like the Academy of Sciences. Authority over public health was in the hands of local officials and, increasingly, the central government. Bewildered by the complexity of most issues, these were becoming more and more dependent on medical experts in various medical and scientific institutions. Hospitals were controlled by religious orders and local political authorities; within them, the role of medical practitioners, particularly surgeons, was becoming significant although their authority remained limited.

The eighteenth century saw increasing, if still tentative, governmental efforts to reorganize the health domain under state bureaucratic control. The Edict of Marly (1707), while ratifying the existence of medical corporations, tried to introduce greater uniformity in the requirements for provincial medical degrees.[4] Surgery after 1720 was significantly consolidated (and its status raised) in the hands of the King's First Surgeon; teaching chairs in surgery were established by the state at the Paris College of Surgery (1724); a Royal Academy of Surgery was created in 1731 to advance practical knowledge, and a royal declaration of 1743 required candidates for the Parisian surgical mastership to take an arts degree from a French university.[5] A parallel effort in 1732 by the Kings's First Physician, Pierre Chirac, to bring greater unity to medicine by creating an Academy of Medicine ended in failure.[6] But the state bureaucracy's need for technical expertise, which expanded quite substantially during the last decades of the century, led to the establishment in 1776 of the Société Royale de Médecine (also led by members of the court medical service) and the centralization in its hands of many traditional research and public health tasks.[7] It was patterned after the several royal academies established since the seventeenth century in order to organize scientific and cultural life under royal patronage and control;[8] it embodied a statist rather than corporate conception of medicine and provoked the intense hostility of the Paris Faculty of Medicine.

Behind the effort to expand the state's role in medical care was the vision of a reorganized medical domain at once unified and oriented toward public health. Such concern with the health of populations was characteristic of most European nations and was justified by a set of policies that characterized monarchical despotism and that have come to be known as cameralism or mercantilism; these sought to increase the productive capacities of the nation through direct state intervention.[9] Prussia and Austria were, in fact, considerably ahead of France in laying the groundwork for a comprehensive reorganization of public health.[10] In France the scope of public health seems to have been defined primarily by the existence of traditional areas of public intervention: epidemics, health care programs for the destitute, the licensing of secret remedies and mineral waters. The Enlightenment belief in reason and human perfectibility together with the expansion of the state bureaucracy added new dynamism to traditional notions of health "police." It also added new themes like hospital reform, training for midwives, and special care for the insane.[11] Toward the end of the eighteenth century, spokesmen for medicine and the state administration began popularizing reform programs to rationalize these activities with the aid of science and affirming the powers of the state at the expense of traditional corporate groups.[12] As Keith Baker has perceptively suggested, the state's need for scientific expertise during the late ancien régime was not merely instrumental; scientific expertise provided powerful legitimation for expanded bureaucratic authority.[13]

A key aspect of the public health program was the creation of institutions to produce, coordinate, and sanction new medical knowledge, as both the Société Royale
de Médecine and Académie Royale de Chirurgie had attempted to do. There was no
sharp distinction between research and public health in the minds of medical reformers of the era. The association of the two tasks would apply to medicine the
pattern established in the Academy of Sciences which combined the production and
sanctioning of knowledge with the provision of technological expertise to the state.
Improving the people's health required major advances in medical science, as it demanded a body of experts to choose, from among the contradictory welter of medical
systems and opinions, principles of administrative action. Simultaneously, the production of new knowledge was dependent on reorganizing the medical profession
into a huge network of information collection, the results of which were to be processed, analyzed, and eventually applied by a Parisian elite. This was the reasoning
behind the establishment by the Société Royale de Médecine of a network of over a
thousand provincial correspondents making use of channels of royal bureaucracy to
send observations and information to Paris.

In the course of the French Revolution, this institutional system was largely
swept away. The new one established piecemeal during the following decade, after a
brief experiment with unregulated practice, owed much (including some of its key
personnel) to the ancien régime; in many ways it carried eighteenth-century tendencies to their logical conclusion, but it was notably streamlined, with power becoming
concentrated in the hands of representatives of the state. Hospitals in each city were
consolidated under the jurisdiction of local administrations.[14] Only three state-run
schools of medicine (called "faculties" after 1803 and integrated into the Imperial
University in 1808) could offer complete training to all future doctors of medicine
and surgery. The diplomas they granted also served as licenses to practice throughout the nation. Disciplinary authority over the profession, previously vested in
corporate bodies, was never fully restored. Authority over both public health and
the advancement of medical science was included among the responsibilities of the
medical faculties, particularly the Paris Faculty of Medicine, which, to better cope
with these tasks, was permitted by the government to establish an academic society
around itself by adding thirty-two associate and adjunct members.[15]

Prerogatives this vast were in many respects unenforceable. A variety of institutions sprang up to fill the many gaps in the faculties' activity. Since provincial
medical elites insisted on offering courses of medical training, informal schools centering on the local hospitals developed in many cities. Their precise function within
the official system was a subject of some dispute until the 1820s, but they were primarily occupied with the training of low-level *officiers de santé* meant to work in the
rural countryside. Departmental juries, made up of faculty professors and representatives of the local medical profession, examined and licensed *officiers* and other
low-level practitioners such as midwives. They also played a minor and not always
satisfactory role in regulating local practice by inspecting pharmacies and combating
illegal practice.

In the three faculty cities, Paris, Montpellier, and Strasbourg, a variety of private
teaching institutions sprang up to remedy the manifest inadequacies of faculty teaching. Private instruction in Paris was especially rich and diversified. After 1811 the

Parisian hospitals began playing a significant role in medical education by offering courses. Hospitals everywhere, moreover, developed internships and externships (akin to clerkships in British hospitals) which provided the brightest medical students, chosen by public competitions, with invaluable practical training and experience. Through this institution, education for the future medical elite became centered in the hospital rather than in faculty courses. Military physicians and surgeons were also trained in an autonomous system of military hospitals, despite faculty efforts to share in this role.[16]

Medical research of one sort or another took place in a variety of teaching and therapeutic institutions. But only the Paris Faculty of Medicine and the Academy of Sciences could claim *formal* authority to direct and validate the search for new medical knowledge. Similarly, from the purely juridical standpoint, the faculty monopoly over education and licensing was more or less complete, even if unenforceable.

In the public health and sanitation spheres, administrative responsibilities were badly defined because of conflicting ministerial jurisdictions and because of the multiplicity of functional and regional bodies concerned with such matters.[17] But the state at least attempted to direct activities in a wide variety of spheres and was in constant need of technical expertise. The various ministries playing a role in the health sector were largely dependent on the advice of the Paris Faculty of Medicine. The faculty, in fact, was regularly bombarded with requests for information and advice about epidemics, epizootics, secret remedies, and mineral waters; other requests came from judges, prefects, and local authorities.[18] Professors were sent on missions to study epidemics in the provinces and abroad. In 1805–6 the Ministry of the Interior established a network of epidemic doctors distributed throughout the country. Incumbents were expected to direct medical work in the event of epidemic outbreaks and, in the aftermath, to submit reports that were to be studied by the Paris faculty.[19] The administrators of hospitals and dispensaries frequently called upon the faculty to recommend physicians for medical appointments.[20]

All this activity created enormous strain on the faculty's resources. Consequently, by the end of the Empire there arose, among both administrators and professors, the idea of transforming the Society of the Faculty into a larger and better endowed society along the lines of the old Société Royale de Médecine and Académie Royale de Chirurgie.

The task of advancing medical knowledge was in some respects even more of a problem. The Faculty of Paris counted some of the best known medical scientists in the world among its staff. However, neither the faculty nor its society appeared particularly successful *as institutions* in either stimulating and directing medical research or resolving the many doctrinal disputes characteristic of this period. Its monthly bulletin was exceedingly thin and was distributed as a supplement to another medical journal. To contemporaries, the activities of the society did not seem very significant in view of the enormous power and resources at the faculty's disposal.[21]

The predominance of the Faculty of Medicine, it must be emphasized, was vehemently opposed by many segments of the medical profession. In 1797–98, for instance, the school of Paris was violently criticized in legislative debates concerning the future reform of medicine. The legislature's Commission of Public Instruction proposed to introduce a far more decentralized system, making the advancement of science uniquely a responsibility of the Institut de France (which included the Academy of Sciences), and cutting back significantly on the Paris faculty's resources, staff, and facilities.[22]

In 1801 representatives of the defunct Académie Royale de Chirurgie announced to the new first consul, Napoleon Bonaparte, that they were resuming their activities, and they requested official governmental "protection and succour" as well as a return to the corporate divisions of the ancien régime.[23] That same year, the very progressive Société de Médecine de Paris responded to Napoleon's invitation to submit a proposal on methods of combating charlatanism by insisting on the necessity of reestablishing medical corporations "freed of their ancient abuses and of everything that could offend the constitution. . . ." These corporations or colleges had to be numerous enough to ensure that current medical anarchy not be replaced by "a no less dangerous aristocracy; that henceforth, no form of despotism weighs down on citizens who cultivate the art of healing, not even that of talent which is not the least dangerous."[24]

The government of the Empire ignored these arguments. Accepting the views of such political figures as Jean-Antoine Chaptal, François Fourcroy, and Pierre Cabanis, it opted for a unified profession and administrative centralization. It seems to have been motivated by the prevailing beliefs that (1) a single medical science now underlay all forms of medical practice; (2) the faculty really did represent the elite of medical science and practice; and (3) the government's need for expert information could be met with greater ease by a centralized institution like the Society of the Faculty than by a number of distinct corporations.[25]

Consequently, the authority of the School of Paris grew enormously during the first years of the Empire. The law regulating medical practice in 1803 accorded the faculties a monopoly over the granting of the doctorate. It was widely recognized that both medical education and the organization of the profession needed drastic overhauling. But the government generally appointed Parisian professors to the commissions discussing reforms.[26] It is thus not surprising that opponents of the faculty abandoned the strategy of direct assault. Until 1814 they waited for better days or sought to establish themselves in areas where the faculties' hold was weak. Most important for our purposes, a number of medical societies set themselves up as unofficial competitors of the Society of the Faculty and sought to win official recognition from the government.

Medical societies, which began to proliferate after 1796, represented above all the attempt at reorganization by medical groups that had lost their traditional corporate structures during the Revolution. Some were concerned predominantly with professional affairs; others, notably the Société Médicale d'Émulation, were primarily interested in advancing medical knowledge. Two in particular brought together many of those seeking to challenge the powers of the Paris Faculty of Medicine.

The Société de Médecine de Paris was the first medical society established after the Revolution (1796). Many of its founding members had formerly been members of either the Société Royale de Médecine or the Académie Royale de Chirurgie and viewed the new society as the legitimate successor to these institutions. It maintained regular contacts with authorities, especially those of the Paris region, on all matters relating to public health and occasionally sent commissions to study epidemics. It offered free consultations to the poor and became closely linked with the semiofficial Commission of Vaccination founded a few years later. It sought to advance medical science by offering prizes for written works and published the distinguished *Journal général de médecine française et étrangère*. By 1801 it had 444 members and 100 correspondents.[27]

The society played a significant public health role in the Paris region by acting as technical adviser to the prefect of the Seine, yet it was not taken seriously by the central government. In fact, Napoleon's 1801 request for ideas promoting the repression of charlatanism provoked the society to scarcely concealed euphoria. After years of being completely ignored by the government, the society stated in its response, the first consul had finally "consecrated its legal existence."[28] Its suggestions, as we saw, were not implemented, and the society appears to have concentrated exclusively on its scientific and public health activities until the fall of the Empire.

A second society, the Académie de Médecine de Paris, was founded in September 1804 by a group of regent-doctors of the eighteenth-century Faculty of Medicine, including the famous Joseph Guillotin, who had headed the health commission established by the National Constituent Assembly in 1790–91.[29] The society's stated goal was to bring doctors together in order to raise the status of medical practice. The choice of the name "Académie" reflected its pretension to semiofficial status. At its second meeting, in fact, it passed a motion requesting the emperor to grant it the title Académie Impériale de Médecine.[30] Its request was ignored and it was soon forced to change its name to the less official-sounding Société Académique. Its membership was dominated by members of the defunct faculty; it admitted the graduates of the postrevolutionary schools of medicine but deprived them of influence by setting up an elaborate system of hierarchical distinctions.

Although it performed several useful activities, offering, for instance, free medical consultations to the poor, its chief goal seems to have been the restoration of the corporate trappings and privileges of the old faculty. At an early meeting, it was decided that disciplinary surveillance over members would be maintained.[31] In this way, it was seeking to reestablish corporate powers by extralegal means and was insinuating itself into the realm of professional discipline where the vacuum created by the Revolution had never been filled. In a variety of public statements, representatives of the society admitted that their goal was to raise from the ashes the old Faculty of Medicine.[32] This ambition, however, was undermined by internal dissension. From 1809 to 1811 the society split.[33] A splinter group led by Antoine Portal of the Collège de France seceded from the parent Société Académique to create the Cercle Médical, a name Portal chose after being denied permission by the government to use the title Académie de Médecine and to exercise disciplinary power over members.[34]

The failed efforts of the Société Académique and the Cercle Médical to undermine the Paris Faculty of Medicine reflect the impotence of opponents of the faculty during the Empire. Despite its widely recognized inability to fulfill all its multiple roles, the faculty was an integral part of the general system of centralized power developed by the regime.[35] It was thus futile to attack it directly. The alternative was to seek symbolic titles and, on a small scale, corporate disciplinary powers, or, like the Société de Médecine de Paris, to carve out an autonomous niche by assuming public health and scientific functions. The fall of the Empire, however, entirely transformed political conditions.

Restoration and Conflict

Soon after setting foot on French soil on April 19, 1814, Louis XVIII received a statement of welcome from the Faculty of Medicine assuring him of its loyalty.[36] Despite the well-known Bonapartist sentiments of certain professors, the new government was not disposed to take action against the faculty. The minister of the interior, the Abbé de Montesquiou, in fact, expressed interest in expanding the Society of the Faculty into a full-fledged academy.[37] The idea was not a new one in administrative circles.[38] As has so often been the case in France, a change in regime seemed like an opportune moment to introduce long-contemplated institutional reform. Such a measure may have appealed to France's new rulers because it emphasized and appeared to renew the monarchy's traditional concerns with the health of the nation.

At about the same time, a group of Parisian surgeons presented the new king with a petition calling for the reestablishment of the Collège de Chirurgie and Académie Royale de Chirurgie as well as the return of their building and facilities now in the hands of the Faculty of Medicine. They emphasized the superiority of medicine under the ancien régime and the need to restore legitimate institutions destroyed by revolutionary usurpers.[39] But their arguments do not appear to have carried much weight at the ministry, more heavily influenced by a report prepared by the Faculty of Medicine.[40] This defended the current unity of medicine and surgery and proposed the establishment of a single Royal Society of Medicine and Surgery to respond to governmental inquiries about epidemics, epizootics, legal medicine, secret remedies, and mineral waters.

In justifying its proposal, representatives of the faculty also emphasized the continuity of their institution with those of the ancien régime. But they stressed even more that the government would find a single institution to which it could address itself far more efficient and convenient: "[R]elations will be much more prompt, much more sure than if it had been necessary to consult two groups." It would also be considerably less expensive than two societies, the dean emphasized.[41]

These were powerful arguments for an administration which contained many holdovers from the Empire and which was seeking to promote the reconciliation of pre- and postrevolutionary elites. In a report to the king, the minister of the interior essentially swallowed whole the arguments of the faculty.[42] The Society of the Faculty, he asserted, "now replaces the former Société Royale de Médecine and Académie Royale de Chirurgie." It could, however, render even greater service if the king agreed to extend its attributes and organize it on a stable footing. Soon after, however, Napoleon returned for his final hundred days. When the dust had settled after his conclusive defeat, the position of the Faculty of Medicine had deteriorated singularly.

Ultraroyalists opposed to reconciliation with the notables of the Empire found themselves immeasurably strengthened; they won a resounding victory in the legislative elections of August 1815, which produced the intransigent Chambre Introuvable and a more right-wing government. As a product of the Revolution and Empire, which had, moreover, compromised itself by publicly welcoming the "usurper" after his return from Elba, the faculty was viewed with considerable suspicion by royalists. Those traditional opponents of the faculty, the surgeons of Paris, now had allies in a number of important medical societies: the Société Académique de Paris representing the regent-doctors of the old faculty; the more modern Société de Médecine de Paris; and Portal's Cercle Médical. These groups could rally behind a new seat of institutional medical power: the physicians and surgeons of the royal court. They could also pursue their aims within a political system that was relatively more open than that of the Empire and that allowed greater scope to pressure group politics.

A court medical service had been maintained by Napoleon throughout the years of the Empire. But it was dominated by professors of the Paris faculty,[43] who made no claim to constitute an autonomous center of institutional power. On his return to France, Louis XVIII reestablished a wide variety of traditional court positions for his loyal supporters. Among them were many medical titles, often carrying generous stipends. The leading court physicians began claiming for themselves an independent institutional existence and authority rooted in royal patronage and proximity to the king's person. The King's Chief Surgeon was Père Elisée (Marie-Vincent Talachon), a secularized member of the Frères de Saint-Jean de Dieu who had emigrated in 1791 and become surgeon to the future Louis XVIII. The man appointed as the King's First Physician at the end of 1815 was none other than Antoine Portal, anatomist at the Collège de France and president of the Cercle Médical. Elisée, in particular, is supposed to have been granted authority over medical affairs by the king. His interventions were especially intolerable to professors because he lacked a medical degree and was considered little more than a charlatan.[44] Portal was an eminently more respectable figure whose tactics were less confrontational and frequently involved the appropriation of official titles. His stationary, for instance, began to sport the heading "Service de Faculté du Roi" making it resemble the stationary of the Ministry of the Interior. "Faculté du Roi" had been a traditional though by no means common title for the court medical service in the eighteenth century and Portal's rehabilitation of it was clearly meant to give this service a status comparable to that of the Medical Faculty of Paris.

The campaign to separate surgery from medicine appears to have been launched by a report to the king written by Elisée criticizing the Faculty of Paris in virulent terms and recommending the institutional separation of medicine and surgery. Professors responded with their own pamphlet based on their report to the Ministry of the Interior the year before. In November 1815 the king appointed a special commission to examine the state of medicine. This unleashed a torrent of pamphlets and articles which did not begin to dry up until after 1817.[45]

The main issue, as Paul Delaunay wrote in 1931, was control of medical institutions.[46] Those without power were demanding either a share in or domination of elite medical institutions. The unity of medicine and surgery was associated with and had in fact been used to justify the administrative centralization imposed under the Revolution and Empire. It was thus an obvious target for critics of the faculty. The only reason that professors defended the unity of medicine, declared the majority report of the royal commission on medical reform, "is that they wish to retain the administration of the schools, the accumulation of places, their salaries and this absolute empire over all branches of the healing arts which they have exercised for the past twenty years."[47]

However, the separation of medicine and surgery did not imply a simple return to local and corporate forms of authority. It was used rather to justify a variety of distinct and irreconcilable programs and interests. Elisée's position cannot be understood apart from the fact that the King's Chief Surgeon during the eighteenth century had accumulated virtual dictatorial powers over surgery in France. Elisée's goal thus seems to have been continued centralization but along different lines. Many opponents of the faculty, on the other hand, wished to create corporate bodies giving ordinary practitioners greater influence over medical institutions.[48] Questions of authority were complicated by charges that the faculty was guilty of disloyalty to the monarchy and by claims and counterclaims about who really represented continuity with the traditions of the Société Royale de Médecine and Académie Royale de Chirurgie. There were also vigorous debates about which system would cost the government less money. But two more substantive issues also shaped debate: the nature of knowledge and practice in medicine and surgery and the performance of the Paris faculty in fulfilling its educational, scientific, and professional functions.

In the view of many opponents of the faculties, repeating the conventional wisdom of previous centuries, a common education for physicians and surgeons was inappropriate because both their tasks and the knowledge on which these tasks were based were separate and distinct. The work of the physician, according to this view, was one of observation, meditation, discernment, and calculation of probabilities in order to grasp the nature of illnesses that were beyond view. It was necessary to observe and then "to go back, through rigorous reasoning, to the causes which become the bases of directions for cure."[49] Surgery, in contrast, was a simpler and more accessible activity based on the application of well-known methods. The senses, experience, dexterity, boldness, and the capacity to ignore the pain of others were paramount. Consequently, the education each required was very different. The physician, having to understand changes in the body during illness, needed to study a broad range of scientific subjects and, above all, needed to "learn at the sickbed the causes, symptoms, progress, the different terminations of illnesses and the curative means indicated by experience." The surgeon required a more profound knowledge of anatomy, some knowledge of mechanics, and, above all, familiarity with operating procedures; his studies therefore needed to be largely practical.

Defenders of the faculty recognized that surgery and medicine were distinct activities; but both, they insisted, were based on a body of medical knowledge that was indivisible. They claimed as well that the vast majority of practitioners ordinarily combined the two activities; surgeons especially could not earn a livelihood by limiting themselves to major operations. It was thus necessary to teach all future practitioners both the medicine and surgery they would require in their practices.[50] An intermediate position recognized that medicine and surgery had to be based on a common foundation but argued that it was dangerous to allow surgeons to practice without a somewhat more elaborate practical training and without passing special examinations.[51]

There was fairly widespread agreement that medical education was not functioning properly. Some professors (especially the elderly) did not teach a normal load;[52] courses were often too short and subject matter incompletely covered; examinations were lenient so that diplomas were granted with too much facility; the Faculty of Medicine had not succeeded in fulfilling its public health and scientific roles. Everyone agreed that too many medical graduates were flooding into the largest cities. For faculty spokesmen, the problem lay with faulty regulations which did not specify the tasks of professors, did not allow for retirement, and did not grant the faculty sufficient resources. These could be remedied easily by a prudent reform of medical institutions which, for all their weaknesses, had never enjoyed so much international recognition, or produced so many fundamental discoveries.

Opponents of the faculty, in contrast, argued that French medicine had manifestly declined since the golden days of the ancien régime. Abuses were not the result of regulations but of a fundamentally bad system of organization which allowed a small minority to control institutions. Consequently, competition necessary for improvement could not develop while all manner of patronage and abuse flourished. Untrained practitioners now flooded the countryside in excessive numbers because training was inadequate and because it was in the interests of professors to grant as many degrees as possible since fees for diplomas were appropriated by the faculty. The solution, therefore, was to return to a proven system of corporate control of educational institutions.

Whatever the principles at stake, the outcome of events depended primarily on the type of political support which each side was able to mobilize. Opponents of the Paris faculty could count on the personal influence Elisée seems to have exercised over Louis XVIII, widespread suspicion about the loyalty of the faculty to the monarchy, and their superior claim to embody the best traditions of the ancien régime. Nevertheless, the campaign to restructure medical institutions never seems to have gained much support among the political classes, even the ultraroyalists among them.[53] The faculty, in contrast, managed to retain the firm backing of administrators in the Ministry of the Interior and the education system. Furthermore, Louis XVIII and his government were committed to a course of political moderation incompatible with any serious effort to return to the institutions of the past. Most important, the centralized structures developed during the Empire were supremely useful to a fundamentally despotic government like that of the Restoration.[54] In the particular case of the Ministry of the Interior, the far-reaching powers of the faculty seem to have been viewed as a necessary means of bringing order and control to the chaotic world of medical practice. Reforms were clearly imperative, but they would move toward more rational forms of centralization rather than decentralization or the concentration of power in the hands of an erratic royal favorite.

In actual fact, the creation of a commission to reform medicine was vigorously supported by the two administrators chiefly responsible for medicine at the Ministry of the Interior, J.-G. Hyde de Neuville and Edouard Laffon de Ladébat.[55] Assured that the Council of Ministers was firmly opposed to the separation of medicine and surgery, they attempted to construct a reform commission dominated by the faculty. However, they appear to have seriously misconstrued the mood at the royal court. In November 1815 the king did indeed appoint a commission to examine medical institutions—but it was dominated by opponents of the faculty.[56]

In May 1816 the reform commission produced a report, or rather several reports, for it did decide in favor of the separation of medicine and surgery, but only by a vote of eight to six. A majority report called for separate schools of medicine and of surgery controlled by the doctors and surgeons in each city.[57] The minority, favoring the continued unity of teaching, divided on details and produced three separate minority reports.[58] That the faculty felt seriously threatened is indicated by the concessions which its dean Jean-Jacques Leroux and the professor of surgery Guillaume Dupuytren offered to make in their minority report. They admitted that regulations governing medical education had isolated the faculties from the corps of physicians and surgeons: "[I]t was forgotten that they [the faculties] were only the agents of the medico-surgical corporations. They were given too much latitude, too much independence, too much power because this power was not grounded on the corporations."[59] To correct this imbalance they suggested that two new institutions be established, one to handle professional discipline and another responsible for the advancement of medical knowledge. They insisted, moreover, that these be institutionally distinct from each other *and* from educational institutions. By abandoning the position that the faculty dominate any academy of medicine, Leroux and Dupuytren seem to have been guarding against the threat that the faculty would come under the jurisdiction of a new disciplinary or academic institution. "The teaching corps cannot be dependent on its equals," they insisted. It could only be subservient to the minister and the educational administration.[60]

The government did not in the end act to implement the commission's recommendation. The diversity of opinion within the medical world would certainly have made any attempt at implementation politically hazardous. Action became even less likely when a new minister of the interior, Joseph-Louis Laine, solicited the opinion of the Commission de l'Instruction Publique officially administering the education system. The response in January 1817 was an unequivocal recommendation to disregard the majority report, which was said to be based on "false principles and consequences deduced even more falsely, extreme exaggeration in the reproaches addressed to existing institutions, ignorance of facts, [and] absence of method in the plan presented as in the reasoning. . . ."[61] Soon thereafter Elisée died and was replaced as the King's Chief Surgeon by Guillaume Dupuytren. The movement to topple the medical elite thus lost its last bit of influence within the royal court. By 1818 the Paris Faculty of Medicine felt secure enough to seek to reinforce its teaching monopoly; it petitioned the minister of the interior to put an end to the private clinical teaching going on in the Paris hospitals.[62]

The Creation of the Academy of Medicine

The issue of a public health-research institution, we saw, was near the center of the debate over the separation of medicine and surgery. While the necessity of establishing one or more institutions of this type was clear, the details remained in question. Would it extend the powers of the Paris Faculty of Medicine, or would it constitute an autonomous and competing center of power?

Once the campaign for separation fizzled out, leadership of the opposition to the faculty fell to Antoine Portal, named the King's First Physician in late 1815. He was to abandon the strategy of direct assault pursued by Elisée in favor of more indirect, devious tactics. Even during the debates of 1815–16 he had played a curious role. As a member of the reform commission he had finally voted with the majority in favor of the separation of medicine and surgery. But before doing so, he submitted a strange report in which he took a strong stand in favor of a single unified system of education for physicians and surgeons.[63] He did, however, implicitly call into question the faculties' dominance over the public health-research sphere by suggesting that a system of academies or colleges be set up in each department to direct the advancement of medical learning. Although he was willing to forsake titles currently monopolized by public institutions (like "academy"), he insisted that these societies include all practitioners in an area while exercising disciplinary authority over members. Portal's subsequent actions make it evident that he saw his own Cercle Médical as the core of a Parisian society that would coordinate and lead provincial societies.

By 1818 it was common knowledge that the government planned to create some kind of academy of medicine.[64] The Paris Faculty of Medicine, in particular, had every financial reason to welcome a change. Between 1814 and 1817 the annual allocation to the faculty declined from 111,000 to 55,000 francs, making it impossible to support the activities of the Society of the Faculty. The minister agreed to the dean's request for a special subsidy of 9,000 francs to cover the society's expenses for two years. He emphasized, however, that "the Faculty of Medicine should not count on the renewal of this subsidy; and I invite it to search immediately for the means to meet, through its own resources, the expenses of the society it has formed in its midst."[65]

It was Portal, however, who precipitated matters. In 1819 he engineered a reconciliation between the Cercle Médical and the Société Académique, which had been separated for nearly a decade. Soon after, he published the essay he had submitted to the reform commission of 1815, calling for the creation of a system of official medical societies. He then sent this essay to the king, along with the request that the reunited Cercle Médical be permitted to assume the title Cercle Royal de Médecine. This petition led to the decision to establish the Academy of Medicine.

Several interpretations have been offered for the government's decision to create the academy in 1820. According to one account, Louis XVIII was inspired by some features of the proposals submitted by Elisée and Portal in 1815 and merely waited until the passions aroused by the campaign against the faculty had abated before implementing them.[66] A more sophisticated analysis offered by Huard and Imbault-Huart recognizes that the proposal to establish an academy predated Elisée.[67] The government finally decided to act, according to this view, because the political situation had badly deteriorated as a result of the *complot de l'est*, assassination of the duc de Berry, and agitation against the electoral law. It finally settled the issue of the academy in order to resolve its difficulties with the intellectual bourgeoisie. There is, however, no evidence to suggest that anyone connected with the creation of the academy linked it in any way with such political difficulties. I would therefore suggest a somewhat different line of argument.

The government in 1820 was interested in establishing an academy for exactly the same reasons that had prompted its initiatives in 1814. Its growing involvement in health care required a centralized institution that could develop and transmit the specialized knowledge required for effective state action. Furthermore, creating an academy with much fanfare and publicity could provide badly needed legitimation for the government by highlighting the monarchy's humanitarian commitment to the welfare of its people and to the best features of the ancien régime. There existed a virtual consensus about the need for some institution of this sort. But, as we saw, its advocates were divided into two camps. The government might have imposed a compromise before 1820 except for the fact that the proposal to establish an academy independent of the faculty was swallowed up in the far more radical campaign to separate surgery from medicine and to dismantle the existing institutional machinery. This was unthinkable even for the most conservative of Restoration ministries, which those of 1815–19 most definitely were not. After 1817, however, the proposal for an autonomous academy became gradually disentangled from the radical assault on the faculties. Presented in moderate fashion by Portal, a man close to the royal court and with impeccable scientific credentials, the plan attracted support in royalist political circles, which were becoming increasingly hostile to the education system. The personnel of the Ministry of the Interior and the Paris Faculty of Medicine were opposed to Portal's vision of an academy independent of, if not actually dominating, the faculty. But the former, confident of their ability to determine the outcome of events and desperate to put the public health-research tasks of the faculty on a sounder financial footing, pressed ahead for a resolution to the stalemate. This permitted the government to impose a compromise.

The ministry's insistence on forging ahead at all costs duplicated its obstinacy in convening a reform commission in 1815. Indeed, the same individual, Laffon de Ladébat, helped define policy in both cases. By 1820, however, the ministry had a number of additional motives for precipitating events.

First, the government had since 1817 been attempting to decide how best to react to the epidemic of yellow fever raging across the border in Spain. The Paris Faculty of Medicine had been consulted in 1817, a commission was sent to Cadiz in 1819, and in November 1820, about one month before the appearance of the ordinance establishing the academy, the government appointed a Central Sanitary Commission to propose appropriate sanitary legislation. The result was the passage of the Sanitation Law of 1822 and the creation several months later of a Superior Council of Health to oversee the apparatus of quarantine, disinfection, and *cordons sanitaires*.[68] Consequently, the creation of the academy must also be seen in the context of a wide-ranging effort to cope with epidemics.

Second, the creation of the academy can be seen as part of an even broader strategy to reorganize and centralize health care under the national government. Laffon de Ladébat had for several years been working with the alienist Jean Esquirol to establish lunatic asylums controlled by the central government in place of the locally managed asylums then in existence.[69] But the most critical part of the task was to reorganize the system of medical education and professional regulation. The government was already in the midst of planning legislation to this effect; it would be introduced in the Conseil d'État less than a year after the creation of the academy.[70] (Two political figures, Georges Cuvier and Joseph-Marie de Gérando, played a major role in developing both proposals.) The foundation of the academy was seen as a crucial first step in the restructuring being envisaged, as is suggested by the opening remarks of the ordinance creating that institution:

> It being our intention to grant as soon as possible regulations to perfect the teaching of the healing art and bring an end to the abuses which have been introduced into the exercise of its different branches, we thought that one of the best means of preparing this double benefit was to create an academy especially charged with working to perfect medical science. . . .[71]

In March 1820—soon after the fall of Elie Decaze's liberal ministry and replacement by the more conservative Richelieu government—Portal petitioned the king, asking that the word "Royal" be added to the name Cercle Médical.[72] The king ordered Portal to address himself to the minister of the interior, indicating that he himself was favorably disposed to the request—or so it seemed to functionaries of the Ministry of the Interior, who learned of the petition immediately. Within two days, the two officials responsible for medical institutions, Baron Guillaume Capelle and Laffon de Ladébat, prepared a report to the minister[73] that firmly opposed Portal's request on the grounds that allowing a private society to assume the title "royal" might compromise the ministry's plan to establish a genuine royal society.

When Portal finally got around to sending his proposal to the Ministry of the Interior[74] he was conciliatory. His letter spoke of the need for an academic society with powers of professional discipline and surveillance in addition to its responsibility over public health and medical science. He suggested that a special commission be appointed to discuss the most appropriate form for such a society. He did insist, however, that the commission be broadly representative of the profession, bringing together "the sometimes opposed interests and pretensions of the various medical functions." He proposed a commission of eight members on which professors were a minority.

Despite fears regarding Portal's intentions and influence at court,[75] Baron Capelle chose to utilize Portal's request in order to further his own plan for an academy of medicine. On April 27, he and Laffon de Ladébat submitted a report to the minister[76] advising that the Cercle Médical not be granted use of the term "royal" and insisting on the need to establish a new institution. A sly effort was made to placate Portal by suggesting that the presidency of the body be conferred on the King's First Physician. To implement their suggestion, the authors proposed the nomination of a special commission. Of the nine members suggested and soon after appointed (under the chairmanship of Georges Cuvier), only Portal and the councillor of state, de Gérando, were not members of the Society of the Paris Faculty of Medicine.[77]

This flurry of activity was only the first round in an intense process of political maneuvering. Portal sought without success to get a more representative commission.[78] As a result of his failure, the commission's report, completed in July 1820,[79] faithfully reflected the views of the faculty. Claiming to have achieved unanimity on all major points, the commission refused to accord the title "royal" to either the Cercle Médical or the Society of the Faculty on the grounds that a successful academic society needed to be "a creation of the government." It thus proposed the founding of a Royal Academy of Medical Sciences composed of distinct sections of medicine, surgery, and pharmacy. The commission made no provision for a permanent president (inevitably Portal), calling instead for an annual presidency rotating among the three sections. It also argued for a small academy with a membership of 180 (not including correspondents and adjuncts) on the grounds that the academy should not be a representative college but, like the academies of the eighteenth century, a working corps. Finally, it stipulated that however nominations were to be effected, all faculty professors and all associates and adjuncts of the Society of the Faculty were to be admitted as members.

Capelle transmitted the commission's report to the minister with his own warm endorsement.[80] He also suggested a procedure for nominations that would protect the government against charges of favoritism. The king would name a portion of the members, who would proceed to elect their remaining numbers. He was, however, very specific about the fifty-six to be named: twenty-four professors of the Paris faculty, twenty members of the Society of the Faculty, six professors of the Paris School of Pharmacy, two professors of the Collège de France (including Portal), and four secretaries of authorized medical societies.

Portal's response to the minister insisted only that the new institution be large and representative of Parisian medicine.[81] However, the political situation was evolving in his favor. After the assassination of the duc de Berry, the influence of the ultraroyalists grew apace, culminating in the formation of the reactionary Villèle ministry in December 1821. Hostility to the Faculty of Medicine was increasing as well, partly as a result of the general tendency to abandon the policy of reconciliation with the notables of the Empire and partly due to widespread student disturbances directed against the electoral law. Matters would reach a head in 1822 when the government closed the Paris Faculty of Medicine; it was reopened several months later minus eleven professors, who had been dismissed from their posts and replaced.[82] At the end of 1820 things had not yet deteriorated so dramatically. But especially after the victory of the ultraroyalists in the legislative elections held in November, a mild gesture repudiating the Faculty of Medicine must have seemed attractive to many.

On December 19, 1820, the faculty acknowledged Portal's growing influence by recommending that he be named as an associate of the Society of the Faculty.[83] The next day a royal ordinance established the Royal Academy of Medicine. Seven days later the first members were appointed by the king.[84]

The statement of introduction to the ordinance of 1820 essentially repeated the rationales elaborated in all the earlier recommendations for the creation of an academy. The long-range goal was "to perfect the teaching of the healing art and to end the abuses introduced into the exercise of its different branches." The more immediate task was to respond to questions from the government "concerning everything relevant to public health."[85] It was also to concern itself with all research that might contribute to the progress of medicine. The ordinance called for an academy made up of three sections, medicine, surgery, and pharmacy, of unequal size.[86] These were to meet regularly in separate session and more infrequently in combined session. Members were divided into five hierarchical categories, with decision-making powers concentrated in the highest rank, *titulaire*.

The ordinance differed in several respects from the proposal submitted by the Cuvier commission and Baron Capelle. The new institution was to be called Academy of "Medicine" rather than "Medical Sciences," more directly emphasizing its professional character. The King's First Physician was designated permanent honorary president. Most important, Portal had his way with respect to size: the academy was to be composed of 285 members (in addition to an indeterminate number of corresponding and adjunct members) rather than the 180 recommended by Cuvier and Capelle. The full significance of this figure becomes more evident if we note that there were only 571 physicians and surgeons and 197 pharmacists officially registered in the Paris region in 1820.[87] The huge membership was due essentially to a decision to swell the ranks of the honorary members and associates. While this would bring a swarm of Parisian practitioners into the academy, its effects were to be practically offset by the fact that neither category was supposed to have decision-making powers over internal affairs.

The ordinance of December 27 nominating the first cohort of members (which was to elect the rest of the membership) also differed significantly from Capelle's proposal, which would have given the faculty overwhelming preponderance. Contemporaries believed that the faculty named half the members while Portal named the other half. This seems a reasonable supposition given the results. Faculty professors obtained twenty-one of sixty-nine appointments, with another nine chosen from among professors in the School of Pharmacy. No less than ten other appointees were associated with the royal medical corps. Political considerations do not seem to have played a determining role in these nominations. If well-known monarchists like Esquirol and Hallé were appointed, so too were figures identified with the Empire like Corvisart and liberal opponents of the monarchy like Broussais. The government at this stage seems to have accepted choices made by the faculty and by Portal based on nonpolitical criteria.

While clearly a slap in the face for the faculty, this initial selection allowed the faculty to retain significant influence. Only the forty-four men named as titular members were to elect the remaining members. Professors in the Faculty of Medicine and School of Pharmacy constituted exactly half of these *titulaires*. Another six, moreover, were associates or adjuncts of the Society of the Faculty. Power was divided evenly enough in the new academy to provoke brutal conflicts over the details of institutional organization and structure. In July 1821 one medical journal reported:

> What things have occurred since the creation of the new Academy! What agitations, what schemings, what intrigues! All the passions have been aroused at the same time; egoism, beneath the mask of the public good, has been agitating with convulsive violence, impatient with all restraints, and burning to overrun everything. . . . [O]ne came, one went, one met in committees; the Minister of the Interior was importuned with recriminations of all sorts, and sat on the fence uncertain about which party he should favor.[88]

Some of the conflicts were about basic principles. Several members, for instance, tried to convince their colleagues to return to the original idea of a unified academy divided into disciplinary sections but meeting as a single body.[89] But either because they agreed with arguments that specialized discussions would be impossible if all members met or because they were simply unwilling to challenge the original governmental guidelines, academicians did not act on this passionately argued proposal.

Most of the intrigue had to do with the struggle for power between the faculty and the King's First Physician.[90] Portal bombarded the Ministry of the Interior with letters seeking support for his efforts to assume all the traditional attributes of a King's First Physician. The ministry seems to have gone along with his unilateral hiring of a secretary to handle the academy's correspondence (against the objections of the faculty). Portal also seems to have been successful in efforts to have all correspondence between the academy and the government channeled through his office. He failed, however, to keep the academy physically separate from the faculty. When the promise of space at the Louvre was not honored, the president tried to arrange for meetings to be held at the Paris City Hall rather than at the faculty.[91] But he was unsuccessful and most of the academy's meetings during its first four years took place in the uncomfortable (in all respects) premises of the faculty. Professors also succeeded in setting up an administrative structure for the academy that controlled day-to-day activities independently of the permanent president and that was dominated by the faculty. Initially, moreover, the voting core of the academy was successfully kept small. A precipitate vote to elect the rest of the titular members in the winter of 1821 excluded and enraged the honorary members, who protested vehemently but ineffectually.

The Conflict Abates

By late 1823 most of these issues had been resolved and the academy was functioning with some success. Many academicians remained hostile to the faculty and would have been happy to turn the academy into an alternative source of institutional power. But they made few efforts to realize their aspirations. With hindsight one can suggest several reasons for their caution.

First, the day-to-day activities of the academy quickly became routinized and time-consuming; they left little latitude for controversial issues of medical power. Structural constraints were magnified by the fact that opponents of the faculty lacked effective leadership. Portal was tireless in protecting the formal symbols of his authority. He was, however, eighty years old in 1822 and participated only rarely in the academy's activities. During most of the 1820s he appears in the archival record almost exclusively to defend the prerogatives of the academy against some government slight. In 1823 the government appointed Etienne Pariset as permanent secretary of the academy, despite the fact that regulations specified that this position be filled by election. The office might have become a power base but Pariset lacked the intellectual stature to overcome his irregular appointment and to assume significant influence.

Second, and most seriously, there was little that could be done in the face of the government's unwillingness to consider the academy in terms other than narrow technical expertise. A body of modest experts could be useful to the government, whereas one with excessive administrative pretensions was likely to be a political embarrassment. The government found this out in 1827, when it asked the academy to evaluate Nicholas Chervin's documents purporting to demonstrate the noncontagiousness of yellow fever. When it became apparent that the academy was going to decide that these documents seriously called into question the government's quarantine policy, the minister firmly reminded that institution that it had been asked to make only a scientific and not an administrative judgment.[92]

Even in less controversial situations, differences in expectations were striking. In 1828 the ministry asked the academy along with the medical faculties to evaluate proposed legislation to reform the organization of medical practice. The academy appointed a commission to study the matter; it was led by François-Joseph Double, who made it clear that he was in no hurry to respond. He envisaged an exhaustive study of medical practice in France and asked the minister to arrange for the academy to receive complete statistical information on the number of medical practitioners in each department. The chief administrator for medical affairs at the ministry, Etienne Tessière de Boisbertrand,[93] wrote to the president of the academy to urge the committee to speed up its work "and restrict itself to responding to the questions which have been submitted to it, leaving to the administration the task of reconciling the opinions of the Academy with the administrative documents which exist or which arrive." The letter concluded with an expression of concern that the commission would, by taking too long with its work, prevent the government from introducing its proposal at the next legislative session. Double, however, did not flinch. The commission, he said, believed that "it would work quickly enough if it worked well; it will thus continue its work according to the plan it has adopted."[94]

By this time, relations between the academy and the government had reached a nadir. A year earlier, de Boisbertrand had written to the academy suggesting that the decline in the numbers of vaccinations being performed by the academy indicated that some reorganization of the vaccination committee was in order.[95] More significantly, he sent out two missions in 1828, one to analyze a mineral water in situ and another to report on a local epidemic; none of the individuals involved were members of the academy, which was not consulted on either matter. These acts, perceived as a usurpation of academic prerogatives, prompted the academy to send a vigorous protest to the ministry. De Boisbertrand responded in the name of the minister by telling the academy in no uncertain terms that a consultative *corps savants* "cannot take part in administration." The mandate of the academy was to respond to requests for advice, but this did not mean that the minister was obligated to ask only the academy; "he has complete liberty to make his way as he thinks appropriate, and to designate the men whom it pleases him to employ."[96] At the start of 1829 the academy was conspicuously omitted from a ceremony in which major institutions delivered new year's wishes to the king. A protest managed to extort a belated invitation.[97]

This conflict undoubtedly expressed political tension between the increasingly right-wing government and the academy, which contained a number of prominent liberals. But it also reflected a more basic divergence between administrative perceptions of the academy and the aspirations of academicians. And these transcended political regimes. On at least two occasions administrators under the more liberal July Monarchy behaved very much like their Restoration predecessors. In 1831, for instance, hackles were again raised in the academy. The ministry requested the academy to prepare practical instructions for dealing with the cholera epidemic that was then expected. Instead of waiting for the academy to complete its work, the ministry sent out a circular suggesting preventive measures; the circular was based on the advice of Alexandre Moreau de Jonnès, a member of the government's Superior Council of Health who was neither a physician nor a member of the academy. Although it had not yet begun its own discussion of this issue, the academy decided that "the executive bureau of the Academy should pay a visit to the Minister in order to resolve everything connected with this affair."[98]

Four years later, a new minister of the interior, Tanneguy Duchâtel, consulted the academy about the possibility of organizing a commission to try a number of remedies in a cholera epidemic that had broken out in the Midi. When the government sent its own medical representative to Marseilles to treat the outbreak, it was widely perceived as a snub to the academy, which hastened to send off a letter of protest. In responding to the protest, the minister carefully explained that the doctor sent to Marseilles to treat the sick had nothing to do with the original proposal. Nevertheless, he repeated with some emphasis the comments made by de Boisbertrand six years earlier, to the effect that the government was not obligated to solicit or take advice from the academy.[99]

A major reorganization of the academy in 1829 was recognized to be an effort by the government to gain greater control over the somewhat recalcitrant institution. One medical journalist predicted that it would mean the end of the academy as a scientific body and its reduction "to the narrow limits of a consultative committee, . . . a veritable section of this Ministry [of the Interior]."[100] The reform decree specified that meetings of the academy "will be exclusively devoted to science,"[101] foreclosing the option of discussing issues of medical politics or even public health unless it was invited to do so by the government. A concern to augment effectiveness or perhaps increase control over members was manifested in efforts to cut the academy down to more manageable size. Henceforth, only one in every three vacancies would be filled until the number of titular members fell to sixty, with another forty becoming adjunct members.

As it turned out, the reorganization was not fully implemented. The difficulty of turning titular into adjunct members forced the government of the July Monarchy in 1835 to raise the target goal for titular membership to one hundred. This figure was reached only during the Second Empire so that opponents of the faculty remained strong through much of the 1830s and 1840s. But they were kept in check by administrative pressures to focus on narrow technical issues. As a result, the considerable opposition to the faculty within the academy emerged only sporadically.

In 1825, for instance, the academy discussed a proposal to recommend to the government the establishment of a special school of legal medicine to train forensic specialists. The new school was to be placed under the direction of the academy rather than the Faculty of Medicine. This suggestion can be seen as, in some ways, a return to Portal's original vision of an academy serving as an alternative to the power of the Faculty of Medicine. Not surprisingly, it provoked considerable hostility, but it did not win much support and was quickly dropped.[102] Several years later, however, another controversial discussion succeeded in polarizing the academy.

The Academy Polarized

The ambition to create an academy of medicine, we saw, was inextricably intertwined with a long-standing desire to reform medical education and practice. Solutions might differ from one reform proposal to another but all focused on three major areas of concern. First, how could the twenty or so informal schools of medicine that had arisen around hospitals in provincial cities without faculties of medicine be formally integrated into the system of medical education? Second, what was to be done with the inferior medical degree, the *officiat de santé*, for which local schools prepared many if not most of their students? Some reformers argued for raising educational standards; others insisted on nothing less than the abolition of the inferior degree. Those who argued for maintaining two medical degrees insisted that doctors trained in urban faculties would never agree to settle in the rural countryside, leaving inhabitants at the mercy of charlatans. Advocates of a single medical diploma, including most doctors, claimed that most *officiers* in fact practiced in cities and that doctors would not fail to settle in rural areas once their livelihoods were no longer compromised by the competition of *officiers*.[103]

The third, and most contentious reform issue had to do with the creation of institutions to impose standards of discipline on the medical profession. The corporations of the ancien régime had exercised disciplinary authority over members and there was a widespread sense that reintroducing such authority in a more appropriate form was the solution to the perceived disorder of nineteenth-century medicine. Some administrators saw such disciplinary councils as administrative extensions of the public service. Those doctors supporting the proposal, however, usually visualized disciplinary councils as representative bodies of a medical corps exercising considerably augmented professional autonomy. They were opposed by many, perhaps the majority of doctors, hostile to disciplinary councils in any form, for they feared that such institutions would place them at the mercy of medical competitors and would compromise the dignity of the entire profession by bringing into the open and publicizing professional scandals.

Because of such disagreements, numerous reform initiatives proved unsuccessful before the Revolution of 1848 put an end to legislative efforts to reorganize medicine. In 1825 Minister of the Interior Jacques Corbière introduced legislation to integrate local medical schools into the state system. The academy was studiously ignored by the government on this occasion.[104] Two years later, however, a new minister, Jean-Baptiste de Martignac, asked all major medical institutions, including the academy, to evaluate a legislative proposal that he intended to introduce.[105] While other institutions managed to respond promptly, the academy, we saw earlier, appointed a committee headed by Double to prepare a definitive report. After the exchange with Boisbertrand discussed previously, nothing more was heard from the committee. In 1833—after yet another new minister wishing to introduce legislation requested specifically that the academy respond to the original query—the committee finally reported to the academy. In light of the ministry's desire for a rapid response, the academy decided to meet three times weekly without interruption until a review of the report was completed. The academy met over several months in what was one of the longest and most rancorous debates in a history filled with long and rancorous debates.

The very lengthy report was written by F. -J. Double,[106] a physician without a faculty or hospital appointment who had worked closely with Portal in setting up the academy.[107] His report makes clear that he shared both his mentor's hostility to the faculty and the hope that the academy might become an alternative source of medical power. His aggressiveness may well have been fueled by the recent reorganization of the academy, which represented a major defeat for Portal's broader vision of academic authority.[108] Whatever its source, his open hostility to the faculty seems to have been shared by many academicians.

By the time the report came up for debate, the issue of the local medical schools had already been resolved by their integration into the education system as *écoles secondaires de médecine*, teaching the first two years of the four-year program for the doctorate and preparing future *officiers de santé* for examinations. As for this latter degree, the Parisian medical elite seems to have reached a consensus that it should be eliminated, and this proposal passed without difficulty.[109] Nevertheless, academicians found a great many other subjects to argue about.

One of these had to do with various hostile comments about the faculty that Double insinuated into the report. Professors protested a remark to the effect that examiners for the *officiat* examination (primarily professors) pocketed fees and thus had an interest in passing as many candidates as possible.[110] Double also raised hackles with a bald pronouncement that the state monopoly of medical education was "absurd."[111] Faculty professors, led by Adelon, repeatedly attempted to discuss the overall orientation of the report rather than its specific details but were consistently overruled by a slight majority of academicians.

Double's report recommended that three new provincial faculties be established. This would have cut into the recruitment of the three existing faculties. Despite a debate that was described by one medical journal as "exceptionally stormy,"[112] this proposal was adopted by the academy, provoking a breakdown of the meeting into "tumult and confusion."[113] The recommendation that most directly struck at the faculty insisted that one-third of the members of the juries evaluating the final examinations leading to the doctorate be appointed from among practitioners *not* affiliated with the faculty. The justification for this proposal was that practitioners had the right to assure themselves of the high quality of future colleagues.[114] In the end, with the academy "divided among friends and enemies of the faculty," members voted thirty-five to twenty-seven in favor of an even more drastic measure: that *half* the participants on examination juries had to be practitioners from outside the faculty.[115]

The most sustained debate was about the creation of disciplinary councils in each department to regulate the profession. It quickly became clear that Double and his allies were seeking to give these institutions the widest possible powers while faculty professors, once they failed to vote down the principle of creating them, sought to limit their attributions as much as possible. It is difficult not to see the debate as it was conducted in the academy as anything other than a struggle between the faculty and rival academicians over professional powers.

One proposal that was adopted, for instance, would have transferred the inspection of pharmacies from the schools of pharmacy to the disciplinary councils because, it was explained, the commission "wanted to completely separate the teaching from

the policing of the [medical] art, and to confine the schools to what concerns studies."[116] The academy also voted—against the wishes of professors—in favor of
another proposal which gave councils the power to prevent and settle disputes among
practitioners. Double even succeeded in extending their duties to the activities regulated nationally by the academy. It was decided that councils should prepare and
publish medical statistics and topographies, study local epidemics, and send their results to the academy, in addition to taking responsibility for smallpox vaccinations.[117]
Clearly Double was reasserting and the majority of academicians were supporting
Portal's vision of the academy as the center of a national network of scientific and
professional bodies. Only on the issue of giving councils broad disciplinary powers
over the profession did a narrow majority of academicians (thirty-eight to thirty-
seven) vote against Double because of widespread fear that such bodies would
intensify conflict among doctors and publicize professional wrongdoing.[118]

When debate concluded, Double promised to rewrite the project to take account
of the revisions that had been voted.[119] The revised project, however, never came
before the academy, and it was not sent to the minister until four years later. The ministry thus received the academy's response ten years after its original request for an
opinion.

Opposition to the Paris faculty did not disappear in the following years. If anything, it gained new sources of expression as rank-and-file medical practitioners
organized themselves in medical societies and tried to exercise some influence over
the reform efforts that were going on. Although their hostility to the faculty was
somewhat less intense than that of competing Parisian elites, it was nonetheless substantial. In 1845 the first significant effort at medical self-organization took place in
France. Nearly seven hundred doctors, pharmacists, and veterinarians attended a
medical congress in Paris to demand medical reform. The congress voted, among
other things, to abolish the *officiers de santé* and to create disciplinary councils for
the profession. Most significantly for our purposes, it affirmed the right of all doctors
to freely teach medical students on the premises of the faculty and called for practitioner representation on *concours* juries electing faculty professors. By an "immense
majority" and over the vigorous protest of professors in attendance, the congress also
passed a resolution giving doctors at least half the seats on the juries examining doc-
toral candidates.[120]

Though such demands were being raised, they were no longer being raised within
the Academy of Medicine. In fact, the debate over Double's report was the last major
professional issue to be discussed in the academy until World War I. The academy
never addressed this matter directly, but the most likely explanation for this with-
drawal from professional debate is that the bitter conflicts which they generated were
considered embarrassing and best avoided; at a time when the institution's status was
by no means secure, it may have seemed prudent to avoid questions that caused such
deep divisions, eroded intellectual authority, and diverted the institution from its
primary tasks. This view seems to have been shared by governmental authorities,
which henceforth avoided asking the academy's opinions on controversial issues of
medical politics.

If motives, insofar as we can guess at them, were most probably pragmatic, the
avoidance of medical politics effectively guaranteed the primacy of a narrow vision

of the academy's role. In this vision, the academy was essentially a "scientific" institution, complementing rather than challenging other elite institutions. Whatever their deepest aspirations, opponents of the faculty in the academy seem to have been unwilling to place at risk their newly won status by actively seeking to overturn the existing system of institutional power relations.

The creation of the academy was the culmination of years of struggle among the conflicting segments of the postrevolutionary medical elite. The Paris Faculty of Medicine, which had emerged from the revolutionary decade with enormous institutional powers, suffered a clear defeat as a result of this process. Nevertheless, the existence of the academy ended up reinforcing rather than overturning existing institutional arrangements. At the most banal level, the decision to restrict the size of the academy gradually led to the numerical dominance of the faculty over the institution. By 1914 some 41 percent of the academicians taught at the faculty with another 8 percent at the School of Pharmacy. Four of the five men who served as permanent secretary of the academy from 1873 to 1944 were professors at the Faculty of Medicine.[121]

At a deeper level, the academy became part of, rather than an alternative to, the existing system of power and status distribution. It ended up consolidating the existence of the Parisian medical elite by extending the system of medical authority that had emerged during the Revolution and Empire. The essential reason, one suspects, is that, irrespective of their political orientation, successive French governments were more interested in establishing an effective and pliable instrument of state policy than in power struggles among medical elites. This narrow administrative vision would determine the way the academy functioned during its first century of existence.

NOTES

1. Othmar Keel, "The Politics of Health and the Institutionalization of Clinical Practice in Europe in the Second Half of the Eighteenth Century," in *William Hunter and the Eighteenth Century Medical World*, ed. W. F. Bynum and R. Porter (Cambridge, 1985), pp. 207–56; Laurence W. B. Brockliss, "L'Enseignement médical et la Révolution: essai de réévaluation," *Histoire de l'éducation* 42 (1989), 79–110.

2. Among recent works on the structure of French medicine during the eighteenth century, see especially Toby Gelfand, *Professionalizing Modern Medicine: Paris Surgeons and Medical Science and Institutions in the Eighteenth Century* (Westport, Conn., 1980); Caroline Hannaway, "Medicine, Public Welfare and the State in Eighteenth-Century France: The Société Royale de Médecine of Paris (1776–1793)," Ph.D. diss., Johns Hopkins University, 1974; Matthew Ramsey, *Professional and Popular Medicine in France, 1770–1830: The Social World of Medical Practice* (Cambridge, 1988). Also see Chapters 3 and 4 in Charles C. Gillispie, *Science and Polity in France at the End of the Old Régime* (Princeton, N.J., 1980). Among older works on the subject, see especially Paul Delaunay, *La Vie médicale aux XVIe, XVIIe et XVIIIe siècles* (1935) and *Le Monde médical parisien au dix-huitième siècle* (1906).

3. On this institution, see Colin Jones, "The *Médecins du Roi* at the End of the Ancien Régime and in the French Revolution," in *Medicine at the Courts of Europe, 1500–1837*, ed. Vivian Nutton (London, 1990), pp. 209–61; Delaunay, *Le Monde*, pp. 93–165.

4. Jan Goldstein, *Console and Classify: The French Psychiatric Profession in the Nineteenth Century* (Cambridge, 1987), p. 19. The best overall study of medical faculties during this period is Laurence W.B. Brockliss, *French Higher Education in the Seventeenth and Eighteenth Centuries: A Cultural History* (Oxford, 1987), chap. 8.

5. Gelfand, *Professionalizing Modern Medicine*, pp. 62–67.

6. Pierre Huard and M.-J. Imbault-Huart, "Le Concept d'académie en France au XVIIIe siècle: son évolution face à la médecine et à la chirurgie," in *100e Congrès national des sociétés savantes; histoires modernes et histoires des sciences* (Montpellier, 1975), p. 295.

7. On these matters, see Hannaway, "Medicine, Public Welfare"; Gelfand, *Professionalizing Modern Medicine*; Othmar Keel, "Cabanis et la généalogie de la médecine clinique," Ph.D diss., McGill University, 1977; Gillispie, *Science and Polity*, chaps. 3 and 4.

8. On the academies of the ancien régime, see Roger Hahn, *The Anatomy of a Scientific Institution: The Paris Academy of Sciences, 1666–1803* (Berkeley, Calif., 1971); Daniel Roche, *Le Siècle des lumières en province: académies et académiciens provinciaux, 1680–1789* (1978); James E. McClellan III, *Science Reorganized: Scientific Societies in the Eighteenth Century* (New York, 1985); David S. Lux, *Patronage and Royal Science in Seventeenth-Century France: The Académie de Physique in Caen* (Ithaca, N.Y., 1989); Alice Stroup, *A Company of Scientists: Botany, Patronage and Community at the Early Parisian Academy of Sciences* (Berkeley, Calif., 1990); Bruce T. Moran, ed., *Patronage and Institutions: Science, Technology and Medicine at the European Court, 1500–1750* (Rochester, N.Y., 1991); Robin Briggs, "The Académie Royale des Sciences and the Pursuit of Utility," *Past and Present* 131 (1991), 38–86.

9. Marc Raeff, "The Well-Ordered Police State and the Development of Modernity in Seventeenth- and Eighteenth-Century Europe," *American Historical Review* 80 (1975), 1221–43; George Rosen, "Cameralism and the Concept of Medical Police," *Bulletin of the History of Medicine* 27 (1953), 21–42, and "Mercantilism and Health Policy in Eighteenth-Century French Thought," *Medical History* 3 (1959), 259–75.

10. Johanna Geyer-Kordesch, "Court Physicians and State Regulation in Eighteenth-Century Prussia: The Emergence of Medical Science and the Demystification of the Body," in *Medicine at the Courts of Europe, 1500–1837*, ed. Vivian Nutton (London, 1990), pp. 155–81.

11. Goldstein, *Console and Classify*, pp. 21, 44–47; Dora B. Weiner, *The Citizen Patient in Revolutionary and Imperial Paris* (Baltimore, Md., 1993), pp. 21–44; Thomas M. Adams, *Bureaucrats and Beggars: French Social Policy in the Age of the Enlightenment* (New York, 1990).

12. The emblematic example is F. Vicq d'Azyr, "Nouveau plan de constitution pour la médecine en France," in *Histoire et mémoires de la Société Royale de médecine* 9 (1790), 1–210.

13. Keith Baker, "Scientism at the End of the Old Regime: Reflections on a Theory by Professor Charles Gillispie," *Minerva* 25 (1987), 21–34.

14. On these changes, see Weiner, *The Citizen Patient*.

15. On the establishment of the Society of the Faculty see the dossier in AN: AJ16 6705. All further references to the AJ16, F17, and F15 series are in AN. Also see Pascale Zweibel-Muller, "La Société de l' École de médecine et la santé publique en France de 1801 à 1821," Thèse 3e cycle, École des Hautes Études en Sciences Sociales, no. 1663 (n.d.).

16. Ministère de l'Instruction Publique, *Enquêtes et documents relatifs à l'enseignement supérieur*, 124 vols. (1883–1929), vol. 37 (1890), pp. 23–31; also see the undated report in AN: F17 2107. On the relationship of the faculty to military medicine during the nineteenth century see the anonymous "Le Service de santé militaire et l'enseignement supérieur," *Revue internationale de l'enseignement* 37 (1899), 481–502.

17. Jacques Léonard, *Les Médecins de l'ouest au XIXe siècle* (Lille, 1976), p. 444.

18. For an idea of its manifold tasks see the *procès-verbaux* of the Faculty of Medicine from 1795 to 1807 in AJ16 6226, 6227, F17 6697, and F15 2738; Léonard, *Les Médecins*, pp. 325–28. On its role in regulating secret remedies see Matthew Ramsey, "Property Rights and the Rights to Health: The Regulation of Secret Remedies in France, 1789–1815," in *Medical Fringe and Medical Orthodoxy, 1750–1850*, ed. W. F. Bynum and Roy Porter (London, 1987), pp. 90–92, 99–100.

19. Léonard, *Les Médecins*, p. 447.

20. Dora B. Weiner, "The Role of the Doctor in Welfare Work: The Philanthropic Society of Paris, 1780–1815," *Historical Reflections* 9 (1982), 279–304; *Bulletin de l' École de médecine de Paris*, 1807, no. 1, p. 3.

21. *Journal général de médecine*, 2e sér., 15 (1821), 133–36; Zweibel-Muller, "La Société de l' École." However, M.-J. Imbault-Huart (*L' École Pratique de Dissection de Paris de 1750 à 1822, ou l'influence du concept de médecine pratique et de médecine d'observation dans l'enseignement médico-chirurgical au XVIIIe siècle et au début du XIXe siècle* [Lille: 1975], p.246) argues that this journal was more significant than is generally supposed. That faculty professors were sensitive to such charges is illustrated by a speech made at the turn of the century by B. Peyrilhe, professor of natural history from 1795 to 1804. The subject was "Can the functions of the medical professor be usefully reconciled with the development of literary or academic knowledge?" In AJ16 6705.

22. The relevant documents are reprinted in *Enquêtes et documents*, vol. 28. In response, the faculty published a pamphlet, *Observations adressés par l' École de Santé de Paris au Conseil des Cinq Cents en réponse aux imputations contenues dans plusieurs opinions émises à la tribune, 17 germinal An VI* (1798).

23. *Adresse présenté au Premier Consul par les commissaires de l'Académie de Chirurgie, An IX,* in F17 3679. On barristers' efforts to reconstitute corporate structures, see Michael Fitzsimmons, *The Parisian Order of Barristers and the French Revolution* (Cambridge, Mass., 1987).

24. "Adresse de la Société de médecine de Paris au Premier Consul de la République," *JGM* 10 (1801), 199–200.

25. The thinking of government spokesmen is illuminated by two administrative reports prepared in 1801 and found in F17 3679.

26. In 1811, for instance, the minister named a commission of ten members to regularize the training of *officiers de santé*. The commission included five professors at the Faculty of Paris, two professors of the Muséum d'Histoire Naturelle, and two inspectors-general of the Université (one a professor and the other a future professor at the Faculty of Medicine).

27. On the history of this society see *La Société de médecine de Paris, 1796–1896: Centenaire* (1896). Also see the report by J.-B. Nacquart and J. Sedillot to the prefect of the Seine, reprinted in *JGM*, 2e sér. 3 (1818), 145–56.

28. "Adresse de la Société de médecine," 199.

29. R. Pichevin, "La Première Académie de Médecine de Paris," *Bull. Soc. fr. his. méd.* 12 (1913), 196–231.

30. Minutes of the Académie, 26 vendémiaire, An XIII, AM, Ms. 42.

31. Minutes, February 1805, AM, Ms. 42, p. 9.

32. Pichevin, "La Première Académie," 213.

33. The split is described in Pichevin, "La Première Académie," 219–25, and massively documented in F17 1147, 2738, 2455, 3679.

34. Portal, *Note sur l'Institut de médecine de Paris* and an administrative report to the Minister of the Interior (n.d.), both in F17 2738.

35. The extent of this integration can be gauged by the fact that Napoleon ennobled eight professors of medicine at the Paris faculty and two at the faculty of Montpellier. The list of en-

nobled doctors is in Pierre Huard, *Sciences, médecine, pharmacie de la Révolution a l'Empire, 1789–1815* (1970), pp. 298–303.

36. The most complete study of medicine during the Restoration remains Paul Delaunay, *Les Médecins, la Restauration et la Révolution de 1830* (1931). Also useful is Jacques Léonard, "La Restauration et la profession médicale," *Historical Reflections* 9 (1982), 69–84. Among the many studies of political life during the Restoration see especially Guillaume Bertier de Sauvigny, *The Bourbon Restoration* (Philadelphia, 1966) and Alan B. Spitzer, "The Ambiguous Heritage of the French Restoration: The Distant Consequences of the Revolution and the Daily Realities of the Empire," in *The American and European Revolutions, 1776–1848: Sociopolitical and Ideological Aspects*, ed. Jaroslaw Pelenski (Iowa City, Ia., 1980), pp. 208–26.

37. Letter to the faculty in F17 3680. It is reprinted in *Réflexions sur l'établissement d'une Société Royale de médecine et de chirurgie* (1815), pp. 1–2.

38. Ministerial letter of December 22, 1811, in F17 2455.

39. The petition, along with several more detailed reports and speeches, is in F17 3680.

40. The report is in F17 3680. It is reprinted in *Réflexions sur l'établissement*.

41. Ibid., pp. 17–19.

42. Undated report in F17 3680.

43. In 1811 the emperor's First Physician was Corvisart and his First Surgeon, Boyer. The former was an honorary professor and the latter an active professor at the faculty. Seven of twenty-three lesser physicians and surgeons were professors (Huard, *Sciences, médecine, pharmacie*, p. 326)

44. P. Hillemand and E. Gilbrin, "Le Père Elisée (1753–1817): Premier Chirurgien de Louis XVIII," *Histoire des sciences médicales* 14 (1980), 238.

45. Among the many texts published during this controversy are the majority and minority reports of the reform commission of 1815–16 in *Enquêtes et documents*, vol. 37, pp. 64–166; *Réflexions sur l'établissement*; J.-B. Baumès, *Observations sommaires sur l'écrit ayant pour titre, Réflexions sur l'établissement* (Montpellier, 1816); *Opinion de M. Portal sur l'enseignement de la médecine et de la chirurgie* (1820); Chrétien-Lalanne, *Considérations sur l'état actuel de la médecine en France: présentées par la Société Académique de Médecine de Paris* (1818). Jacques Léonard in "La Restauration," 70, 72, cites many other relevant sources.

46. Delaunay, *Les Médecins*, p. 30.

47. In *Enquêtes et documents*, vol. 37, p. 77.

48. See, for instance, *Opinion de M. Portal* and the majority report in *Enquêtes et documents*, vol. 37.

49. Baumès, *Observations sommaires*, p. 20. Also see *Enquêtes et documents*, vol. 37, p. 71.

50. Among the many statements of this position see *Réflexions sur l'établissement*, pp. 10–14; the report "Note sur la médecine et la chirurgie" by J.-G. Hyde de Neuville and E. Laffon de Ladébat, October 16, 1815, in F17 4467; the ministerial report to the king in 1815 (no month given) in F17 3680.

51. Chrétien-Lalanne, *Considérations sur l'état de la médecine*, p. 188.

52. The existence of these abuses was admitted in 1815 by Georges Cuvier in the Commission de l'Instruction Publique governing the education system. Meeting of September 5, 1815, in F17 1759.

53. Delaunay, *Les Médecins*, pp. 35–36, is incorrect in suggesting that only Elisée's sudden death in 1817 prevented their victory.

54. See Spitzer, "The Ambiguous Heritage," pp. 222–23.

55. Letter dated October 13, 1815, in F17 4467. J.-G. Hyde de Neuville was chief of the third section in the ministry. As his tenure in that post was brief, it is likely that the memo was

actually written by his cosignatory and immediate subordinate, E. Laffon de Ladébat, chief of the Bureau de secours et des hôpitaux.

56. Of fourteen medical members, only three were faculty professors. Nor was the Commission de l'Instruction Publique, the directing body for all public education, consulted about the constitution of the commission. Its protest is in F17 1759, November 14, 1815. Reprinted in *Enquêtes et documents*, vol. 37, pp. 66–67.

57. Ibid., pp. 67–100.

58. Discussions are in ibid., pp. 92–100. One report, by Leroux and Dupuytren, is reprinted in full, pp. 100–165.

59. Ibid., p. 110. For what follows see p. 119.

60. Ibid., p. 121.

61. Ibid., p. 167.

62. For the response of hospital doctors see their pamphlet, de Montaigu et al., *Observations des médecins de l'Hôtel Dieu de Paris sur une réclamation faite au nom de l'École de médecine* (1818).

63. Portal, *Opinion de M. Portal*.

64. See the letter from Duffour to the ministry dated September 3, 1818, in F17 3679.

65. Letter from the ministry dated February 4, 1818, in F17 6705.

66. P. Hillemand and E. Gilbrin, "Le Père Elisée, premier chirurgien de Louis XVIII et la création de l'Académie de Médecine," *BAM* 165 (1981), 23–26.

67. P. Huard and M.-J. Imbault-Huart, "La Première Séance de l'Académie Royale de Médecine," *BAM* 155 (1971), 414–23.

68. On these matters, see Ann F. La Berge, *Mission and Method: The Early-Nineteenth-Century Public Health Movement* (Cambridge, 1992), pp. 89–92, and George D. Sussman, "From Yellow Fever to Cholera: A Study of French Government Policy, Medical Professionalism and Popular Movements in the Epidemic Crises of the Restoration and July Monarchy," Ph.D. diss., Yale University, 1971.

69. Goldstein, *Console and Classify*, pp. 137–38.

70. "Projet de loi sur la profession relative à l'art de guérir," *Enquêtes et documents*, vol. 37, pp. 172–80.

71. *MEM* 1 (1828), 1.

72. Letter of March 15, 1820, in F17 3680.

73. Report of March 17, 1820, in F17 3680. Laffon de Ladébat was still chief of the Bureau de Secours. His immediate superior was Baron Guillaume Capelle, secretary-general of the Ministry of the Interior. Capelle had been ennobled by Napoleon after an administrative career under the empire. He adhered to the Bourbons in 1814 and became a councillor of state in 1816.

74. Letter of April 5 in F17 3679.

75. See especially a remarkable letter from A.-A. Royer-Collard to Cuvier found in the dossier of A. Portal at the Academy of Sciences.

76. In F17 3680.

77. The members were G. Cuvier (president), J. de Gérando, A. Portal, J. Alibert, J.-J. Le Roux, F. Chaussier, A. Richerand, A. A. Royer-Collard, and R. Desgenettes.

78. Letter of May 8, 1820, in F17 3680.

79. In F17 3680.

80. In F17 3680.

81. July 26, 1820, in F17 3680.

82. The most complete discussion of these events is Charles Odic, "Les Événements du 18 novembre 1822," Thèse en médecine, Université de Paris, 1921. Also see P. Menetrier, "Le Centenaire de la suppression de la Faculté de Médecine de Paris," *Bull. Soc. Fr. hist. méd.* 16 (1922), 441–45.

83. In F17 2544.

84. The two ordinances are reprinted in *MEM* 1 (1828), 1–15.

85. Ibid., 1–2.

86. Membership in the three sections was to be on a ratio of 3:2:1.

87. These figures were arrived at by counting the practitioners listed in the *Almanach Royal* of that year.

88. "Lettres médicales sur Paris, No. III," *Revue médicale* 5 (1821), 328.

89. P. J. Pelletan, *Observations sur une Académie des sciences médicales* (1821), and F.-J. Double, *Opinion de M. le Docteur Double sur la question de la réunion ou de la séparation des sections dans les travaux académiques* (1821).

90. What follows is based on the correspondence by Portal and others, with the Ministry of the Interior in 1821 and 1822 that is located in F17 3680. For a partisan account, see R . . . , "Lettres médicales sur Paris, No. III," *Revue médicale* 5 (1821), 328–51.

91. Letter to Baron Mounier, March 7, 1821, partially reprinted in Académie Nationale de Médecine, *Exposition sur l'histoire de l'Académie de Médecine, 1820–1970* (1972), typescript.

92. The letter to the academy dated June 9, 1827, is summarized in *AGM* 5 (1827), 443–44.

93. Etienne Tessière de Boisbertrand (1720–1858) was chief of the "division des hospices" at the Ministry of the Interior. He had been elected deputy from the Vienne in 1824 and held his seat until 1831.

94. The exchange was reported in *JGM*, 2e sér. 9 (1829), 283–84.

95. *JGM*, 3e sér. 6 (1828), 384–90.

96. *JGM*, 3e sér. 8 (1828), 243. The full text of the letter dated October 5, 1828, can be found in AM, Liasse 104. A June 1828 exchange of letters between the academy and the ministry is in F17 3679.

97. "Réclamation de l'Académie," *JGM*, 3e sér. 9 (1829), 281–302.

98. *AGM* 9 (1831), 273. The incident is also discussed in Patrice Bourdelais and Jean-Yves Raulot, *Une peur bleue: histoire du choléra en France, 1832–1854* (1987), p. 203.

99. *Gazette médicale de Paris* 3 (1835), 509–10.

100. Gendrin, "Note de rédacteur sur la réorganisation de l'Académie Royale de Médecine," *JGM*, 3e sér. 12 (1829), 258.

101. *AGM* 7 (1829), 309.

102. G. Dupuytren et al., "Rapport à Son Excellence Monsieur le Ministre de l'Intérieur, sur la proposition de MM. Dariste, Orfila, Pelletier, Caventou et Pelletan, relative à la création d'une École spéciale de médecine légale" in *Enquêtes et documents*, vol. 37, pp. 250–69. *AGM* 3 (1825), 594–600.

103. George Weisz, "The Politics of Medical Professionalization in France, 1845–1848," *Journal of Social History* 19 (1978), 3–30.

104. Protests by academicians are in *AGM* 1 (1826), no. 1, 647, and no. 2, 135, 457.

105. *AGM* 6 (1828), 448.

106. F.-J. Double, "Projet de loi concernant la réorganisation de la médecine—Rapport fait à l'Académie Royale de Médecine," in *Enquêtes et documents*, vol. 40, pp. 100–217.

107. He also took over Portal's seat in the Academy of Sciences. J.-B. E. Bousquet, "Éloge de F.-J. Double," *MEM* 11 (1845), i–xx. P. Bousquet, "Double (François-Joseph)," in *Les Biographies médicales*, vol. 1 (1927), p. 21.

108. After the reorganization was announced Double initially urged the academy to send the minister a letter of protest. But at a subsequent meeting he declined to pursue the matter.

109. *AGM*, 2e sér. 3 (1833), 461.

110. Ibid., 466.

111. Ibid., 470.

112. Ibid., 631.

113. *Revue médicale* (1833), no. 4, 508.

114. Defenders of the measure could point to numerous precedents including the situation in the faculties of the ancien régime.

115. *AGM*, 2e sér. 3 (1833), 631–35.

116. *AGM*, 2e sér. 4 (1834), 151.

117. Ibid., 153–54.

118. Ibid., 155–59.

119. Ibid., 540.

120. Weisz, "Politics of Medical Professionalization," 7–13.

121. The office of permanent president was eliminated after Portal's death in 1832, leaving the permanent secretary as the dominant figure in the academy.

2

The Academy and Its Structures

By the 1830s the academy was a fully functioning institution. In the next three chapters we shall examine its structures and activities from roughly 1830 to 1939. Our approach will be topical rather than chronological. But it may be useful for the reader to keep in mind that three chronological periods define the history of the institution.

During the first period, which lasted until 1870, the academy was a relatively impoverished institution whose intellectual, financial, and symbolic status was low. It was characterized by a certain administrative disorderliness, violent personal passions, and endless argument. And yet it had an intellectual vitality that made it a central institution of French medicine. Medical journalists frequently criticized it vigorously because they observed it so very closely. The passionate debates for which it was best known reflected the strengths, weaknesses, and disarray of medicine in the mid-nineteenth century.

The start of the second period in the 1870s was marked by an intense desire to raise the status of the institution by transforming the academy into a more exclusive and scientific institution. The academy did become more exclusive, limited for all but some marginal fields to the successful survivors of public competitions (*concours*) for hospital and teaching posts. Likewise, the institution's status clearly rose. The Pasteurian debates made it a center of scientific attention for several years. Its role in advising the national government and local authorities expanded significantly. Public and especially private funding increased sharply. An opulent new building consecrated its status as a revered public institution. And yet by the early twentieth century it was losing its central intellectual role in French medical life.

This process accelerated during the third period, which began in the second decade of the twentieth century. The academy abandoned many of its evaluative scientific functions. In fact, it lost its status as a central institution of medical science, becoming a predominantly public health institution. It took a very active role in applying science to state needs. It performed routine technical-administrative tasks and debated public health and professional issues. During this period the academy became an institution of elderly sages representing in public debate the collective wisdom of medicine.

This chapter examines the administrative structures of academic life. We look first at the organizational hierarchies and financial resources that provided the basis for academic activities. We then attend to the academy's physical surroundings, before going on to analyze debates about the categories of medical knowledge utilized to classify members into specialty sections. Next we consider the membership, investigating titular Parisian members and the various categories of associate and corresponding members who linked the academy to medicine outside Paris and to the scientific, administrative, and literary domains. A theme running through the chapter is the importance for academicians of the Academy of Sciences as a model for academic activities and the high social status to which they aspired.

Inner Workings

The Academy of Medicine as it was originally conceived, with its three quasi-autonomous professional sections and a permanent president who owed his power to royal patronage, was in many ways very different from the Academy of Sciences. But a succession of reforms in the 1820s and 1830s brought it increasingly into line with the older institution in its structures and modes of functioning. It met weekly in full session, following a formal order of business almost identical to the one in use at the Academy of Sciences. Like the latter establishment, it held an annual public meeting in mid-December of every year in which the winners of prize competitions were announced and the most eminent deceased members were elaborately eulogized.

As we shall see, the example of the Academy of Sciences with its significantly greater prestige and resources loomed always in the background when the Academy of Medicine contemplated its own structures. Still the medical institution never became a copy of the older scientific body. Not only did it have a far more homogeneous membership centering on the medical sciences (whereas the Academy of Sciences was responsible for all "science"), but the specific kinds tasks it was required to perform for the government dictated an administrative structure that was in some ways quite distinctive.

The office of permanent president was eliminated after Portal's death in 1832, leaving the academy as an essentially collegial institution. Few if any decisions about its inner workings were imposed against the wishes of a significant minority. Most of the important changes in the academy's working regulations, we shall see, were discussed and voted by the entire academy in secret session.[1] Nevertheless, the institution did have an administrative hierarchy which exercised considerable influence.

Managing the academy was an administrative council composed of elected officials. A single permanent secretary (the Academy of Sciences had two) was certainly the dominant member because he spent so much time on the premises handling day-to-day affairs and because he generally served for a considerable period of time. From 1822 to 1944 only seven men served in this position: Etienne Pariset (1822–47), Frédéric Dubois d'Amiens (1847–73), Jules Béclard (1873–87), E. J. Bergeron (1887–1900), Sigismond Jaccoud (1901–13), Georges Debove (1913–20), and Charles

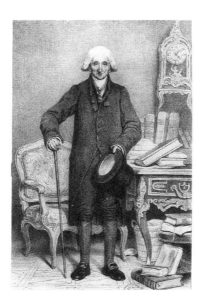

FIGURE 2.1. The academy's first permanent president, Baron Antoine Portal, in 1833.
(Bibliothèque de l'Académie de Médecine)

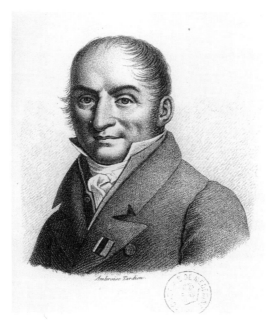

FIGURE 2.2. The academy's first permanent secretary, Etienne Pariset. (Bibliothèque de
l' Académie de Médecine)

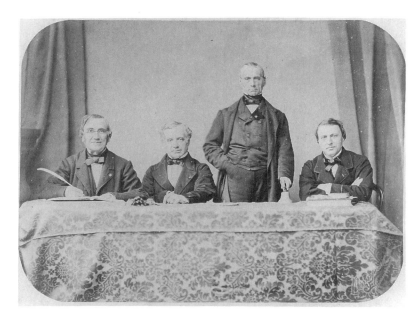

FIGURE 2.3. The officers of the academy in 1862. *Left to right*: Frédéric Dubois d'Amiens, Hippolyte Larrey, Jean-Baptiste Bouillaud, and Jules Béclard. (Bibliothèque de l'Académie de Médecine)

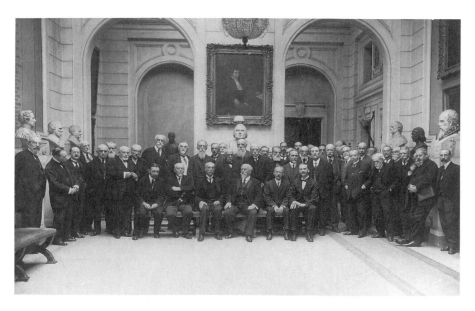

FIGURE 2.4. Members of the academy in 1924. (Bibliothèque de l'Académie de Médecine)

Achard (1921–44). Of these only Pariset was appointed rather than elected. Achard was the first to be elected under a new regime which limited the secretary (now called "general" rather than "permanent") to a tenure of five years, but he had no difficulty winning regular reelection until his death at the age of eighty-four.

The secretary was responsible for the smooth functioning of the academy; his tasks included setting the program of meetings and filtering out any presentations that were unsuitable. He also handled the academy's communication with the government, an increasingly onerous task as the institution's public health role expanded.[2] Dubois d'Amiens, it was said, personally handled the accumulation and deposition of the academy's art collection at mid-century while Bergeron took charge of the exhausting negotiations with national and local authorities which preceded the construction of the new building on the rue Bonaparte. The secretary was also responsible for most of the academic eulogies (*éloges*) honoring deceased members presented at the annual public meetings. More generally the secretary enjoyed substantial autonomy in matters of administration. Many of the changes in procedure which I will describe were introduced by new secretaries at or near the beginning of their tenures. The general deference on such matters is succinctly expressed by a brief entry in the minutes of the administrative council for January 9, 1906: "Monsieur the Perpetual Secretary tells the council about the questions of internal administration to which he has proposed the solution that they appear to require. The council gives its approbation."[3] Although his role was more discrete, the academy's treasurer also served a key function. He was responsible for balancing the small budget, preparing an annual financial report, and keeping track of the investment of bequests that supported the prizes which the academy awarded. He was the only officer beside the permanent secretary to obtain an annual subsidy of one thousand francs. Competent men tended to be reappointed and only ten men served in the post between 1821 and 1955. One of these, A. Hanriot, served from 1896 to 1933.

The administrative council was composed of these two figures, several members at large, including the dean of the Paris Faculty of Medicine, and elected annual officers. An annual secretary assisted the permanent secretary and read at the annual public meeting the report on the results of the prize competitions; it became traditional for him to then say a few words about the members who had died during the course of the previous year. Also on the council were the annually elected vice-president and president.

The vice-president was president-elect and his main task was to take over in the president's absence. The presidency, however, was probably the third most important position in the academy. The incumbent's principal function was to chair meetings, a difficult task during some of the more stormy debates of the mid-nineteenth century. He also was the chief spokesman for the academy at all formal occasions. At the beginning of each new academic year the outgoing president presented a fairly lengthy review of the previous year's activities. The incoming president also made a shorter and more mundane speech. In the last decades of the nineteenth century the president's traditional announcement of the recent death of a member turned into a summary review of the deceased member's career. Around mid-century the journalist Louis Peisse devoted several pages to the many different qualities a president needed to possess.[4] These included wide medical and scientific knowledge, firmness,

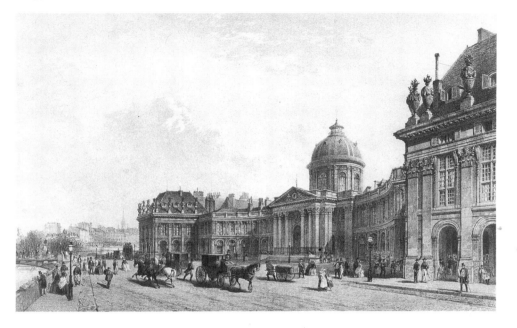

FIGURE 2.5. The Institut de France (home of the Academy of Sciences) in the early nineteenth century. (Lithograph, Musée Carnavalet)

gravity, and impartiality. In fact, longevity and the ability to avoid alienating too many peers seem to have been the major criteria for election.[5]

The academy was never a well-funded institution. Its budget for everything but prizes was allocated by the central government. In 1828 the academy received 40,000 francs from the government. A full quarter of that went toward the rental of the building it occupied. During the next three decades, budgets fluctuated between 43,000 and 53,000 francs.[6] In contrast, the Academy of Sciences in the early 1860s had a state allocation of 188,500 francs, four times that of the Academy of Medicine. To this one should also add one-fifth of the 82,000 francs earmarked for expenses common to all five academies of the Institut de France.

Things improved somewhat in the 1870s when the academy's budget, reflecting similar investments in all scientific and educational institutions,[7] rose to 75,000 francs. About 40 percent of this increase went initially to pay for the purchase of the library belonging to the medical historian Charles Daremberg. But once this was paid, there was considerably more money for academic activities. The academy's funding, however, stagnated for the rest of the century and went up only slightly before World War I (to 84,300 francs in 1910). After the war budgets rose, but they couldn't keep up with galloping inflation. Lack of adequate financing became a frequent theme of academic discourse during the 1930s.

Thus throughout its first century the academy's finances remained modest. And the discrepancy with the finances of the Academy of Sciences remained large since

that institution's budget rose even more substantially during the early Third Republic to nearly 280,000 francs in 1885.[8] These discrepancies are particularly telling in
their details. One of the Academy of Medicine's most stable expenses was the financial compensation provided members who attended meetings and commission
sessions. During the first two-thirds of the century the academy spent from 15,000 to
20,000 francs annually on this, issuing tokens that could be exchanged for money
(three francs a session); from the 1870s the annual figure was 20,000 francs. Divided
by roughly one hundred members, the funds did not allow even the most assiduous
participants in academic activities to earn more than a few hundred francs each year.[9]
In contrast, the Academy of Sciences paid each of its sixty-eight members a subsidy
of 1,500 francs annually. This disparity seldom received comment and would have
doubtless been rationalized by the large earnings which medical practitioners, unlike
scientists in state institutions, were able to draw. But the derisory sums paid out did
little to encourage busy medical practitioners to attend meetings, which may explain
why attendance was frequently low.[10]

The only academician to earn a substantial amount of money was the permanent
secretary. In the 1820s his annual salary was 3,000 francs; in the following decades
an additional 1,000 francs in salary and a housing allowance worth the same amount
were gradually added. Taken together, the salary and housing allowance represented
a substantial sum of money, coming close to the 6,000 francs paid annually to each
of the two permanent secretaries of the Academy of Sciences.

The relatively small budget of the Academy of Medicine is undoubtedly indica- *,*
tive of medicine's place among the state's priorities, but the academy did not suffer
overmuch. Its members quickly learned to perform their functions cheaply,[11] partly
by abandoning their initial aspirations to emulate the Academy of Sciences by performing collective research.[12] Its most expensive activity, the awarding of prizes, was
funded by private donations and legacies. The first major legacy, a sum of 12,000
francs, was appropriately enough left to the academy by its permanent president,
Antoine Portal. Many other academicians and nonacademicians subsequently left
various sums of money to the institution. By 1920 the academy had received gifts
from 114 donors;[13] about 80 supported prize competitions which distributed from
120,000 to 130,000 francs annually. Some substantial donations were earmarked for
other needs. In 1877 the academician Jean Demarquay left the academy 100,000
francs to help it find adequate lodgings. Other academicians added to this endow-
ment, which held over 400,000 francs at the end of the century.

This brings us inevitably to the physical plant of the Academy of Medicine. In
only one respect did complaints about finances go beyond routine and somewhat ritualized levels of intensity: the low quality of the academy's installations throughout
the nineteenth century was a major source of discontent. Unlike the academies
making up the Institut, which met in the early nineteenth century at the Louvre before
moving to their permanent home along the left bank of the Seine, the Academy of
Medicine made do with a series of rented spaces, all meant to be temporary. The inadequacies of these various dwellings would achieve near mythic proportions.[14]

The ordinance creating the academy did not provide for space to house the institution. In the first years the members met in the amphitheater of the Faculty of
Medicine and public meetings were held at the Louvre. In 1824 the academy was in-

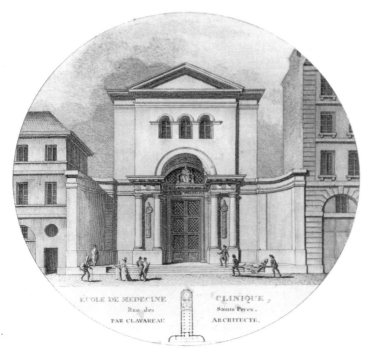

FIGURE 2.6. Architectural rendering of the chapel of the Charité Hospital renovated by Nicholas Clavareau for use as a teaching amphitheater of the Faculty of Medicine. The academy occupied it in 1850. From N. Clavareau, *Mémoires sur les hôpitaux civils* (Paris, 1805). (Bibliothèque Nationale)

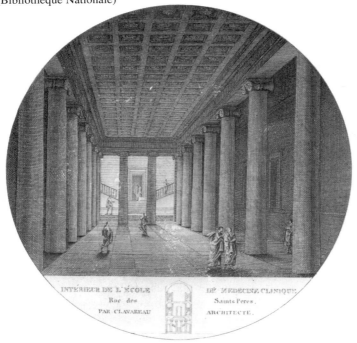

FIGURE 2.7. Architectural rendering of the interior hallway of the Charité amphitheater. From N. Clavareau, *Mémoires sur les hôpitaux civils* (Paris, 1805). (Bibliothèque Nationale)

stalled in a building on the rue de Poitiers where the semipublic vaccination commission had been located.[15] Because of budgetary restrictions, however, the academy could rent only the ground floor. This resulted in a serious shortage of space, making it difficult for more than a handful of visitors and journalists to attend academic meetings. Even so, rent at 10,000 francs per year represented from one-quarter to one-fifth the total annual budget.

In 1848, however, the building's owner decided not to renew the lease. In 1850 the academy moved into the former chapel of the Charité hospital on the rue des Saints-Pères. It remained there for the next half century. The move to a permanent and more grand location represented a step up for the academy, consecrating its status as a public institution.[16] Although the building was rented, the landlord was the Paris hospital administration (the Assistance Publique), making it almost a state building. The rent, moreover, was reasonable at 5,000 francs annually. Its physical appearance was imposing, if not in the same league as the home of the Academy of Sciences. The former chapel of the Charité hospital had in 1797 been converted into a teaching amphitheater of the Faculty of Medicine and had been totally renovated. The architect Nicholas Clavareau had chosen a classical and monumental look inspired by the Temple of Asclepius. Although the most prominent external symbols were the fasces of lictor (beloved by republicans) on each side of the entrance, a small statue of the god of healing sat over the massive door and announced the buildings's medical calling. The structure was clearly understood to be a public monument to medicine, one proclaiming its permanence, dignity, durability, and official status. In the words of a medical journalist of the period,

> Through this official installation in a building of the state, it [the academy] received a sort of new consecration as a public institution. It underwent at the same time, from the decorative point of view, a brilliant metamorphosis. The building of the rue de Poitiers was nothing but a vulgar establishment; the new one is a monument.[17]

The space was considerably larger than that of the rue de Poitiers, with a room for the academy's library and archives. It had been thoroughly renovated according to the design of one of the hospital administration's leading architects. Nevertheless, it was far too small for the academy and an effort was launched almost immediately to find more spacious and appropriate installations. But despite regular visits of commiseration by a succession of ministers, no more suitable lodgings could be found for another fifty years.[18] By 1895 the academy's librarian described the premises as "absolutely insufficient, defective in all respects, unhealthy in most of its parts, a menacing ruin which we occupy at this moment."[19] This is how Sigismond Jaccoud described the academy's ceaseless efforts to find better accommodations:

> [The academy] comes, it goes, it bustles about; with a perseverance that nothing exhausts, a liveliness always being renewed, it knocks at every door; it goes up from ministers to the chief of state, goes back down from the chief of state to the ministers, always listened to, always gaining approval, desires never fulfilled, it readily accepts the fantastic peregrinations that take it virtually from the poste-caserne of the Assumption to the rue de Lille, from the ruins of the Cours de compte to the Montagne Sainte-Geneviève, and exhausted by the battle, it resigns itself in 1883 to accept being carried away to the ethereal regions of the Observatoire.[20]

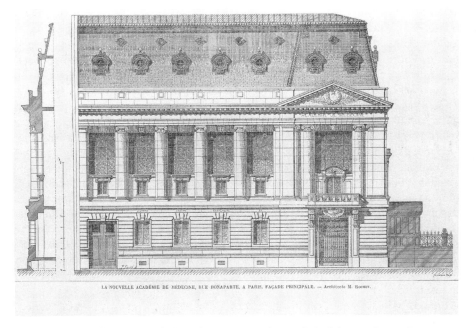

LA NOUVELLE ACADÉMIE DE MÉDECINE, RUE BONAPARTE, A PARIS. FAÇADE PRINCIPALE. — Architecte M. Rochet.

FIGURE 2.8. Architectural rendering of the new Academy of Medicine on the rue Bonaparte. From *L'Architecture* 11 (1902), plate 18. (Collection Centre Canadien d'Architecture/Canadian Centre for Architecture, Montreal)

The last location refers to a piece of land between the avenue de l'Observatoire and the rue Michelet which the government accorded the academy in 1883 after the Assistance Publique announced that it wished to give the building on the rue des Saints-Pères to the Archbishop of Paris. But the price of constructing a building was prohibitive and the land remained undeveloped.

Finally in 1895 the Municipal Council of Paris agreed to transfer to the academy land on the rue Bonaparte next to the École des Beaux-Arts in exchange for the land on the avenue de l'Observatoire and 663,500 francs. The academy paid nearly half of this cost from its own funds accumulated from donations. It took several years for a definitive agreement to be worked out and for construction—which cost another million francs[21]—to be completed. But in 1902 the academy finally moved into its new premises. If the move in 1850 had reflected the rising status of the institution, that of 1902 symbolized its elevated position in society. "The academy is no longer a tenant," said one medical journal; "it is henceforth installed *chez elle*, in a public building that is worthy of it."[22]

The new premises were very impressive indeed. Despite the narrowness of the lot on which it was built, the architect Rochet had found space for offices, laboratories, technical services, committee meetings, a room for medical examinations, and even stables for the calves used to produce smallpox vaccine. The building also represented the last word in hygienically inspired architecture; parquet believed to be "a receptor of microbes . . . was banished" to be replaced by stone and linoleum.[23] Sky-lights provided the main rooms with natural light and an airy feel. In the main meeting hall, each academician had a comfortable leather armchair, a table, and a lamp. There was a balcony for the public and press with a special press room off to the side. In addition to staircases there was an elevator. The only major problem immediately noted had to do with poor acoustics, which made it difficult for those on the balcony to hear speakers. (The problem was exacerbated by the buzz of constant talking in the hall.)[24] Offsetting this inconvenience was the impressive number of bathrooms, one journalist having counted "up to twenty *places assises*."[25]

Aside from pointing out the difficulties under which the academy functioned, this account underscores the academy's relative lack of political clout for much of the nineteenth century. Although the academy's need for better premises was undisputed, somehow nothing could be done. In view of the magnificent if somewhat cramped installations of the Institut, it is hard not to attribute this state of affairs to the lesser estime in which medicine was held. One finds direct confirmation of this lesser status in a matter of protocol. Under both the July Monarchy and Second Empire there was an annual ceremony at which official institutions presented themselves to the ruler. Rigid protocol determined the order of presentation and the academy was chronically disgruntled with its own low ranking. Its representatives periodically made efforts to get it positioned just behind the academies of the Institut.[26]

That a solution to the academy's edifice complex was finally achieved in the last years of the nineteenth century is hardly fortuitous. If it corresponds to a general willingness on the part of government during this period to invest massively in buildings for science and higher education,[27] it also reflects the new status of medicine that followed in the wake of the Pasteurian revolution. The new building signified decidedly that the academy had "arrived" as a public institution.

The Classification of Parisian Members

Aside from the matter of institutional accommodations, only one other administrative issue—the division of full members into sections—seriously agitated academicians during the nineteenth century. Though this concerned primarily changing notions of how medical knowledge and its practitioners should be classified, it too was largely fueled by dissatisfaction with the public status of the Academy of Medicine and desire to emulate the Academy of Sciences.

The reorganization of 1829 attempted and failed, not for the last time, to reduce the size of the academy's membership to sixty titular and forty associate members. It succeeded, however, in dividing the academy into eleven specialty sections. Both sets of numbers would seem to have been efforts to imitate the Academy of Sciences, whose sixty members[28] were then divided into thirteen sections.

All sections of the Academy of Medicine met together as a single body but recruitment was determined by vacancies in particular sections. When such vacancies appeared, the section ordinarily presented a list of candidates to the academy, which voted as a whole to elect a member. The eleven sections were meant collectively to cover all medical knowledge and were a curious mixture of professional and disciplinary categories. They followed a codified order that seems to have reflected the

TABLE 2.1   Sections of the Academy, 1829–1923

Sections	Members
1. Anatomy and physiology	10
2. Medical pathology	13
3. Surgical pathology	10
4. Therapeutics and medical natural history	10
5. Surgical procedure (*Médecine opératoire*)	7
6. Pathological anatomy	7
7. Obstetrics (*Accouchement*)	7
8. Public hygiene, legal medicine, medical police	10
9. Veterinary medicine	6
10. Medical physics and chemistry	10
11. Pharmacy	10
TOTAL	100

organization of chairs at the Paris Faculty of Medicine (see table 2.1). First on every list was the section of anatomy and physiology, in which two of what we would now call basic sciences were brought together. The next four sections divided both medicine and surgery into pathology and therapeutic applications. Next came three categories which did not fit the traditional division between internal medicine and surgery. The more surprising of these is pathological anatomy, not considered a basic science but nonetheless distinct from both medical and surgical pathology. Most likely, pathological anatomy was, like the next two categories, obstetrics and public hygiene, considered an integral part of medicine (in its large sense) but unintelligible in terms of the traditional categories of internal medicine and surgery.

The existence of obstetrics as a special category is less surprising. A variety of institutions, particularly maternity hospitals and faculty chairs, had brought obstetrics as close to specialty status as was conceivable in early nineteenth century France.[29] Public hygiene and forensic medicine also approached specialty status, with faculty chairs, a professional journal, and positions on administrative bodies. This was followed by two professional categories separated from medicine by distinct training schools, diplomas, and professional regulations. Veterinary medicine, which had been integrated into the section of medicine in the organizational plan of 1820, was now given a small section of its own. The section of pharmacy had its own associated basic science section, medical physics and chemistry. That these two disciplines were seen to be associated with pharmacy while medicine was linked with natural history tells us much about the state of medical knowledge in the early nineteenth century.

From the beginning, this new system of sections provoked considerable protest. It was completely arbitrary, complained one medical journalist, separating matters which should be joined.[30] The source of the problem, it was suggested, was the misguided effort to ignore the logic of medical practice and to seek instead to imitate the more abstract categories of the Academy of Sciences or faculties of medicine.[31] On what basis, for instance, could one distinguish between surgical pathology and surgical operations? There was a practical aspect to complaints as well. Vacancies opened regularly in large sections of medicine and surgery but were considerably less frequent in small sections. The issue of waiting time was all the more dramatic during the 1830s and 1840s since only one in three vacancies was filled until membership fell to one hundred.

Unhappiness with the academy's structure soon died down but did not disappear. There is in the academy's archives a detailed proposal to reorganize the academy that dates from mid-century.[32] There is no evidence that it was ever acted upon but it prefigured in many specifics later efforts at reorganization. The central purpose of the document was to integrate the academy into the Institut de France, where it would join the five existing academies, most notably the Academy of Sciences. Among the many rationales offered in defense of this proposal were the following: the academy having become one of the preeminent scientific societies of Europe, the distance separating it from the Institut had been greatly reduced; the move would consecrate the achievements and sacrifices of France's doctors and was warranted by the social importance of medicine; and, most interesting for our purposes, since the internal structure of the academy needed reform anyway, a total institutional makeover was appropriate.

The most salient aspect of this reorganization aside from the attachment of the academy to the Institut was to reduce the membership by more than half. There would be a perpetual secretary plus only forty-five full members divided into six unequal sections which merged together many of the existing categories (see table 2.2, part A). Associate and corresponding categories would also be substantially reduced. The goal would seem to have been to raise the academy's status by making it smaller and more exclusive.

In the wake of the French military defeat in the Franco-Prussian War, when all aspects of science and higher education in France were being questioned, there erupted a more serious movement to transform the academy's structure. Discontent with institutional structure was again fueled by discontent with the academy's inferior public rank. In January 1873 the outgoing president, J.-B. Barth commented on the incongruity between the institution's real social importance and its low official status. The academy, he claimed, was in reality a sixth section of the Institut, occupying "an elevated place . . . in the regions of science" and reflecting medicine's increasing importance for society. But the academy "is not yet officially invested with the rank it deserves among scientific institutions." As proof he cited the almost negligible presence of academicians in the nation's highest political assemblies.[33]

Such aspirations demanded change in the academy's structures, and a year later the academy met in secret session to discuss numerous requests for reform submitted by members. A commission comprised of a representative from each of the existing sections was formed to examine the institution's organizational structure. After five months of deliberations, a report was read to the entire membership by Paul-Émile Chauffard, professor of pathology at the Medical Faculty, whose courses were then being disrupted by students who disapproved of his political and religious views. The commission's proposal had two parts.[34]

TABLE 2.2   Plans for Reorganizing the Sections of the Academy

Sections	Members
A. SECTIONS PROPOSED IN 1856	
1. Human anatomy and physiology, normal and pathological	6
2. Medicine	10
3. Surgery and obstetrics	10
4. Public hygiene, legal medicine, sanitary police	10
5. Medical chemistry and physics, pharmacy	6
6. Veterinary medicine	3
B. SECTIONS PROPOSED BY CHAUFFARD IN 1874	
1. Medicine (medical pathology, pathological anatomy, therapeutics)	17
2. Surgery (surgical pathology, operating procedures, obstetrics)	15
3. Biological sciences (anatomy, physiology, comparative medicine, veterinary medicine)	10
4. Physical and natural sciences (natural history, physics, chemistry, pharmacy)	12
5. Public medicine (hygiene, legal medicine, statistics, medical police and legislation)	6
C. SECTIONS INTRODUCED IN 1923	
1. Medicine and medical specialties	28
2. Surgery, obstetrics, and surgical specialties	24
3. Hygiene	10
4. Biological, physical, chemical, and natural sciences	22
5. Veterinary medicine	6
6. Pharmacy	6

The first, unanimously approved by all the commissioners, called for an end to the existing system of sections. It would be replaced by five much broader sections that did not slice up knowledge in arbitrary ways but rearranged and combined the existing sections (see table 2.2, part B). Medical pathology, pathological anatomy, and therapeutics would be combined in a new section, no longer linked to natural history, whose usefulness for treatment was no longer evident.[35] This new section of medicine would thus bring together the study of disease, both symptomatic and anatomical, with therapeutics. Similarly, surgical pathology was combined with operational procedures and with obstetrics, now defined as a "branch of the surgical art" not different in principle from urology or ophthalmology.[36] This attitude undoubtedly reflected the development of specialization during this decade, which removed much of the professional uniqueness of obstetrics.

Yet another section brought together anatomy, physiology, comparative medicine, and veterinary medicine. The justification was the experimental character of all these disciplines based on dissection and vivisection.[37] The inclusion of veterinary medicine in this category, clearly controversial, was defended on the grounds of common methods and concepts, as well as the fact that most veterinarians in the academy were in fact physiologists.[38]

Natural history (detached from therapeutics) was attached to another large section, composed of medical physics, chemistry, and pharmacy. Justification for the union was that all these categories were devoted to the agents of cure.[39] There is little mention of natural history in all this, suggesting that it was thrown into this section only because outright elimination was not possible. The last category was the old section of public health, legal medicine, and medical police enlarged by two new terms, population statistics and legislation. The first was a specific form of knowledge while the second proclaimed the academy's advisory role in drawing up public health legislation.[40]

Chauffard emphasized that there was nothing revolutionary about his classification; for the most part it reorganized the academy's traditional categories. "We have not had pretensions of starting from scratch, but of arranging in a larger more rational way the existing elements and supplementing them by the addition of new elements. . . ."[41] But these were not just mechanical groupings; each category was described by a generic term meant to encapsulate what was common to the original categories retained in a subtitle. Thus the first section was called simply "medicine" and the second "surgery," while anatomy, physiology, comparative medicine, and veterinary medicine were combined under the generic term "biological sciences." The introduction of such general terms had practical implications; these sections were not limited to the old categories since the new generic terms were very broad indeed; they opened up the possibility of recruiting from a much vaster terrain of emerging medical science. As an example, Chauffard suggested that under the general term "medicine" one might include, for purposes of recruitment, history and philosophy of medicine. "Biological sciences" might include general anatomy, general biology, or even anthropology.[42]

The ability to introduce new disciplines, as well as the fact that the subcategories had no specified quota of representatives, created the possibility, even probability, that the current distribution of members according to subjects would be transformed. There were, however, two exceptional subcategories whose numerical representation was specified: obstetrics and veterinary medicine. Chauffard suggested that both involved practical and theoretical training that was distinctive. More to the point, he added that "they [the members] represent in the section to which they belong a large profession whose dignity will suffer if they do not have a sufficient almost official number of representatives in the academy."[43] In other words, these two sections had refused to agree to the reorganization unless they were assured of keeping their share of seats.

Few questioned the need to reorganize an existing structure of sections recognized to be inappropriate. But there was opposition to Chauffard's proposal from members of some of the existing sections in danger of losing their place in the academy. (Veterinary medicine was frequently mentioned by medical journals.) Others, in contrast, felt that certain disciplines had been slighted. Some members of the reform commission, according to the editor of *L'Union médical*, who warmly supported their views, were unhappy that a section of medical history and philosophy (in which editors of medical journals would presumably be well represented) had been rejected.[44] But it is unlikely that reorganization would have provoked enough opposition of this nature to prevent its implementation.[45] There was, however, a much more controversial, though by no means original, proposal in the re-organization package—reducing the membership of the academy from one hundred to sixty.

Chauffard insisted that the large size of the academy was responsible for low scientific standards because criteria for recruitment were not stringent enough. The Academy of Sciences, which covered the entire gamut of the sciences, had only sixty-six members and none of the other academies of the Institut had more than forty. Effective academies had to constitute "an elite that is zealous and small in number."[46] The problem he believed was that professional distinction, even in the absence of scientific accomplishment, was sufficient for election to the Academy of Medicine. This institution should not be

> an eminent and honored representative of the profession but a purely scientific in-stitution. . . . The extension of science, the increasing difficulty of research, no longer permit one to divide oneself equally, and without being diminished as a result, between scientific life and professional life; one of the two must dominate or obliterate the other; there will be either men of science or men of practice. The acad-emy must be constituted above all with a view to the first.[47]

There were simply not enough men "dedicated to an austere science" to fill an acad-emy with one hundred members. By eliminating purely professional criteria for election, the academy would achieve new stature. "Its judgments will be listened to more; the discussions which it relishes will be more intimately associated with the preoccupations of contemporary science."[48]

But haunting Chauffard's report was the specter of the Academy of Sciences. It was more than just an example of the small institution which the Academy of Medi-cine should become; it represented the high status associated with dedication to "science." In his closing remarks, Chauffard pointed out that when the Institut had been created to represent human knowledge, medicine had not been thought worthy of constituting an entire academy; it received only "as through grace" a poor and small section in the "vast" Academy of Sciences. And when a new academy was added to the Institut in 1832, it was not one of medicine but of Moral and Political Sciences. "Our academy remained isolated, apart from this movement of representa-tion, as if one was afraid to acknowledge or increase its role, and the rank which it occupies in the theater of human knowledge."[49] By limiting the academy to ardent workers of science, this exclusion might be lifted, Chauffard concluded portentously, at least for the academicians of the future.

Chauffard's report was dealt with by the academy in "secret session." This did not prevent medical journals from reporting rumors of intense disagreements within the academy. They also participated in the debate by expressing vigorous opposition to the cutback in membership. Several made impassioned pleas for the centrality of medical practice within the academy.[50] Normal business was temporarily paralyzed as the reorganization controversy held center stage. In December 1874 the acad-emy—by one vote, according to one journal—rejected the reform proposal.[51] Although the commission was supposed to produce a revised proposal, none was forthcoming in the following months. The academy thus remained saddled with a system of sections that was recognized to be seriously inadequate.

It was not until forty years later, in the midst of World War I, that the academy resumed its discussions of structural reorganization, again in "secret session." We know little of what transpired beyond the fact that Charles Achard prepared three different proposals, none of which was able to win sufficient support from academicians.[52] In 1923 Achard, now permanent secretary, managed to get agreement for a new structure that was quickly approved by the minister of public instruction.[53] The silence of medical journals about this reorganization presents a striking contrast to their active participation in discussions fifty years before.

The new classification was similar to and yet quite different from the one proposed by Chauffard (see table 2.2, part C). It had an extra section and no effort was made to include all the old sections among the new categories. A development which had only begun to assume importance in the 1870s, clinical specialization, was clearly recognized in the new scheme of things. The link between pharmacy and the physical sciences was broken as the latter was lumped together with the biological sciences to constitute an effectively experimental section.

The lack of controversy surrounding this reform was undoubtedly due to its dissociation from plans to reduce the size of membership. By the twentieth century increasing exclusiveness in this way no longer commanded support. For even without a radical reorganization, the academy had in fact gradually transformed itself into a highly exclusive institution.

Parisian Membership

The reforms of 1829 and 1835 granted honorary and associate members titular status, creating a single category of Parisian members that gradually shrank in size from 210 in 1829 until it reached the mandated figure of 100 in the 1850s. This shrinkage of membership had major consequences for the institution. Designed originally as a compromise to bring together the various sectors of the medical domain, the academy, as the nineteenth century advanced, became increasingly dominated by professors in state or semipublic schools of medicine and science, particularly the Paris Faculty of Medicine. The proportion of professors (or their equivalent in certain institutions) among academicians rose from 47 percent in the cohort of 1820–21 to 76 percent in that of 1935. And those who were not professors were increasingly likely to be only a rung or two below on the medical career ladder.[54]

By far the largest group at the academy taught at one time or another at the Paris Faculty of Medicine (see Table 2.3). Appointment to a professorial chair at that institution virtually guaranteed eventual election to the academy.[55] The number of faculty professors was artificially large among academicians in 1821 because of demographic and political factors. Many of those appointed to the newly created academy in 1820–21 were already quite old and were replaced at the faculty during the next decades by younger academicians. The purge and replacement of eleven professors in 1823 also helped to swell the ranks of faculty professors at the academy. Consequently, in the following generation the proportion of professors among the academicians of 1861 was somewhat lower; it rose steadily, however, in our two twentieth-century populations, as the staff of the Faculty of Medicine expanded in size.[56]

TABLE 2.3   Professors in the Academy of Medicine, by percent[a]

Institution	1821	1861	1901	1935
Faculty of medicine	34	28	38	46
School of pharmacy	6[b]	6	8	8
Science and research	9	7	19	22
Other medical education	5	6	11	17
Other	1	3	1	—
Without professorship	53	47	36	22

[a] Includes professorships obtained after the sample date. Individuals may appear in more than one category.

[b] Includes a professor at the medical faculty who was also director of the School of Pharmacy (Vauquelin).

Professors at the Paris School of Pharmacy made up a much smaller cluster of academicians, which grew little during the period being examined. Unlike the staff of the Faculty of Medicine, which expanded throughout the nineteenth and twentieth centuries, that of the School of Pharmacy remained stable. There were ten professors and senior administrators in 1832 and only two more in 1904. Pharmacist-academicians without professorships, common enough in the early nineteenth century, disappeared in the twentieth.[57]

The group that expanded most rapidly during the latter half of the nineteenth century, becoming in the process quite heterogeneous, was composed of professors in the institutions of science and medical research. In the early nineteenth century, individuals in this category worked in three institutions, the Collège de France, the Muséum d'Histoire Naturelle, and the Science Faculty of Paris. These institutions continued to serve as major sources of academicians; over 10 percent of the membership in both 1901 and 1935 taught at one of them. However, another 10 percent or so in both these populations now worked in a number of newer institutions: the école des Hautes Études, the more directly medical Institut Pasteur, and the Institut de Radium. In 1935, six academicians worked at the Institut Pasteur and three others were at the Institut de Radium.

Another fairly heterogeneous group at the academy taught at other medical schools. During the first half of the century this meant essentially the military training school at Val-de-Grâce and the veterinary school at Alfort. The number of academicians in the latter institution fluctuated from a low of two in 1821 to a high of five in 1861. The number of academicians at Val-de-Grâce increased from three in 1821 to six in 1935. This was not due to any rise in the number of military doctors in the academy. On the contrary, the number of academicians who spent at least a decade in the military declined quite dramatically.[58] The growing dominance of Val-de-Grâcians among these military academicians reflects changes in the academy's recruitment criteria. In the early nineteenth century, it was possible to be appointed or elected to the academy as a result of a career in military medical practice or administration. Increasingly from the mid-nineteenth century a career in research and teaching was also demanded.

A handful of new job possibilities existed among academicians of 1935. Colonial expansion led to the creation of an Institut Colonial where tropical medicine was

TABLE 2.4.   Age of Academicians

Academicians	1821	1861	1901	1935
Average age at election				
(yrs)	53.2	44.8	48.4	6.5
% under age 40	—	23	12	1
% over age 60	—	1	2	35
Average age in that				
year (yrs)	53.2	62.1	61.4	69.6
% less than age 60	71	37	47	5
% over age 70	16	25	18	45
Mean age at death (yrs)	72.0	75.2	75.9	82.2

taught by one academician. A private school of dentistry, which opened its doors at the end of the nineteenth century, provided a position for another. One member of the academy even taught in Brazil before World War I. Such positions, however, were not sufficient for appointment to the academy; they were ordinarily held before or simultaneously to appointment to a chair in a more prestigious Parisian institution.

A category that declined gradually but relentlessly during the course of the nineteenth century was made up of individuals without professorships in teaching or research institutions. The academicians in this category, moreover, were increasingly likely to have attained at least the intermediate levels of a common medical hierarchy. Among those appointed to the newly created academy in 1820–21, more than half of those without professorships (28 percent of all academicians) held neither hospital posts nor the *agrégation*, the most important junior teaching post at the Faculty of Medicine. Some were named to the academy by virtue of positions that had been held during the ancien régime. Many others were simply well-known practitioners or members of the Royal Medical Service. Among academicians of the late nineteenth and twentieth centuries, few were without either the *agrégation* or hospital posts.[59]

The shift to an academy of professors was largely completed by the end of the nineteenth century. However, in one important respect—the age of academicians—recruitment to the academy continued to evolve during the early years of the twentieth century. Academicians in both the 1861 and 1901 samples were elected fairly young (see table 2.4). On average, they were in their mid- to late forties, at the peak of their careers. They were from seven to ten years younger than medical appointees to the Academy of Sciences. Members in 1935, however, had been appointed late in their lives (at an average age of 56.5). The rising age of academicians reflects the increasing competitiveness for elite medical positions that characterized Parisian medical institutions in the early twentieth century. Only one academician in 1935, Arsène d'Arsonval, had been appointed to the Academy of Medicine before the age of forty, and he was a relic of an earlier era, having been elected in 1881. In contrast, 35 percent of the academicians in 1935 had been over sixty at the time of their election to the academy. Furthermore, academicians in the twentieth century lived longer than their predecessors (see table 2.4). The average age at death of academicians, stable during much of the nineteenth century, rose by more than six years from the sample of 1901 to that of 1935 (to 82.2).[60]

Both of these factors had important consequences for the age structure of academicians (see table 2.4). In the populations of 1861 and 1901, the average
academician was in his early sixties. In 1935 the average age was nearly seventy,
making the academicians a gerontocracy. Nearly 40 percent of academicians in 1861
and almost half in 1901 were less than sixty years old. The figure in 1935 was only
5 percent; nearly half the membership in that year was over seventy. The great age
of many members had visible effects on the academy's activities, as we shall see.

The consolidation of Parisian members into a single category did not do away
completely with membership distinctions. The academy sought to keep up links with
medicine outside Paris, both French and foreign. It also sought to maintain ties with
nonmedical science and the state administration concerned with health care and prevention. It needed, finally, to take account of various nontraditional medical domains
that emerged during the course of the nineteenth and early twentieth centuries. Two
kinds of membership assured these links: associate status was the more selective and
prestigious while corresponding status was more easily accessible.

Non-Parisian Members

Non-Parisians constituted the most important categories of nontitular members. They
were perceived to be the basis of that national network of medical information and
research that was one of the original raisons d'àtre of the academy. They also contributed in important ways to the intellectual activities of the academy. A handful
eventually moved to Paris and were promoted to full membership in the academy,
but this was a very rare occurrence.[61]

The original ordinance establishing the academy appointed thirty-two "nonresi-
dents" to the academy. About half were professors in a provincial medical school of
medicine or pharmacy. Five others worked in civil or medical hospitals and four were
inspectors of mineral waters. This association with the public system of medical institutions meant that most associates lived in relatively large cities; the two cities with
medical faculties, Montpellier and Strasbourg, contributed fourteen individuals.

In 1824 thirty-one more associates were elected by the academy in the context of
a worsening political situation. Before approving the academy's choices, the government requested police reports about the political reliability of those elected.[62] The
vast majority of these, including one characterized as "très mauvais" were confirmed.
But five others received very negative reports and were not appointed. (The academy
eventually elected all five to the lesser position of corresponding member.[63]) The new
crop of associates was somewhat more disparate than the original group. Eight were
faculty professors while five others worked and taught in military hospitals. Although
the new associates were somewhat less concentrated geographically than their predecessors, the majority nevertheless lived in cities.

The non-Parisian associates (there were only 53 left in 1828) were not sufficiently
numerous to constitute that scientific network which the academy was supposed to
coordinate. Consequently, in 1825 another nonresident category was created, that of
national correspondent. No less than 462 individuals were appointed to the academy
in this capacity during the first year. One cannot say much about individuals in this

group since most were too obscure to be included in the usual biographical sources. Eight men were or became corresponding members of the Academy of Sciences. We know from other sources that about half of all correspondents lived in towns or cities that were administrative centers of their department (*chef-lieu de département*)[64] but this left quite a number in the smaller towns of France.

For all of these non-Parisians, membership in the academy constituted a significant professional honor. The academy received many requests for membership, and meetings at which elections were held were not infrequently lively affairs. Usually a commission was formed to prepare a list which would then be voted on by the entire academy.[65] Every academician had friends, relatives, or former students living in the provinces who could be made very happy by election to the academy. One journal reported on a particularly animated meeting to elect correspondents with the wicked comment: "In order to complain about the neglect which befell their friends and protégés, academicians have rediscovered that ardor and that enthusiasm which they rarely bring to scientific discussions."[66] The number of places available was small in relation to demand. By the 1850s, when the number of corresponding members was beginning to shrink, thirty-three men applied for corresponding membership between July 1854 and November 1857. Only three of these were ever elected, in two cases ten years after this application and in the third case twenty-five years later.

Faced with such candidacies, academicians seem to have looked primarily for scientific and literary accomplishments; but there was until the 1870s agreement that superior practitioners should also be considered. Efforts were also made to achieve geographical balance. Above all, there was a strong tendency to favor those who actually contributed work to the academy,[67] for non-Parisian members were an important source of scientific activity. The papers, reports, and longer works which provincial doctors submitted to the academy in the hope of eventually becoming academicians were the basis for much of the activity of intellectual evaluation carried out in that institution. And, once elected, a goodly number of correspondents and associates did in fact participate in academic discussions either through the mail or by attending the occasional meeting.

The growing homogenization which increasingly characterized Parisian academicians at the end of the nineteenth century applied as well to non-Parisian members. More and more corresponding and associate members came to represent official medicine, particularly medical education in the provinces. Furthermore, from a vast network of essentially low-level information gatherers, they were transformed into a considerably smaller group of more highly trained and active medical researchers who happened to live outside the capital. Underlying this transformation was the growth of medical education in the provinces, particularly the creation of four new provincial faculties in the last decades of the nineteenth century. This created a large and thriving sector of official medicine in the provinces.

In 1900 there were only twenty national associates in the academy. Nine of these were professors in a medical faculty (with that of Lyon contributing five) while seven others taught in a secondary school of medicine, a school of pharmacy, or a school of veterinary science. Every single one had originally been elected as a correspondent and had then been appointed to associate status. Like Parisian members, associates in the twentieth century were increasingly elderly. Only one of the nineteen associates in 1935 was less than sixty years old. Nine others had passed their seventieth year.[68]

The number of corresponding members shrank even more precipitously than did the number of associates; already down to 135 in 1861, it fell to 97 in 1900. About half held teaching posts in a faculty or secondary school of medicine. Most of the others had an administrative connection of one sort or another; seven men were in the army, four worked in hospitals, and seven others were epidemics doctors or inspectors of mineral waters or public health. A consequence of this changing professional profile is that corresponding membership became predominantly urban-based. All of those who would go on to associate status and about three-quarters of the rest lived in cities, particularly those with medical faculties.[69]

The new scientific status of these members was recognized by the Academy of Sciences. Among the first cohorts appointed to the Academy of Medicine in the 1820s, some 11 percent of the associates and less than 1 percent of the correspondents were elected corresponding or full members of the Academy of Sciences. Among those of 1900, the figure was 25 percent for associates and 7 percent for correspondents in spite of the increased competitiveness of election to this academy.

One consequence of this change of status is that provincial members in the early twentieth century were much more likely than their predecessors to be posthumously recognized with necrological notices by their Parisian colleagues. Among the original cohorts of the 1820s, only three associates and no correspondents were acknowledged in the academy by eulogies or necrological notices; this gives some indication of how distant they were from the central concerns of the Parisian medical elite. Among the members of 1900, in contrast, all associates and all but ten of the correspondents were remembered with necrological notices.

There were certainly political reasons for the growing recognition of non-Parisians by the academy. The public combativeness of professors in certain faculties, particularly that of Lyon where anti-Parisian feeling was vigorously expressed,[70] made it increasingly difficult to ignore them. There were also changes in academic procedure (discussed in Chapter 3) that made such recognition more feasible. But the basis of this more equal treatment, I suspect, is that non-Parisians no longer followed career paths very different from those of Parisian members. Rather than being seen primarily as *practitioners* and producers of low-level information to be processed in Paris, they tended increasingly to be urban medical teachers and researchers.

Foreign Members

In 1825 the academy appointed nineteen foreign associates. Eight of them were already or would become corresponding or associate members of the Academy of Sciences. Germany provided eight members, the largest contingent of foreign academicians, followed by Italy with four and Great Britain with three. Surgeons were the largest professional grouping represented (with five) followed by physicians (four), botanists (three), and anatomists (three).

In 1835 the academy created another more inclusive category, foreign corresponding members. By 1861 there were eighty-one correspondents, far more than regulations allowed. By not replacing all deceased members, the academy managed to reduce the number to forty-one by 1900. Associate status, in contrast, was somewhat ignored during the second half of the century; there were only thirteen associates in 1861 and five in 1887. Just before the turn of the century an effort was made to rehabilitate this category, with thirteen associates elected in 1900, bringing the total number to eighteen. Four of the eighteen had initially been elected as correspondents before being elevated to the more prestigious associate status. Surgeons continued to be the largest professional group among them but physicians and botanists had been largely displaced by bacteriologists and other experimentalists.

Germany continued to have the largest number of foreign associates (six), but it was now followed closely by Britain (five). Russia provided three associates but one of these, Élie Metchnikoff, was actually living and working in Paris. Scientific stature continued to be the major factor in the election of foreign associates. Four were also correspondents or associates of the Academy of Sciences while five were Nobel laureates. In contrast, correspondents seem to have been elected with political considerations in mind. Belgium, Romania, Switzerland, and Austria each contributed five correspondents while Italy and Germany each contributed four and Britain three. This suggests that an effort was made to ensure the representation of countries within France's linguistic and intellectual sphere of influence.

The decision to reemphasize associate status in 1900 seems to have been part of a concerted effort to increase scientific ties with major foreign powers and to bring international medical science into the academy, most notably under the tenure of Sigismond Jaccoud as permanent secretary (1901–13).[71] Not only was the number of associates increased but more attention was paid to them. Only one of the foreign associates of 1825 received a eulogy after his death. And this was the Italian anatomist Antonio Scarpa, trained in France. Such neglect of foreigners continued throughout the nineteenth century but was reversed in the twentieth. Ten of eighteen foreign associates of 1901 were honored with necrological notices. This was the first generation of foreign members to be so honored.

In spite of the increased attention paid to them after the turn of the century, foreign members did not contribute significantly to the academy. They presented the academy with books or articles that might not have come to its attention otherwise, but it is doubtful whether any important discoveries were made in this way. The main purpose of having foreign associates was to maintain France's place in an international network of medical science. Foreign memberships increased the visibility of the academy abroad and also increased the possibility that French scientists would be appointed to similar positions in foreign societies. During World War I the academy expressed its patriotism by expelling German and Austrian foreign members.[72]

Associés libres

Perhaps the most interesting and complex of the associate categories was that of *associé libre* (AL). Eleven men were appointed to this level of membership in 1820 and another seventeen were elected three years later. The first group included some of the most eminent scientists of the period. Nine of the eleven were members of the Academy of Sciences. A few of these men had degrees in medicine (Claude Berthollet) or pharmacy (Jacques Thénard), but most did not. Many of these scientists were, as was common during this period, also active in politics or administration. But there is little doubt that this category of membership was meant primarily to align the new Academy of Medicine with the Parisian scientific elite.

Although we do not know how or on what basis they were appointed, it is likely that Georges Cuvier, who played such a critical role in setting up the academy, also loomed large in these scientific appointments. (The most common institutional affiliation of these members was the Muséum d'Histoire Naturelle, Cuvier's own institution.) Nevertheless, we cannot dismiss these choices as unrepresentative of medical opinion. Four of the nine scientists were the subjects of academic eulogies (*éloges*) after their death, an even higher proportion than was the case for full members. The *éloges* of Berthollet and Cuvier were among the lengthiest presented during the first half of the nineteenth century. It would seem that at this early stage in the academy's existence, both associate membership in and posthumous recognition by the academy tended to recapitulate success within the larger Parisian scientific community.

Only two of the original members did not fit this scientific mold. Duc François de La Rochefoucauld-Liancourt was undoubtedly being honored for his work in propagating Jennerian vaccination and his activities in hospital administration. (He resigned in 1824.) The politician Count (later Baron) de Gérando was probably being rewarded for his work on the commission which created the academy as well as for a modest scientific reputation.

Of seventeen new ALs elected in 1823, nine were eminent scientists and members of the Academy of Sciences. It may be that the ranks of eligible Parisian scientists had been depleted by the first wave of nominations since some of these newcomers were in fields quite remote from medicine including mineralogy (Alexandre Brongniart), physics (Pierre-Louis Dulong), and mathematics (Jean Fourier). As a result, only one of the nine, the naturalist Henri de Blainville, was the subject of a posthumous *éloge*. Another seven associates came from the administrative and political sectors. In some cases, notably that of Baron Capelle, the academy was discharging debts of gratitude for work in setting up the academy. In other cases, including those of the minister of the interior, Count Jacques-Joseph-Guillaume Corbière, and the prefect of the Seine, Count Gilbert-Joseph-Gaspard Chabrol de Volvic, the academy was likely attempting to stroke men of power whose goodwill was desirable.

The most striking change during the next few decades was the declining importance of the scientific elite among ALs and their replacement by individuals following a wide range of somewhat marginal medical careers. Of the seventeen ALs in the academy from 1861 to 1870, only six were members of the Academy of Sciences, including four with posts at the Muséum. Five others were in medical administration. A new group appearing in this cohort were five medical writers and journalists, including Émile Littré, best known for his dictionary and edition of the Hippocratic texts, and Amédée Latour, editor of a medical journal and leader of the movement for professional association among doctors.

The proportion of scientists held steady in the next generation. Of the nineteen ALs between 1891 and 1901, seven were members of the Academy of Sciences; the most notable was Louis Pasteur. While most taught at the Muséum and the Sorbonne, two were at the recently created Institut Pasteur. The group included only one journalist and one health administrator. On the other hand, public health assumed a much more prominent role. One member of the military medical corps and another member of the colonial medical service, both strongly oriented to public health, were in the academy, as were four physicians known mainly for public health activities. Associate status remained a way of recognizing marginal medical fields; one AL, Théodore Hamy, was an ethnographer instrumental in founding the Musée de l'Homme at Trocadero. But this category of membership was also beginning to serve to reward men following more conventional elite medical careers. Ernest Mesnet, for instance, was a neurologist with a hospital post, while Victor Galippe was a stomatologist best known for toxicological research. Émile Roux, director of the Institut Pasteur and an eminent bacteriologist with an MD degree, did not have a substantially different profile from other colleagues at the Institut Pasteur who were full members of the academy. This suggests that this category of membership was beginning to be used as a way of bringing new members into the academy when no vacancies existed for titular members.

As the twentieth century progressed, those elected as ALs came from increasingly diverse fields. The world of science did not quite disappear from the academy but its place was further reduced. Only three of the sixteen ALs elected from 1925 to 1935 were members of the Academy of Sciences. (Two of these were associate rather than full members there too.) One of these three was Jean-Baptiste Charcot, son of the famous neurologist and not your run-of-the-mill career scientist; his fame rested on his journeys of scientific exploration to Antarctica in the early twentieth century. The other two members of the Academy of Sciences were Gaston Ramon and Félix Mesnil, both of the Institut Pasteur. In fact, the most famous representative of Parisian science in the Academy of Medicine was Marie Curie, who was, remarkably, never elected to the Academy of Sciences.[73] There was one other AL who worked at the Institut Pasteur (Gabriel Marchoux). But most associate members were, like Jean Charcot, doctors who had gained fame or distinction in other fields: politics (Georges Clemenceau), journalism/belles lettres (Paul Le Gendre and Maurice de Fleury), medical art (Henri Meige and Paul Richer), and anthropology (Louis Capitan). A small number of nondoctors whose work was in one way or another relevant to the academy's work were also elected. These included Marie Curie, the politician Paul Strauss, medical administrator Gustave Mesureur, and psychologist Georges Dumas.

Given the diversity of ALs, participation in academic affairs was uneven. Nearly everyone submitted works or read papers in order to be considered for election. Once elected, few ALs crossed the threshold of the academy (which did not distinguish them from many full members). Some ALs, most notably Louis Pasteur, did work that was of direct relevance to academic concerns, presenting many papers and participating frequently in discussions. A handful even served on permanent committees. But overall, and excepting Pasteur, ALs probably did not substantially affect the nature or substance of academic activity. On the other hand, the gradual addition of doctors to this category made a few ALs virtually indistinguishable from full members. This was recognized by the reorganization of 1923, which changed the title from *associé libre* to *membre libre* and increased their formal institutional prerogatives.

Of the various categories of members examined in this section, most had come by the early twentieth century to resemble the full members in the growing uniformity of their professional profiles. The single exception is the category of *associés libres*, which made room for a heterogeneous collection of professional medical careers that emerged during the course of the nineteenth century and that did not conform to the rigid criteria that governed full memberships. Its evolution also suggests a growing separation between the medical elite and the world of nonmedical science so closely interwoven in the early nineteenth century. This separation will be largely confirmed in Chapter 9 when we examine another facet of this traditional connection: medical membership in the Academy of Sciences.

The diverse meanings of the word "structure" have permitted us to recount a number of quite different stories in this chapter. Although their plots vary, most point to important changes that took place in the later decades of the nineteenth century. With the example of its rival model, the Academy of Sciences, constantly before it, the Academy of Medicine sought to raise its status by becoming a more exclusive scientific institution. A magnificent new building and significant private donations suggest successful movement toward this goal. Changes in the recruitment of Parisian and provincial members transformed the academy into an institution for professors and medical scientists. But other forces were undermining the scientific vocation of the academy. Representatives of nonmedical science were increasingly excluded from the institution. During the interwar years, the rising age of members turned the academy into a gerontocracy. A desire for institutional exclusiveness delayed until 1923 the reorganization of membership sections into categories adapted to modern notions of medical science.

NOTES

1. Unlike the minutes of the "secret sessions" of the Academy of Sciences, which have been preserved, those of the Academy of Medicine cannot be located.

2. Charles Achard, "Cent ans d'éloges à l'Académie de Médecine," *BAM* 86 (1921), 358–75.

3. AM Liasse 15.

4. Louis Peisse, *La Médecine et les médecins; philosophie, doctrines, institutions, critiques, moeurs et biographies médicales,* 2 vols. (1857), vol. 2, pp. 153–62.

5. From one-quarter to one-third of all academicians were elected to the office of president.

6. Budgets until the 1870s are from AN F17 3692–96. For later years they are taken from the annual budgetary reports presented by the Ministry of Public Instruction to the legislature.

7. George Weisz, *The Emergence of Modern Universities in France, 1863–1914* (Princeton, N.J., 1983).

8. This excludes the sum devoted to common services of the Institut.

9. In 1829, for instance, Adelon, serving as acting permanent secretary, accumulated 240 *jetons*, worth 720 francs. The next two best paid academicians earned 480 and 450 francs respectively. In subsequent years the amounts individuals earned fell: in 1840 only about a half dozen academicians received more than 300 francs for the year (AM Liasse 198).

10. E. De Lavarenne, "La Séance annuelle de l'Académie de Médecine," *Presse médicale*, 10 (1902), 1226.

11. In 1847 a minor scandal erupted when a medical journal reported that the academy was not in fact spending its entire budget and had invested nearly 10,000 francs. Bureaucrats at the Ministry of Public Instruction became extremely agitated and demanded explanations. The relevant documents are in F17 3692.

12. Budget report dated January 28, 1828, in F17 3692.

13. Donors are listed in Maurice Hanriot, "Les Bienfaiteurs de l'Académie," *Centenaire de l'Académie de Médecine, 1820–1920* (1921), pp. 212–13.

14. The following account is based on Dr. A. Dureau, "Les Vicissitudes du logement de l'Académie de Médecine," *Chronique médicale* 2 (1895), 157–203; S. Jaccoud, "Un adieu à la rue des Saints-Pères," *BAM* 40 (1906), 1–30; Paul Ganière, *L'Académie de Médecine: ses origines et son histoire* (1964).

15. The move was bitterly opposed by the head of the vaccination commission, the eminent philanthropist duc de La Rochefoucauld-Liancourt, and it required the direct intervention of the king to get the commission to abandon the premises. La Rochefoucauld eventually resigned his membership in the academy.

16. Peisse, *La Médecine*, p. 301.

17. Ibid.

18. As early as 1859 the academy's permanent secretary, Dubois, responded to a ministerial inquiry about the needs of the academy with a long report indicating the features it needed in a building. The report is in F17 3681.

19. Dureau, "Les Vicissitudes," 158.

20. Jaccoud, "Un adieu à la rue des Saints-Pères," 2.

21. J. Noir, "La Nouvelle installation de l'Académie de Médecine," *Progrès médical* 3e sér., 16 (1902), 425–27.

22. *Gazette des hôpitaux* 133 (1902), 1315.

23. L.-C. Boileau, "La Nouvelle Académie de Médecine," *L'Architecture* 15 (1902), 83.

24. *Progrès médical*, 3e sér. 16 (1902), 462; De Lavarenne, "La Séance annuelle de l'Académie de Médecine," 1226.

25. *Gazette des hôpitaux* 133 (1902), 1318.

26. Meetings of the administrative council, January 2, 1844 (AM Liasse 13) and January 3, 1857 (Liasse 14).

27. Weisz, *Emergence of Modern Universities*.

28. Membership would soon be raised to sixty-six.

29. George Weisz, "The Development of Medical Specialization in Nineteenth-Century Paris," in *French Medical Culture in the Nineteenth Century*, ed. Ann F. La Berge and Mordechai Feingold (Amsterdam, 1994).

30. *AGM* 7 (1829), 309.

31. Ibid.; and *JGM* 3e sér. 12 (1829), 260.

32. In F17 3681. This proposal is undated but would seem to correspond with a plan that was first proposed in 1847 according to J. Cheymol, "Histoire de l'Académie Nationale de Médecine," in Académie de Médecine, *La Médecine et notre temps* (1980), p. 265.

33. J.-B. Barth, "Compte rendu des actes de l'Académie," *BAM* 2 (1873), xxvii–xxviii.

34. Chauffard's report is in *BAM* 3 (1874), 1041–72.

35. Ibid., 1044.

36. Ibid., 1045.

37. Ibid., 1048.

38. Ibid., 1049.

39. Ibid., 1045.

40. Ibid., 1050.

41. Ibid., 1052.

42. Ibid., 1055.

43. Ibid., 1064.

44. *Union médicale*, 3e sér. 18 (1874), 729, 741–42.

45. *Union médicale*, for instance, felt that points of detail aside, the principle of the reform commanded general assent. Ibid., 729.

46. Chauffard, *BAM* 3 (1874), 1059.

47. Ibid., 1060.

48. Ibid., 1067.

49. Ibid., 1068.

50. *Union médicale*, 3e sér., 18 (1874), 742. Also see *Gazette des hôpitaux*, 47 (1874), 1113, 1138.

51. *Gazette des hôpitaux* 47 (1874), 1138.

52. *Index biographique des membres, des associés et des correspondants de l'Académie de Médecine, 1820–1900* (1991), p. x.

53. In his memoirs, Achard presents the reorganization as something he arranged personally with the minister. This is plausible, since the only trace of the reform in *BAM* is the minister's letter agreeing to the changes. Charles Achard, *La Confession d'un vieil homme du siècle: souvenirs du temps et de l'espace* (1943), p. 80.

54. What follows is based on a prosopographical study of the membership of the academy that will be more fully discussed in Chapters 10 and 11. It examines four populations of academicians, in 1821, 1861, 1901, and 1935.

55. The few exceptions either died shortly after their appointment to the faculty or were political appointees never accepted by the medical elite.

56. There were twenty-six chairs at the faculty in 1845 and forty-six chairs in 1930.

57. There were a half dozen or so pharmacist-academicians who never became professors at the School of Pharmacy in both the populations of 1821 and 1861. There was only one in this category in 1901 and none in 1935.

58. There were sixteen, ten, seven, and six among our populations of 1821, 1861, 1901, and 1935 respectively.

59. Those without either title made up only 8 percent and 2 percent respectively of the academicians who were without professorships in 1901 and 1935.

60. Longevity seems to have been characteristic of doctors generally during this period. The age of death of a random sample of nonacademician Parisian doctors in practice for thirty years or more in 1935 was similar to that for academicians (84.2).

61. Those in this category include Th. Laënnec, J. Cruveilhier, Ph. Ricord, and A. Chauveau.

62. The report from the director of police in the Ministry of the Interior is dated April 27, 1824, in F17 3683.

63. Four were elected in 1825 and the fifth in 1840.

64. Patrice Bourdelais and Jean-Yves Raulot, *Une peur bleue: histoire du choléra en France, 1832–1854* (1987), pp. 201–2.

65. For the purposes of electing and organizing associate members the system of sections did not apply. In the case of corresponding members, the eleven sections were combined into four megacategories which presented lists.

66. *AGM*, 4e sér. 16 (1848), 268–69. Also *AGM*, 2e sér. 5 (1834), 314–15.

67. Bousquet, "Rapport de la commission des élections pour les correspondants nationaux," *BAM* 1 (1836–37), 171–76.

68. The mean age was sixty-eight.

69. In 1900 Lyon had fourteen corresponding members, Bordeaux eight, and Montpellier and Marseilles six each.

70. Weisz, *Emergence of Modern Universities*, pp. 151, 322–24.

71. P. Ménétrier, "Éloge de François-Sigismond Jaccoud (1830–1913)," *BAM* 104 (1930), 589; Menetrier's remarks as incoming president, *BAM* 103 (1930), 14; Jaccoud, "Un adieu à la rue des Saints-Pères," *BAM* 40 (1906), 6.

72. *BAM* 81 (1919), 297–304.

73. Her single candidacy is discussed briefly in Maurice Crosland, *Science under Control: The French Academy of Sciences, 1795–1914* (Cambridge, 1992), pp. 234–35.

3

Academic Functions and Genres: Communication, Evaluation, and Debate

This examination of the academy's activities begins with two quotations. The first is from the initial article of the ordinance that created the academy and clearly stated its mandate:

> This academy is instituted especially to respond to the requests of the government for everything that concerns public health, and principally epidemics, the illnesses specific to certain regions, epizootics, the different cases of legal medicine, the propagation of vaccine, the examination of new remedies and secret remedies, both internal and external, mineral waters that are natural or artificial, etc.
>
> It will be responsible, furthermore [*en outre*], for continuing the work of the Société Royale de Médecine and the Académie Royale de Chirurgie. It will occupy itself with all the objects of study and of research which may contribute to the progress of the different branches of the healing art.[1]

The wording indicates clearly that the primary function of the academy in the minds of its organizers was to respond to questions from the government regarding public health. There is a list of matters regarded as especially important, including collective diseases and the regulation of certain forms of therapeutics traditionally under the jurisdiction of the central government. The second paragraph suggests a distinct and perhaps even secondary task for the academy (depending on how one translates *en outre*): contributing to the "progress" of the different branches of medicine.

Thus the functional distinction that marked the history of the academy appeared at its very inception. The development of medical science might very well be considered a precondition for fulfilling public health tasks, but the two activities nonetheless obeyed very different sorts of logic. The relative weight placed on each could also vary quite significantly from one historical period to the next. In the 1870s, the scientific role clearly preoccupied academicians,[2] whereas public health predominated in the 1920s and 1930s.

A second quotation appeared in a promotional prospectus which J.-B. Baillière, publisher of the academy's *Bulletin* circulated during the 1850s as a way of boosting circulation:[3]

> This official *Bulletin* renders an exact and impartial account of the meetings of the Imperial Academy of Medicine; in rendering an accurate tableau of its work, it offers the entirety of all the important questions which the progress of medicine can bring to life. The academy having become the center of a nearly universal correspondence, it is through the documents transmitted to it that all doctors can follow the movement of science in all the places where it may be cultivated, and can learn about inventions and discoveries, almost from the moment of their birth. . . . Thus every correspondent, every doctor, every savant who submits any writing whatsoever to the academy can follow the discussions [of it] and know exactly what judgment has been rendered on it.

The claim of academic authority and of intellectual interest for the journal in this advertisement rests on the breadth of information represented by the contents. Furthermore, anyone submitting a piece of writing to the academy could hope to read the academy's discussion and judgment of it in the journal.

Advertising hyperbole aside, this text is suggestive of the academy's role in processing and disseminating a large body of information and medical knowledge. In the present chapter we will examine some of the ways in which the academy fulfilled this role. Since we are dealing with textual records of these activities, we are, I think, using more than figures of speech in referring to academic "genres" as well as activities. In examining the academy's functions we will be particularly attentive to the ways in which the institution combined its various roles: providing expert knowledge to public authorities and developing medical science; communicating the results of members' research and evaluating the work of nonacademicians; examining issues of public health prevention; and encouraging innovation in clinical therapeutics.[4]

Communicating and Evaluating

The weekly Tuesday afternoon meetings of the Academy of Medicine followed a pattern reminiscent of, and probably modeled after, the Monday sessions of the Academy of Sciences. Correspondence was dealt with first, followed by the reading of academic reports; then came oral presentations first by members and then by nonmembers. Within this common general framework, some important divergences reflected the differing functions of the two institutions.[5]

In the early and mid-nineteenth century, the weekly meeting of the Academy of Medicine typically began with a reading of the minutes of the previous meeting. The permanent secretary would then publicly discuss the correspondence that had been received. First to be examined was the "official correspondence," consisting of messages from a ministry or other government body. These could be administrative announcements, requests forwarded on behalf of third parties for authorization of mineral waters or secret remedies, and, occasionally, a ministerial inquiry about an issue of public health. In the latter case, the academy would usually strike a special commission to draft a response.

During the academy's first half century, ministers frequently passed along manuscripts and therapeutic appliances that had been sent in by individual doctors and laymen. These did not differ substantially from the materials sent directly to the academy by individuals and listed as "manuscript correspondence." In the case of both "official" and "manuscript" mail, materials regarding epidemics, vaccinations, mineral waters, and secret remedies were sent to the appropriate permanent commission for processing, as were submissions for the growing list of prize competitions. The operation of these commissions will be described in Chapter 4. Works sent in on behalf of a candidacy for membership in the academy were passed on to the appropriate election commission. Sealed letters transmitted to the academy as a means of eventually demonstrating scientific priority were filed away until the sender requested that they be opened.[6] Submissions by nonmembers that did not fit any of these categories were, if they were deemed serious, forwarded to ad hoc committees of from one to three academicians that were supposed to prepare evaluative reports for discussion and vote by the entire academy.[7]

In sending work of this latter sort to the academy, an author might seek either scientific recognition and eventual election to the academy or endorsement for a product or procedure. The major difference between "official" submissions and "manuscript" correspondence was that the former could not be so conveniently filed away and forgotten. Ministerial inquiries thus produced lengthy discussions of such weighty matters as hernia trusses, mustard, and nutritive biscuits.

That such products received serious attention in so august a body was a source of some consternation. The medical journalist Louis Peisse charged that the pressures of responding to ministerial demands interfered with the scientific tasks of the academy. In one article he complained that meetings were so dull because of the amount of time spent on trivial questions from the government.[8] In another article, he asked rhetorically:

> Are academies not made to advance science, to pose new questions, to expand the sphere of knowledge? Why not follow the example of your colleague in the Academy of Sciences, whose reports written by the Cuviers, the Aragos, the Gay-Lussacs, the Poissons are texts of such rich development and virtually small luminous treatises on specific questions? Why restrict yourself with respect to mustard to what is known and said by an apothecary who did not claim to speak scientifically about it but only to sell it?[9]

In addition to such manuscript submissions, the academy also received published works. These were ordinarily sent to the academy's archives without comment, acknowledged only in a list appearing at the end of each issue of the academy's *Bulletin*. The mandate of the academy to evaluate medical science did not apply to published work that was already in the public domain.

Once the manuscript submissions had been distributed, and institutional business like elections and commission reports taken care of, a typical academic meeting usually went on to hear scientific papers. Titular members of the academy who presented papers might provoke discussion, but as proven masters of science they were not subject to formal evaluative reports.[10] Their presentations were routinely reproduced in full in the *Bulletin*. Outsiders to the academy were also permitted to make oral presentations. But like manuscript submissions, these talks were required to be evaluated by ad hoc committees, whose conclusions were voted by the entire academy. In fact, like manuscript submissions, the vast majority of presentations by nonmembers never received the required report. Once presented, such papers appeared in summary form (consisting in some cases of little more than a title) in the *Bulletin*. For both members and nonmembers, it was frequently the case, at least before 1870, that speakers failed to submit written texts so that published accounts had to be reconstructed by the permanent secretary from memory or from the accounts of medical journalists.[11]

Throughout the nineteenth and early twentieth centuries, the academy distinguished between two types of oral presentations: *lectures* and *communications*. In the mid-nineteenth century, *lectures* were more formal presentations based on a written text. *Communications* were less formal and almost always involved the presentation of something—an instrument, an anatomical preparation, or, frequently, a patient. (There was considerable opposition to the presentation of patients but the practice continued.[12])

Titular members of the academy were equally likely to present *communications* and formal *lectures* whereas nonmembers most often presented *lectures*.[13] The latter did so because they were in many cases seeking election to the academy, which required formal presentations.[14] Furthermore, the official requirement that papers by outsiders be evaluated, even if frequently ignored, made it desirable to present a written text to the evaluating committee.

In the 1850s nonmembers delivered nearly three times as many presentations as did members. This testifies to the widespread desire to be elected to the academy; it also suggests that election removed a major stimulus to such presentations. Academicians did not necessarily stop working. But election brought other sorts of responsibilities and other occasions to make known one's views or research results: reports on the work of nonmembers, the annual reports of permanent commissions, interventions in the many discussions and debates of the period. The surgeon Alfred Velpeau, for instance, published a good many of his articles in the *Bulletin* before his election to the academy; subsequently, however, his list of publications was made up almost exclusively of academic interventions and reports.[15]

The reports presented at academic meetings were of various sorts. Permanent commissions presented the academy with elaborate annual reports and periodic short reports about administrative decisions. Large special commissions, appointed to respond to a ministerial inquiry, to a large influx of submissions on a subject, or to controversial issues which emerged during discussion, would sporadically present a frequently lengthy report, almost always provoking intense discussion. During the 1850s there were two commissions looking into cholera and others examining medical electricity, mortality statistics, and the link between goiter and cretinism, to name but a few.

The most common type of report had to do with the evaluation of nonmembers' manuscripts or oral presentations. Despite the fact that they were supposed to be the work of a small committee, they were characteristically the work of a single academician. On occasion during this period they were quite lengthy. A conscientious reporter might do original research testing the claims of the work he was judging. A report might be very critical of or very favorable to the work under discussion, but the final conclusions ordinarily thanked the author, advised that more research be done, and, in the case of submissions received by mail, recommended that the work be honorably placed in the academy's archives. If a committee was especially favorable, it might advocate that the work be considered for publication in one of the academy's journals. It might even go so far as to recommend that an author be included on the next list of candidates for corresponding membership. This was a controversial practice, however, since it limited the maneuvering room of election committees. If formal conclusions were usually bland, the body of the report was frequently quite piquant. And the need for the academy to collectively vote even bland conclusions brought out all the debating instincts of the members. Consequently, such reports provided the starting point for many academic discussions.

Most of the time, of course, reports were not presented. Only about 13 percent of the oral presentations and 10 percent of the manuscript submissions sent to committees between 1854 and 1857 were evaluated.[16] The failure to complete the vast majority of reports prompted furious letters of protest and sometimes published attacks from slighted authors.[17] Some academicians were also unhappy with this state of affairs, believing that it cast discredit on the academy. But efforts to tighten the procedure were not notably successful.[18]

We do not know the exact proportion of reports completed in the Academy of Sciences but Maurice Crosland's recent book suggests that, at mid-century, reports were even less likely to be completed there than in the Academy of Medicine. Busy scientists deeply resented the obligation to evaluate so many works; by the late 1860s the reporting system had been virtually abandoned.[19] One sees little overt resentment of this sort in the Academy of Medicine in spite of the fact that it was dealing with a huge medical profession whose members were more than willing to share their latest therapeutic triumph, however dubious. Academicians and their correspondents, I suspect, were united by a passionate concern with the practicalities of diagnosis and therapeutics that rendered the evaluative process less onerous for academicians.

Consequently, in spite of the fact that most evaluative reports were never completed, they played a significant role in the Academy of Medicine. They were emblematic of its status as an official tribunal of medical science; they made it possible to recognize especially good work and to dissociate the academy from bad work. This was of some significance because a recurring concern was that poor or potentially dangerous oral presentations would appear to have the imprimatur of the academy in which they were presented.

In the later decades of the nineteenth century, the basic structure of academic meetings remained largely intact. But a number of important changes were introduced during the 1870s, when the desire to make the academy more "scientific" was at its height. "Official" and "manuscript" correspondence remained the first order of business. The government still sent manuscripts and apparatuses for evaluation but these were almost always shunted off to the secret remedies commission, which dealt with them expeditiously and spared the academy the embarrassing debates that had so upset Peisse. The correspondence was followed by a new evaluative practice introduced in the early 1870s. Authors of published books or articles sent their work to an individual academician who would formally present it to the academy. At first this was done without comment; gradually the presenting academicians began summarizing and even praising the works in question. This process did not involve any collective judgment by the academy, so more senior individuals could make their work known with minimal risk of rejection. By the 1890s many unpublished works were also being presented in this way.

As in the past, the next order of business was the presentation of papers. By the later decades of the nineteenth century the distinctions between *lectures* and *communications* had become rigid. *Lectures* were now exclusively reserved for nonmembers. They were summarized very briefly (often with nothing more than the title) in the *Bulletin* and were, like the manuscripts sent by mail, passed on to a committee for evaluation. Although most presentations and submissions were, as in the past, never formally evaluated, the genre of evaluative reports made something of a comeback with more than thirty published annually in the *Bulletin* in the mid-1890s.[20] Nearly 40 percent of those presenting *lectures* were eventually elected to the academy.

Communications, in contrast, were now exclusively reserved for current members. Reproduced in full in the *Bulletin*, they represented more substantial research than in the past. Members were at this time extremely active in presenting *communications*. It is not always easy to distinguish these presentations from longer interventions in debates. But what the index of the *Bulletin* called *communications* considerably outnumbered the *lectures* by nonmembers (eighty-six to sixty in 1892; sixty-one to fifty-two in 1894), reversing the situation of the 1850s.

This format remained substantially the same during the 1920s, with two major changes. First, starting in the years before World War I, academicians presented considerably fewer papers than they had in the 1890s, reflecting the advanced age of many and the large number of alternative forums to present and publish research. Whereas academicians had complained in the late nineteenth century of having too many papers to listen to, they complained in the twentieth about the absence of papers by academicians, particularly the surgeons among them, who were publishing in more specialized journals.[21] The *lectures* of nonacademicians took up the slack to some extent and became the most frequent form of scientific communication in the academy as a result of procedural changes introduced in 1913. Following a meeting in secret committee on October 21, 1913, the *Bulletin* one week later ceased summarizing *lectures* and began printing them in their entirety.[22] Simultaneously, the academy eliminated the requirement that these presentations by nonmembers be subject to evaluation by members.

This procedural modification, which followed the recent election of Georges Debove as permanent secretary, was never explained publicly. However, we know from later statements that it reflected a desire to make the *Bulletin* a more attractive place to publish in order to increase the number of submissions.[23] One can readily follow this reasoning if one notes that the number of annual presentations by members declined from eighty-three in 1892 to fifty in 1910 to just forty in 1912 without any appreciable increase in the number of papers by nonmembers.[24] The new regulations had the desired effect since the number of papers presented annually by nonmembers approached and sometimes exceeded one hundred during the 1920s.

Whatever the motives behind it, the elimination of this form of evaluation finally gave expression to new scientific realities. Nonmembers were by now fellow medical scientists using the academy as a forum to present research results. They were also frequently candidates for membership who accounted for a large proportion of the oral presentations. Formal evaluation was thus redundant because the election process itself was a form of evaluation.[25] Academicians no longer felt quite so responsible for what was said in the academy, reasoning that all scientific work was subject to possible refutation.[26] They remained, however, distressed by the exploitation of presentations to the academy for commercial purposes and thus retained considerable control over what was said in the institution. Before each meeting, the administrative council decided which of the proposed papers would in fact be presented with a view to excluding papers whose purpose was to make commercial claims under academic auspices.[27]

Less officially, many of the same changes occurred in the treatment of unpublished manuscripts. By the 1920s the evaluation of manuscripts had became a rare occurrence.[28] Formal academic evaluation in the twentieth century thus gradually became restricted to the annual prize competitions, as we shall see in the next chapter.

The papers presented at the academy do not invite simple categorization. But overall it would be fair to say that they were overwhelmingly dominated by practical clinical concerns. Chief among the subjects of presentations in nearly every sample year chosen for examination were therapeutics of one sort or another. These changed quite dramatically over time. Bleeding, blistering, and mercury were replaced by chemical preparations, serotherapies, extracts prepared from animal organs, electricity, and radiation. But the goal remained the same: to add to medicine's arsenal of effective remedies. The second most frequent subject of presentations were specific diseases that might be discussed in a variety of ways (anatomical, histological, physiological, statistical) in order to illuminate issues of etiology, diagnosis, symptomatology, and therapeutics.[29] There is nothing surprising about this. The academy was conceived as a practically oriented institution. Opponents of Émile Chauffard's proposal of 1874 to reorganize the academy specifically made the point that its practical medical mission would be compromised if its links to the medical profession were broken.[30] Still, given the fact that from one-quarter to one-third of the full members of the academy in the early twentieth century were laboratory scientists, one would expect to see considerably more papers in a physiological or immunological vein. One would also expect to see presentations reflecting the central role of public health in the academy's activities.

Insofar as public health is concerned, we shall see that there was considerable activity in this domain outside the framework of oral presentations, notably within the permanent commissions. Furthermore, the subject matter of presentations did in fact undergo change; by the 1920s papers by academicians on matters of public health were far more common than they had been in the nineteenth century.[31] The increasing importance of public health issues in the twentieth-century academy will be discussed in the section on debates, where it manifested itself far more dramatically.

The simple explanation for the lack of papers in what we would call the biological sciences is that academicians in these fields did not present their work to the academy or publish in the *Bulletin*. They might participate in discussions and committee work but their research results were ordinarily presented in different institutional frameworks. A striking example is provided by the great physiologist

Claude Bernard. According to the exhaustive bibliography prepared by Mrko Grmek,[32] Bernard published or presented 249 papers of one sort or another. The majority of these papers were presented to the Academy of Sciences or the Société de Biologie; only one was presented at the Academy of Medicine.[33] What makes Bernard's publishing strategy even more remarkable is that during the 1860s he actively sought to promote physiology and experimental medicine more generally.[34] He published accordingly in general intellectual and scientific journals and less frequently in medical journals. The failure to present anything to the academy to which he was elected in 1861 is eloquent testimony to his sense of its irrelevance to his scientific aspirations. The contrast between Bernard and Louis Pasteur, who, although only an associate member of the academy, nonetheless devoted enormous effort to convincing academicians of the pertinence of his discoveries to medical concerns, is a striking example of Pasteur's political genius. But it reflects equally well the essentially *practical* and applied character of Pasteur's scientific corpus, which fit well with the academy's fundamental orientation.

Bernard was not alone in his lack of participation in academic affairs. The great neurologist Jean-Martin Charcot seems never to have spoken in the academy and, according to one academic spokesman, neither did about half the surgeons who were members in the nineteenth century.[35] A handful of laboratory scientists did play a more active part in academic life. But their presentations to the academy tended to focus largely, though not exclusively, on practical medicine and therapeutics. A good example was the chemist Armand Gautier, elected to the academy in 1874 and named to the chair of medical chemistry at the Faculty of Medicine in 1884. Gautier was a prolific writer; his bibliographer lists 610 published works divided into a wide range of categories.[36] Although the majority were presented either to the Academy of Sciences or to the Société Chimique de Paris, forty-nine were read in the Academy of Medicine. Gautier had exceptionally wide-ranging interests but his contributions to the academy clustered in a number of areas. Twenty-one of these presentations were devoted to studies of therapeutic substances. Another eight were devoted to public health in one form or another. Thirteen are listed under the category "biological chemistry" and are primarily concerned with various more or less surprising substances produced or absorbed by human and animal bodies. They are hardly irrelevant to medicine but they do not conform to the very narrow practical focus of the majority of presentations. They remind us that the academy's predominantly practical medical orientation did not completely exclude work in what we would consider the basic sciences.

Still, if such work was not absent from the academy, it was for the most part overshadowed by practical medicine. It was not that the techniques of laboratory science were ignored, but they were ordinarily co-opted in the service of practical medical questions. Academicians understood this well enough and were unapologetic. The outgoing president for 1928, Antoine Béclère, noted matter-of-factly that few major biological questions had come up before the academy. "This is something which one might regret, but it is necessary to recognize that the new facts and ideas produced around the problems which agitate biologists go naturally to the specialized societies, like the Société de Biologie and the younger Société de Chimie biologique. . . ."[37] Exactly thirty years later, another president, Robert Debré, re-

minded the members of the academy of Pasteur's efforts to transform their institution into one devoted exclusively to science:

> In truth, the academy had to choose to a certain extent another orientation. Most
> often, the exposition of new facts in all domains of biology is better suited to a
> public restricted to savants devoted to the study of a particular discipline. . . . On the
> contrary, the work to which it [the academy] would like to contribute is the practi-
> cal application of the acquisitions of biology to prevention or therapeutics.[38]

Within this generally practical orientation some genuinely pathbreaking work
was presented to the academy during its first century of existence. Manuscript submissions seem to have been of fairly low quality while the oral presentations were
clearly very uneven. But at various ceremonial occasions academic spokesmen had
little difficulty in pointing to that institution's association with important and even
pathbreaking work:[39] Pierre Bretonneau's proclamation in 1829 of the contagiousness of typhoid fever; Jean Villemin's papers in 1865 and 1866 on the inoculability
of tuberculosis; Casimir Davaine's papers in 1868 and 1870 on anthrax; Alfred
Fournier's papers on parasyphilis and the syphilitic origins of tabes and general paralysis. Louis Pasteur presented the academy with many of his most notable results,
including those for the famous experiments at Pouilly-le-Fort on the effects of anthrax inoculation (1881) and those reports on the treatment of Joseph Meister with
rabies vaccine (1885). To be sure, Pasteur frequently reported his results first to the
Academy of Sciences, but this did not detract from the luster reflected on the Academy of Medicine. In the twentieth century it was possible to cite the papers
presenting Albert Calmette and Jules Guérin's BCG (*Bacillus Calmette-Guérin*) vaccine (1920, 1924), and Gaston Ramon's diphtheric and tetanic anatoxins (1930).
Outside the field of bacteriology one could refer with pride to a great many surgical
innovations presented to the academy, including some of Alexis Carrel's work on
tissue preservation (1909, 1912). Although it was not cited in the early twentieth century, probably because no practical use had yet been found for them, modern
historians would probably consider notable several instruments to measure physiological processes presented by E. J. Marey to the academy, as well as his more
general "graphic method" (1863, 1878).

But for virtually all academic spokesmen, the actual presentation of these research results was only a small part of the academy's contribution to medical science.
It was the discussions and debates that followed the papers, clarified issues, and
forced innovators to strengthen their arguments which constituted the essence of the
academy's scientific role. Before examining this topic, we shall briefly survey the
publications in which papers and subsequent discussions eventually appeared.

Publication and Diffusion

Submitting a manuscript or presenting a paper to the Academy of Medicine could be
a stressful experience.[40] Nonmembers left themselves exposed to severe criticism or,
worse, being ignored. A frequent theme of presidential speeches was the need for
academicians to pay attention to speakers.[41] Why then did so many individuals send

or present their thoughts and research results to the academy and why did academicians take so much time to discuss this work?

There is no single answer to the question. Many individuals were fulfilling requirements for election to the academy. Others had more commercial aims and hoped that academic approval would prove lucrative. Even if approval was not forthcoming, the examination of a product or procedure by the academy could be used in advertising. Those with state positions, like inspectors of mineral waters, epidemics doctors, or public health inspectors, were, as we shall see, pretty much bullied or coaxed into sending regular reports and statistics that could be utilized by the permanent academic commissions.

The periodicals of the academy were also relatively good places in which to publish. The *Mémoires*, established in 1828, appeared somewhat irregularly and printed each year only a small number of lengthy essays. The *Bulletin* devoted to the academy's regular proceedings had a checkered publishing history. In contrast to the *Comptes Rendus* of the Academy of Sciences established in 1835 as a weekly publication, the *Bulletin* founded one year later appeared monthly. The number of subscriptions to the *Bulletin* was never high. According to its publisher, Baillière, the number of individual subscriptions to the *Bulletin* declined from a high of 269 in the mid-1840s and hovered around 200 during the next two decades. By 1871 the figure was down to around 120. The publisher furnished another 200 copies to the academy (first gratis, then from 1850 at less than half the subscription price). These went to all titular members, leaving 50 copies or so that were sent to major institutions and journals.[42]

Despite this limited circulation, presenting a paper or conveying an opinion at the academy in the mid-nineteenth century provided a unique means of making something known throughout the medical profession, since academic proceedings were widely reported in the medical press with presentations frequently reproduced at some length. I have compiled a list of twenty-five Parisian medical journals published during the period 1854–56, excluding those devoted to the proceedings of a single society. Most journals on the list reprinted the odd paper read in the academy or published an occasional commentary on the institution and its activities. No fewer than twelve, or nearly 50 percent, regularly printed summaries of the academy's meetings, including accounts of papers read and major discussions.[43] Of the ten journals that appeared more frequently than once a month, no fewer than nine contained summaries of meetings. It is likely that many Parisian doctors obtained much of their knowledge of recent medical news from such weekly, semiweekly, or biweekly publications. Consequently, an oral presentation at the academy would be extremely well diffused; this undoubtedly constituted one of the academy's chief attractions as a scientific forum.

In 1871 a second series of the *Bulletin* was launched in collaboration with a new publisher, Masson. The general enthusiasm for science and medicine characteristic of the period seems to have infected the new publisher, whose financial investment in the journal enabled it to appear bimonthly. In 1873 the academy obtained increased government financing that nearly tripled its annual expenditure on the journal (from 2,400 to 7,000 francs).[44] As a result, the third series of the *Bulletin* began appearing weekly in April 1873. Since academicians were supposed to receive the proceedings of the last meeting before the next one was convened, the quality of discussion was improved. The weekly appearance of the journal also guaranteed that a presentation would appear in print very rapidly, though it put pressure on speakers to speedily submit manuscripts and correct proofs. Academic spokesmen expected the new arrangement to have even more significant benefits: "it will contribute to the creation of new readers for us, to publicize our activities more widely, and to thus augment the legitimate influence of the academy."[45] Soon after, the academy's president was in fact able to report that subscriptions had risen in a few months from 120 to 800.[46] This itself ensured that many more people would see academic papers. In addition, Masson doubled the number of complimentary copies sent to the academy; these were usually exchanged for other journals, making it considerably easier for periodicals to publish the proceedings of the academy.

The wide dissemination of academic proceedings continued at the end of the nineteenth century. The great Pasteurian debates created widespread public interest in academic proceedings, which were frequently covered by the popular press. And this interest carried over in some respects into the early twentieth century. One medical journalist justified a plea for improved facilities for journalists at the new premises of the academy on the grounds that most medical and many nonmedical journals and newspapers sent reporters to cover meetings.[47]

Examined more closely, however, the situation appears in a less positive light. To be sure, medical journals continued to cover the meetings of the academy. Of twenty-two weekly medical journals published from 1900 to 1905 that I have identified, eleven were available for examination in Montreal. Of these, ten carried summaries of the sessions of various scientific and medical societies. Eight of these summarized Academy of Medicine sessions consistently. But a number of other societies enjoyed similar coverage in the medical press. The meetings of the Société de Chirurgie were also reported in eight journals, while those of the Société Médicale des Hôpitaux and Société de Biologie were covered in seven. Only three summarized those of the Academy of Sciences on a regular basis.

One sees more direct signs that interest in the academy was in fact slipping. The editor of one journal admitted somewhat sadly in 1902 that summaries of the academy's proceedings now lacked the details that had been the rule in earlier years. And, he added, they were becoming more and more impersonal; one now rarely found the criticism of speakers that had reflected passionate interest in the proceedings.[48] The length of summaries, which had frequently been many pages in the 1850s, was seldom more than a page or two in the early twentieth century. This can be attributed to some extent to the large number of societies now being covered. (Approximately 20 percent of the content of most journals which I examined was now devoted to summaries of the proceedings of scientific societies.) But it is more difficult to explain away the fact that reports about the Academy of Medicine were frequently quite a bit shorter than those for some of the major scientific and medical societies.

In the venerable *Archives générales de médecine* between 1902 and 1905 the proceedings of the Société de Biologie took up 19 percent of the space devoted to such proceedings (measured by the number of lines) while those of the Société Médicale des Hôpitaux took up 17 percent. Those of the Academy of Medicine took up only 9 percent. In the bimonthly *Revue de thérapeutiques médico-chirurgicales*, the Société de Chirurgie took up 45 percent of the space devoted to societies, the Société Medi- cale des Hôpitaux 21 percent, and the Academy of Medicine 13 percent. In the prestigious *Presse médicale*, the academy took up only 9 percent of the space for summaries while the Société de Chirurgie and the Société Anatomique took up 24 per- cent and 20 percent, respectively.[49] Each journal had its own preferences in covering scholarly societies but devoting limited space to the Academy of Medicine was common to them all.[50]

While the twentieth-century academy clearly remained a major medical institu- tion in France, one cannot avoid the impression that the papers which it heard and discussed no longer commanded the same level of attention as they had in the previ- ous century; the intellectual content seems to have become somehow less relevant than those of societies with a more specialized and well-defined mandate. Academic spokesmen recognized that a loss of scientific influence had occurred. They admitted that attracting good material had become something of a problem and complained that even academicians chose to publish in other journals. Active steps, we saw, were taken to make submission of papers more attractive to nonmembers. Subsequently, the format of the *Bulletin* was blamed for a lack of submissions. There was limited space for lengthier contributions, it was suggested, and little capacity to publish the reproductions and illustrations becoming common in medical publishing.[51] In the early 1930s necessary funds were found to introduce a new and larger format. By 1935 the general secretary, Charles Achard, could report to the academy that the *Bul- letin* had become an "honorable publication," the elevator had finally been fixed, and the art collection would soon be cleaned.[52]

It was not just academic papers that attracted little attention. Neither did the acad- emy's internal politics. Such administrative changes as the removal in 1913 of the obligation to evaluate presentations by nonmembers or even the reorganization of the sections carried out in 1923 received little comment in the medical press. On the oc- casion of the centenary of the academy in 1920, many medical journals reprinted the major speeches delivered at the ceremonies, but few journalists provided the kind of in-depth evaluations or overviews of the academy and its activities which such occa- sions had provoked during the nineteenth century.[53] One cannot avoid the conclusion that despite or perhaps because of its unquestionably "establishment" status, the academy was no longer central to the concerns of the medical profession.

Academic Debate and Public Health

Whatever prestige the Academy of Medicine enjoyed internationally in the nineteenth century owed less to the papers and reports read within its walls than to the epic dis- cussions and debates which, erupting periodically, "place the academy in the first rank of scholarly societies in Europe. . . ."[54] Public disputations of this sort were based on the view that scientific truth emerged through dispute while public knowl- edge of such conflict was in no way demeaning to the status of science. This was not a universal view; many British learned societies of the period, including the royal so- cieties of London and Edinburgh, sought to prevent disagreements that might "undermine the public image of natural science as straight-forward and objective knowledge"[55] by proscribing discussion following papers.

There also seems to have been relatively little formal debate in the Paris Academy of Sciences, although major scientific disagreements could develop in other contexts. This resulted, at least in part, from principled opposition to public debate, which was thought to inhibit institutional consensus.[56] That the French medical elite embraced official debate reflected a certain tolerance for the disagreements and polemics that characterize medical science. It also expressed a strongly hierarchical view of medical science in which leaders of the profession were expected to legislate matters of controversy.

Debates were oratorical events that have come down to us in the form of texts. Accounts reproduced in the *Bulletin* of the academy are presented as pretty much verbatim accounts and will serve as our primary source for the discussion that follows. They certainly omit a great deal of information which an observer might take in at a glance. But since major inaccuracies were usually rectified at subsequent meetings, one can suppose that these accounts are accurate enough for our purposes.

A discussion in the Academy of Medicine could last for a few minutes or go on for many months. It could involve two or three or twenty members. It might get started in any number of ways. The attempt to cope with a request for advice from a ministry was a frequent cause. Disagreement was periodically generated in the course of the academy's evaluation of the scientific work of nonmembers; such debates were not infrequently about the report evaluating the work rather than about the work being evaluated. Presentations to the academy by members were not subject to reports or votes but could nonetheless give rise to lengthy discussions.

Even when a formal vote was required, substantive conclusions were voted only for a minority of debates. Most discussions ended when the academy passed formulaic resolutions thanking the author, encouraging further research, and occasionally suggesting that the work be considered for publication. The preference for avoiding definitive judgments about controversial medical work had a number of sources. The most important was an acute awareness that the academy would lose credibility if it condemned what might someday be viewed as a major medical innovation or strongly supported what might turn out to be useless or dangerous. Furthermore, what could collective judgment actually mean when academicians disagreed among themselves about virtually everything? The surgeon Velpeau raised both issues in arguing against the conclusions of a report that condemned the use of pessaries for uterine deviations:

> No. One must beware of these sorts of judgments; they compromise academies. Here, we discuss scientific questions, we offer our opinions, and the public which listens to us, here or elsewhere, comes to decisions on the basis of the impressions it gets from our discussions. Finally, when one speaks of the opinions of the academy, one means at most the opinion of such-and-such a member.[57]

The prudent response was thus to encourage more research and to allow clinicians to experiment with an innovation. Its therapeutic value would eventually become apparent.

Second, the nature of therapy during this period favored tolerance or agnosticism toward therapeutic innovations. Few therapeutic measures were effective under all or even most conditions. Medical experience was that therapies worked for some patients at some times and did not work for others or at other times. Doctors concluded that each patient and case of disease was highly individualized. Almost anything, therefore, could be useful under the proper circumstances and for the right patient; only experience would determine what those conditions might be. Thus any innovation which expanded the range of therapeutic alternatives available to physicians was to be encouraged. The academy's role was not to legislate therapeutics but to offer informed judgments about innovations:

> Enlightened by this judgment, practitioners remain free in the cases submitted to their care, to reject or accept the diverse efforts of those seeking to enrich the healing art with new procedures. They [practitioners] then act at their own risk and peril, without the academy's intervention.[58]

Academicians might reach specific decisions affirming the freedom of doctors to utilize and judge innovations. In an 1857 debate about the administration of anesthesia, the academy overrode pressure to regulate anesthetic procedures and voted that these should be left to the discretion of individual practitioners.[59] Therapeutic freedom was not merely a prudent response to uncertainty but a deeply held medical value.[60] Only if a procedure seemed positively harmful in some way—preventive syphilis vaccination, for instance, which was condemned by the academy in 1852[61]—or if the innovation claim involved the *rejection* of accepted practice (the case of tubage as a replacement for tracheotomy discussed in Chapter 7) did the academy feel called upon to collectively reject an innovation or choose among alternatives.

Such tolerance, it should be noted, did not apply to the submissions of nonmedical laymen, whose works were usually sent off to the secret remedies commission to be peremptorily dispatched, or to those numerous submissions by doctors that seemed to be attempts to exploit academic endorsement for commercial purposes. Most public health debates also required firm conclusions, either because a ministry posing a question expected a clear response or because the subject demanded some more or less urgent public action.

If academic debates resulted only occasionally in concrete judgments (and these mainly in matters of public health), what then was their role in medical science? Contemporaries had few doubts on this score. A useful debate was one in which the issues and disagreements were clearly stated, the evidence on each side systematically marshaled, and the areas requiring further research precisely articulated. As one academic spokesman put it in 1872:

> In is in effect rare that scientific questions are resolved by scholarly assemblies. The Academy of Medicine, like the other academies, is an arena where the facts converge, where the most diverse appreciations are produced, where contradictory opinions enter in combat. From this shock, there shoot forth lights which illuminate the questions and prepare their evolution.[62]

In many cases, in fact, formal conclusions were unnecessary because one side or another had visibly dominated the proceedings or enough doubt had been cast on a fashionable procedure to shake the confidence of enthusiastic practitioners.[63]

A second benefit the historian with hindsight can discern involves the interdisciplinary quality of the debates. The academy was one of the few forums where surgeons, internists, physiologists, chemists, and veterinarians could bring their different perspectives and expertise to bear on the same problems. Such multiple perspectives occasionally cast problems in ways that were new and innovative.

Academic debates could not only clarify an issue; they could also disseminate very widely the views that emerged, for the many medical journals which covered academic proceedings usually gave prominent coverage to debates. This does not mean that doctors accepted the academy's verdicts in all instances. Debates were sometimes inconclusive and were in any case filtered through the opinions of the journal editors. With all these reservations, we are still dealing with a capacity to diffuse ideas that was matched in nineteenth-century France only by the Academy of Sciences.

As important as the capacity to diffuse a particular point of view was the ability to capture medical attention and stimulate research. A frequent result of lengthy debates was the reception by the academy of numerous letters, research notes, and articles on that subject from across France. These might be integrated into the debate and would continue to trickle in after discussion had ended. As a consequence of academic discussion, one academician suggested, the attention of "a throng of young doctors" was focused on a specific issue; "they become the source of new works that have not been dreamed of."[64]

I do not mean to suggest that all debates were illuminating or even interesting. Many failed to clarify issues or meandered aimlessly because academicians could not agree about the most basic presuppositions. Debates which hinged on matters of theory were especially likely to get bogged down in irreconcilable disagreements. Occasionally, personal animosities seem to have been paramount. Nonetheless, academic debate was a significant medicoscientific genre in the nineteenth century.

Let us look more closely at the longer debates (arbitrarily defined as discussions that went on for four or more meetings) which occupied the academy during the 1830s and 1850s. During both decades there were on average two or three such debates a year. In both decades two sorts of issues predominated. Most numerous were discussions of therapeutic innovations, which might turn into discussions of all therapeutic alternatives for a particular condition. Usually this meant methods of cure or relief but occasionally discussion focused on diagnostic methods or even prevention. Eleven of twenty-four debates during the first decade were devoted to therapeutic issues, as were fourteen out of twenty-six during the second decade. Another related category of debates had to do with specific illnesses or conditions. Such debates tended to be quite wide-ranging, encompassing etiology, causation, transmission, and diagnosis; but these too dealt frequently with therapeutic issues. There were four such discussions during the 1830s and eight during the 1850s. In both decades there was also an occasional discussion of an issue or procedure of forensic medicine.

In both decades there were fundamental disagreements of medical philosophy. During the 1830s the academy discussed systems of medical thinking like phrenology, Broussaism, homeopathy, therapies that challenged medical orthodoxies like animal magnetism (which was discussed three times during the 1820s and 1830s), and basic issues of scientific methodology like the role of statistics and animal experimentation. During the 1850s few of the therapies discussed challenged the basic principles of medicine, possibly because the membership was smaller and less heterogeneous and possibly because of the influence of a clinical empiricism impatient with theory, exemplified by Armand Trousseau. Still, even the most concrete issues frequently gave rise to discussions of basic medical philosophy: notably vitalism versus organicism, the role of parasites in disease, and the role of the microscope in the diagnosis of cancer.

During both decades relatively few debates dealt with public health and professional issues in spite of the fact that the provision of public health expertise was one of the primary rationales for the existence of the academy. During the 1830s, four out of twenty-four debates were devoted to such issues; during the 1850s, the number was only two out of twenty-six. To be sure, all debates, even the most theoretical, were potentially useful to public health authorities. Furthermore, academic debate did occasionally sway public policy. The academy's support for Chervin's anticontagionism had significant influence on public and medical opinion in the 1820s and 1830s.[65] Its conclusions about plague quarantine in 1846 had an even more direct effect on health policy, prompting the government to shorten the quarantine period while establishing a network of inspectors in foreign ports.[66] Nevertheless, the dearth of explicit debate about matters of public health demands explanation.

The simplest explanation is that there was limited need for the expertise of the academy in this domain because the public health activities of the French state at mid-century remained restricted.[67] Such need as there was could be satisfied by the academy's permanent public health commissions. Consequently, the various ministries of government only occasionally consulted the academy about major public health matters; when they did, they requested expert advice on narrow technical questions rather than guidance about broad policy issues.

More surprising in light of widespread rhetoric about the social role of medicine is the fact the academy rarely initiated public health discussions. It was motivated by a combination of diffidence and political prudence. Unlike scientists, medical men did not have a long tradition of service to the state. During the early decades of the academy's existence, they appear to have been uncertain about their roles and prerogatives. It was thus common for academicians to cut off discussion on a point of administration or politics on the grounds that the government had not specifically requested an examination of this issue. Frequent changes of regime during this period further fostered political prudence and hesitation about entering controversial domains without explicit invitation. The debate of 1827 on the contagiousness of yellow fever, in which the academy seriously displeased the Restoration government by arriving at anticontagionist conclusions, demonstrated what a perilous minefield public health could be.

As far as public health was concerned, the diffidence of academicians began to dissipate by the early 1860s. Like the educated bourgeoisie more generally, the academic elite during the last decade of the Second Empire exhibited a new self-confidence in demanding institutional reform. With no prompting from the government, the academy during these years discussed in considerable detail hospital hygiene and infant mortality. In both cases academic deliberations seem to have been instrumental in provoking wide-ranging debate and, eventually, reforms. Academicians began to insist that the academy should make its voice heard not merely on traditional questions of public health but on all matters relating to "the advancement of the sciences which have humanity as their object, and to the improvement of physical and moral conditions of modern societies."[68]

During the following decades the academy's public health activity accelerated as the very domain of public health expanded. The defeat at the hands of Germany in 1870, followed by the insurrection of the Paris Commune, created a sense of crisis that encouraged academicians to bring medical expertise to bear on larger social issues.[69] Whereas public health discussions had traditionally been about contagious diseases or questions of administration, debates on population decline and alcoholism brought the academy into the intimate realms of personal behavior.

Professional issues, however, remained unexplored by the academicians. The debate over the reorganization of medicine in 1833, as we saw in Chapter 1, brought out many of the internal conflicts dividing the profession; it also ended formal discussion of such issues until after World War I. All the major deliberations of the nineteenth and early twentieth centuries about professional legislation and medical education were virtually ignored by the academy. Individual academicians in their other institutional capacities actively debated such issues. But there seems to have been a tacit understanding that the academy as an institution should stay away from the more controversial questions agitating the medical profession.

Debates which took place during the next decade examined (1875–85) were dominated by the repercussions of the bacteriological revolution. No less than thirty-seven long debates took place during this decade, eleven more than during the 1850s. The number would have been higher still had I not counted as a single unit the debates about anthrax which flared up sporadically over a five-year period. The vast majority of these discussions had to do with the impact on etiology, diagnosis, and therapeutics of the germ theory. Pasteur himself recognized the importance of the academy to medical acceptance of his views and frequently attended and spoke out during academic deliberations. Most of the objections to his views came from only a few individuals, notably the veterinarian Gabriel Colin and the very elderly Jules Guérin, who were the main targets of Pasteur's polemical wrath. Overall, acceptance of the main principles of Pasteurism (if not all the details or consequences) seems to have occurred fairly early among most members of the Parisian academic elite. Still there was an epic quality to many of these debates. Whereas only 8 percent of the debates went on for fifteen or more meetings during the 1850s, some 16 percent of the debates during this next period were that long. The number of meetings taken up by debates in the latter decade went up 38 percent from the earlier decade.

Despite the predominance of Pasteurian issues, there were a number of nonbacterial innovations also discussed, including Marey's graphic method, the dangers of chloroform administration, and the therapeutic effects of salicylates. Public health debates also assumed greater importance, with five debates dealing explicitly with public health regulations and with perhaps two others focusing on issues having public health implications.

Nevertheless, despite the increased public health activity of the academy, that institution had little to do with the major medical legislation of this period, the law reorganizing the medical profession in 1892, the medical assistance law of 1893, and the public health law of 1902. In the case of both the laws of 1893 and 1902, the academy was consulted only about the contagious diseases requiring obligatory declaration to administrative authorities; it was not asked about the principle of obligatory declaration. Public authorities continued to limit the role of the academy to the provision of specialized expertise.

Toward the end of the century, academicians occasionally made efforts to extend debates to the principles and details of legislation. A debate on preventing syphilis quickly became, under the influence of the venereologist Alfred Fournier, a discussion of the reform of laws controlling prostitution. Not everyone was happy with this broad interpretation of the academy's mandate. Some academicians were opposed on the grounds that such discussions extended beyond the scientific competence of the academy. Among those most insistent on this point were some of the academicians most active in the public health bureaucracy.[70]

Many academicians were members of consultative commissions set up by national or local authorities. A handful also held paying positions within the public health bureaucracy. Both commissions and posts increased in number during the course of the nineteenth and twentieth centuries. The participation of academicians reflected this expansion, but in unexpected, surprising ways. The proportion with such public health appointments rose from 25 percent among academicians in 1821 to 34 percent among those who were members in 1861. But the proportion remained virtually unchanged among academy members in 1901 and declined to 25 percent among those of 1935, despite considerable expansion of the public health apparatus. In both of the later populations, however, there was now a small group of a half dozen or so men who held at least three positions in the public health bureaucracy and who were thus something like professionals of public health. The most influential of these was certainly Paul Brouardel (1837–1906), professor of legal medicine, dean of the Faculty of Medicine, and president of the Consultative Committee of Public Hygiene, the preeminent advisory body for matters of public health. Brouardel played a unique role in shaping public health in France in large part because he successfully bridged the worlds of the Parisian medical elite, the public health bureaucracy, and national politics.

How did Brouardel respond to the increased role of the academy in the legislative and administrative spheres? He certainly paid lip service to the expertise of the academy and, like Théophile Roussel, who introduced the law on infant protection in the legislature, claimed academic inspiration for many of the measures he introduced. But in actual fact he consulted the academy when it was useful to add the weight of authoritative science to his projects. Let me give just one example.

In 1885 the Committee of Public Hygiene under Brouardel's leadership voted the proposition that the addition of large amounts of potassium sulfate to wines during the production process posed a danger to the health of consumers; it should thus be restricted to a maximum limit of 2 grams per liter of wine. In the face of massive resistance from the wine industry, the committee repeated its advice two years later and also recommended that the question be sent to the academy for an authoritative scientific opinion. A commission was appointed by the academy to study the matter; one-third of its members were also members of the Committee for Public Hygiene (including Brouardel). The commission produced an exhaustive report on all the research done on the subject and came to exactly the same conclusions as had the Committee of Public Hygiene. The use of potassium sulfate should be restricted to a maximum limit of 2 grams per liter of wine.[71] Regulations to this effect were incorporated into a law passed in 1892.

But academic assertiveness in matters of public health policy could also be unwelcome and on several occasions Brouardel had to dampen the enthusiasm of academicians for making policy. In 1887, for instance, a commission named by the academy to study preventive measures against syphilis produced a report calling for, among other things, the introduction of a new law mandating stricter and more effective regulation of prostitution. The report was quite detailed in its legislative and judicial recommendations. In subsequent discussion several academicians expressed reservations about the way in which the academy was going beyond its medical expertise into areas of jurisprudence. The most influential of these was Brouardel, who disagreed with the content of some of the proposals and who argued on principle against the presentation of specific legislative and judicial proposals. It emerged in the course of discussion that he was himself preparing to draft a law regulating prostitution. He thus requested that the academy remain "on medical terrain" by calling in general terms for a sanitary law to regulate prostitution. Such support for his own agenda is more or less what he got from the academy's final proposals.[72]

During the decade from 1900 to 1909 academic debates seem to have changed in character and to have declined in importance. Only twenty-one debates took place with only two extending to ten or more meetings. The number of meetings devoted to long debates declined by 63 percent. This decline stabilized during the decade of the 1920s when twenty-one debates took place. However, the time spent in debate as measured by the number of pages in the *Bulletin* which debates occupied continued to decline.

More meaningful than simple quantitative measurements are the changes in content. Academic debates about medical science and practice were increasingly being displaced by discussions of public health and professional issues. During the decade 1900–1909, for instance, seven, or one-third of the debates, were about public health issues with two others containing a strong public health component. The remaining debates were occasionally controversial, particularly the ongoing discussion of appendectomy. On the whole, however, discussions of medical science tended to be about details. One finds none of the discussion of fundamental principles characteristic of earlier debates and few deliberations at the cutting edge of medical science.

It is during the 1920s that we find clear evidence that academic debate had been transformed beyond recognition. Only four of twenty-one debates during that decade related to traditional therapeutic or etiological issues. Ten were about public health while seven concerned professional or ethical questions, including two about the system of national health insurance that was being introduced and another concerning the regulation of midwifery. Such discussions of professional issues had been absent from the academy for nearly a century. Put simply, academic debates seem to have lost their significance for medical science and practice and to have become increasingly geared to public health and professional regulation. "We are," said one outgoing president, "above all a Society of Public Hygiene."[73] What is more, to academicians unfamiliar with the past, the predominant public health orientation was now a longstanding institutional tradition.[74]

This development can be perceived in two ways. It can be viewed as the logical culmination of the academy's efforts during the past half century to assert its right to influence public policy. Statements about the social role of the academy were certainly more aggressive and insistent during the 1920s than they had been earlier.[75] The validity of academic activity in this domain seems to have been finally accepted by government, which initiated some of these discussions. But the academy did not shrink from energetically offering advice even when none was solicited. There are many possible reasons for this new social activism. It was undoubtedly fueled in part by the heightened status of medicine fostered by scientific developments. That the medical elite had clearly become part of the state "establishment" also helped advance the social claims of the academy. The germ theory of disease opened up new possibilities for public action in the name of health, as did the increasingly medical definition of an ever-growing list of social problems. The social crisis of the interwar years provoked demands for state intervention in health care, which brought politics into the very heart of clinical medicine. Whatever the reasons, there can be no doubt that academicians saw themselves and were perceived by politicians in a new way; they were no longer just scientific experts but also repositories of the social wisdom of medicine. As the president of the academy stated in 1925, the academy brought to the legislative proposals of politicians both scientific guarantees and moral authority.[76]

There is also a second avenue from which to approach this transformation of academic debate. The emphasis on social and public health matters in academic discussion was possible because debates about therapeutics and etiology were being severely cut back. This did not mean that medical science lost its importance in the academy. Even if presentations by academicians about public health became more frequent during this decade, the majority of papers read before the academy continued to be about fairly technical medical questions. Discussion of such papers, however, was characteristically limited to brief exchanges of questions and answers.

Academicians were well aware that a fundamental sea change had occurred. Many would come to see the origins of this shift in Pasteur's famous remark to the academy in 1875. In the midst of a debate about his theories, Pasteur reminded the assembly that several weeks before, the academy in secret session had raised the question of how it "could introduce the true scientific spirit to a higher degree into its activities and discussions." He suggested that this could be achieved if a "moral commitment" was made

> to never call this podium a tribune, to never call a paper [*communication*] presented there a speech, and to never call someone who has just or who is just going to speak an orator. These three words, tribune, speech, orator, seem to me to be incompatible with the simplicity and rigor of science.[77]

There was little immediate reaction to Pasteur's comments. Nevertheless, the desire to make the academy a more scientific institution which he referred to (and exploited rhetorically) gradually had its effect. As early as the 1890s, academic speeches made reference to the scarcity of long debates. They no longer served a purpose, it was suggested, now that experimental "facts" absorbed all attention, reasoning played an increasingly restricted role in academic life, and matters of doctrine inspired "insouciance."[78] This judgment was undoubtedly premature. The decade of the 1890s was not without its doctrinaire debates. But the notion of oratorical debate in medical science was clearly making academicians uncomfortable.

When he reviewed the academy's achievements in 1901, the permanent secretary, Sigismond Jaccoud, felt called upon to defend the debates of the mid-nineteenth century from the claim that they had been dominated by "pure verbiage." He defended their philosophical scope and profundity, as well as their oratorical richness. In so doing, he stated, he was defending the academy's past, "already very remote from us.[79] He did not, however, suggest that such debates might still have their uses.

Even this limited defense of debates gradually disappeared. An outgoing president in 1910 explained the disappearance of the "slightly scholastic" debates of another age by referring to the nature of modern science. "A great number of scientific facts present themselves with such a character of precision that they can be the object of only a simple acknowledgment."[80] A decade later, Anatole Chauffard tried to summarize a century of academic achievement in medicine by contrasting past and present practices:

> There was a period of *doctrinaires*, in the tribune of the academy as in our political assemblies, with long speeches, discussions which lasted months, commissions, agendas for discussion, the entire apparatus of major political debates. . . . [T]he abuse of the word is a poor intellectual discipline. . . .
>
> Today our academic customs have become very calm, much less oratorical; discussions, with the exception of several questions of major importance concerning social medicine, are more rare and less long than in the past, and they remain free of all personal considerations. More facts and less words, is this not the ideal program for all scientific communication?[81]

One need not accept this argument at face value in order to recognize that more than criteria of scientific argument had changed. It was the essential rationale of academic debate which had been overturned.

For much of the nineteenth century, I have suggested, academic debate about medicine was a major scientific genre. It might occasionally determine the validity of new therapies and doctrines, but more often it made widely accessible news of the latest innovations and of the medical elite's reactions to them. And this continued to be the case until nearly the end of the nineteenth century. However much Pasteur attacked oratory, academic debate was a major part of his strategy to win medical support for the germ theory of disease. But the very notion that a medical elite could evaluate new knowledge and techniques was being subverted by specialization in both the laboratory sciences and clinical medicine. Increasingly, medical knowledge of all types was being created and evaluated in specialized journals, within highly formalized articles rather than through the scientific "talking" of a hierarchical elite. Any talking that did occur took place in specialized medical and scientific societies. The shrinking space devoted to academic proceedings in medical journals and the difficulties of attracting first-rate submissions to the academy's *Bulletin*, discussed earlier, here take on their full significance.

The advanced age of academicians may also have been significant in this process. Between 1901 and 1935 the mean age of academicians rose from sixty-one to nearly seventy. The fact that so many academicians were well past their professional prime undoubtedly played a role in this abandonment of the effort to evaluate work at the frontiers of medical science. Whatever the reasons for it, the virtual abdication of the function of scientific debate opened up the institutional space necessary for a new social conception of academic debate to fully emerge.

This chapter has dramatically illustrated the general theme that the academy went through a number of incarnations. In the early nineteenth century it was an active and closely observed scientific body, in spite of the fact that many of its institutional mechanisms did not function very effectively. From the 1870s to the 1890s aspirations to transform the academy into an institution compatible with the norms of modern science brought about extensive change in academic procedures and considerable scientific activity. The academy also began taking a more active role in public health. By the 1920s, however, the academy's scientific role had been severely curtailed as a result of changing norms of scientific practice; deliberations about matters of public health and professional organization now dominated institutional life. Despite or perhaps because of the emphasis on policy issues, the academy's stature within and influence on French medical life seem to have been substantially diminished.

NOTES

1. "Ordonnances portant à la création de l'Académie royale de médecine," *MEM* 1 (1828), 2.

2. See for instance the presidential address by J.-B. Barth in *BAM* 1 (1872), 8, in which the order of the two tasks and their relative importance are reversed.

3. This is bound into the copies of *BAM* in the McGill University Health Sciences Library.

4. Although academicians knew what they meant by "public health," the matter is less simple for historians. When I use the term in this and the following chapters, I refer to preventive or therapeutic activities that require some form of *collective public action* on the physical or social environment.

5. Although the regulations of the Academy of Medicine specified that this order be followed, meetings frequently strayed from the pattern. The workings of the Academy of Sciences are described in Maurice Crosland, *Science under Control: The French Academy of Sciences, 1795–1914* (Cambridge, 1992).

6. The Academy of Sciences also provided this service to scientists.

7. In 1872 fifty-one manuscripts were sent to committees while forty-seven were not deemed suitable for reports. J.-B. Barth, "Compte rendu des actes de l'Académie pendant 1872," *BAM* 2 (1873), xvii.

8. Louis Peisse, *La Médecine et les médecins; philosophie, doctrines, institutions, critiques, moeurs et biographies médicales*, 2 vols. (1857), vol. 2, pp. 143–53.

9. Ibid., p. 166.

10. Corresponding members posed something of a problem since many welcomed evaluations that would publicize their work. The academy was not consistent in dealing with their submissions.

11. J.-B. Baillière and son, *Histoire de nos relations avec l'Académie de Médecine, 1827–1871: lettre adressée à MM. les membres de l'Académie* (1872), pp. 23–24.

12. The practice was prohibited for a time during the early 1840s. In 1855 objections to the practice were again raised, resulting in a decline in the number of such presentations. *BAM* 20 (1854–55), 1178–79.

13. Members presented 39 *communications* and 36 *lectures* during the period 1854–57. Nonmembers presented 158 *lectures* and 48 *communications* during the same period.

14. In thirty-four out of seventy-seven candidacies during these four years, a declaration of candidacy was followed by the presentation of a *lecture*.

15. The bibliography of Velpeau's writings is appended to J. Béclard, "Éloge de Velpeau," *MEM* 29 (1869), 36–43.

16. It helped to be friendly with the reviewer. See the letter from Guersant to Bretonneau regarding the former's review of the latter's work in Paul Triaire, ed., *Bretonneau et ses correspondants*, (1892), vol. 1, pp. 442–44.

17. See, for instance, the footnote in J.-B. De Larroque, *Traité de la fièvre typhoïde* (1847), p. 415.

18. In his speech as outgoing president in 1875, Devergie reported that of fifty-eight manuscripts and oral presentations sent to committees, forty-six were still without a report. Those from the year before still awaiting reports numbered seventy-four. Devergie proposed that everything sent to a commission should get a preliminary report within two weeks indicating whether a full report was worth doing. The suggestion was ignored. *BAM* 4 (1875), 16–17.

19. In that year, he reports, only 6 reports were submitted out of 357 works sent to committees. Crosland, *Science under Control*, p. 269.

20. There were thirty-one in 1894 and thirty-two in 1898.

21. See, for instance, the presidential speeches of Georges Hayem and Edmond Delorme in *BAM* 81 (1919), 16, 32, and that of Léon Labbé in *BAM* 63 (1910), 3.

22. Following standard academic practice, virtually no information about this meeting was provided with the exception of a curt announcement in *BAM* 70 (1913), 282.

23. See the incoming presidential speech by Delorme in *BAM* 81 (1919), 32, and Charles Achard, "Jaccoud à l'Académie," *BAM* 104 (1930), 616–17.

24. The number presented annually ranged from fifty to sixty.

25. At the same meeting which changed the rules about presentations by nonmembers, academicians drew up new guidelines for the presentations which candidates for titular or associate membership were required to give. *BAM* 81 (1914), 413. This suggests that the two issues were closely linked. The proportion of those presenting papers who subsequently became academicians was about 40 percent in 1924. This is close to the figure for 1892.

26. For instance, Sireday in his speech as outgoing president in 1936 stated that the purpose of publication in *BAM* was to make specific work more accessible and thus facilitate its confirmation or rejection. *BAM* 115 (1936), 6.

27. *BAM* 117 (1937), 19. The academy in 1938 set up a special commission with a mandate to find ways to prevent the exploitation of extracts from the *Bulletin* to support commercial claims.

28. In the volumes of *BAM* for both 1924 and 1934 there was only a single report each year on a submitted manuscript.

29. In the four-year period 1854–57, well over half the *lectures* fall into this category. In the first six months of 1924 about half of the presentations by academicians can be classified in one of these two categories. The figure is even higher in the case of presentations by nonmembers.

30. See the discussion in Chapter 2.

31. During the first half of 1924, approximately one-quarter of the presentations by academicians were devoted to some aspect of public health or professional regulation. Presentations by nonmembers, however, continued to be predominantly devoted to therapeutics.

32. M. D. Grmek, *Catalogue des manuscrits de Claude Bernard* (1967).

33. A paper on digestion in herbivores and carnivores originally presented to the Academy of Sciences in 1846 was also presented to the Academy of Medicine. But though mention of the presentation was made in *BAM* (11 [1846], 564), it was not reprinted or even summarized.

34. William Coleman, "The Cognitive Basis of the Discipline: Claude Bernard on Physiology," *Isis* 76 (1985), 49–70.

35. Edmond Delorme, "La Chirurgie à l'Académie, 1820–1920: esquisse historique," *Centenaire de l'Académie de Médecine, 1820–1920* (1921), pp. 202–3.

36. Ernest Lebon, *Armand Gautier: biographie, bibliographie analytique des écrits* (1912).

37. *BAM* 98 (1928), 13.

38. Robert Debré, "L'Académie de Médecine," *Médecine de France* 97 (1958), 4.

39. See especially S. Jaccoud, "Un adieu à la rue des Saints-Pères," *MEM* 40 (1906), 1–30, and the essays in *Centenaire de l'Académie de Médecine, 1820–1920* (1921).

40. An amusing first-person account of Bretonneau's presentation to the academy in 1821 is found in Triaire, *Bretonneau et ses correspondants*, vol. 1, pp. 423–25.

41. Devergie in *BAM* 3 (1874), 5. Pleas for less noise during the reading of papers became highly ritualized parts of the speeches of incoming and outgoing presidents during the 1930s. See, for example, *BAM* 115 (1936), 5, 10; *BAM* 117 (1937), 3, 18. Also see the discussion of this problem in Maurice de Fleury, *Le Médecin* (1927), pp. 22–34.

42. Figures for subscriptions are from Ballière and son, *Histoire de nos relations avec l'Académie*, p. 15; and Barth, "Compte rendu 1872," xi. I have found no trace of those receiving complimentary copies but a report of 1863 lists institutions which received copies of the annual *Mémoires* of the academy. These included municipal libraries in thirty-four French cities, seven European academies of science, four academies of medicine, four medical societies, six European and six French medical periodicals (AN F17 3686).

43. Most of these also published summaries of the meetings of the Academy of Sciences. Provincial journals showed much less interest in the work of the academy; only one of nine covered it constantly, although most others published the occasional paper or commentary.

44. Meeting of the administrative council, January 28, 1873, in AM Liasse 14.

45. Béclard's comments to the academy in *BAM* 1 (1872), 43.

46. Barth, "Compte rendu 1872," xi.

47. E. de Lavarenne, "Le Service de presse de la nouvelle Académie," *Presse médicale* 98 (1902), 1166.

48. Ibid.

49. These figures are calculated from a sample of twelve issues of each journal from this period.

50. To these three journals, one could add *Progrès Médical*, which also devoted relatively little space to the academy.

51. Ménétrier, *BAM* 103 (1930), 16.

52. *BAM* 114 (1935), 451.

53. I have not come across any evaluations of this sort but my search was not exhaustive.

54. A. Devergie, "Lecture sur les travaux de l'Académie impériale de médecine," *BAM* 25 (1859–60), 180.

55. Martin J. S. Rudwick, *The Great Devonian Controversy: The Shaping of Scientific Knowledge among Gentlemanly Specialists* (Chicago, 1988), p. 25.

56. Crosland, *Science under Control*, pp. 112–20. The Cuvier–Geoffroy debate in 1830 took place as an exchange of scientific papers read before the academy while the equally famous Pasteur–Pouchet debate took place within a special commission to examine the experimental evidence.

57. *BAM* 19 (1853–54), 886.

58. C. Gibert, *BAM* 19 (1853–54), 973.

59. *BAM* 22 (1856–57), 1087.

60. For some twentieth-century manifestations, see George Weisz, "The Origins of Medical Ethics in France: The International Congress of *Morale Médicale* of 1955," in *Social Science Perspectives on Medical Ethics*, ed. George Weisz (Dordrecht, 1990), pp. 145–61.

61. *BAM* 17 (1851–52), 1094–95.

62. Barth, "Compte rendu 1872," xxiii. For very similar language several years later see Bouley's address to the academy on assuming the presidency (*BAM* 7 [1878], 3).

63. Vincent Duval, "Coup d'oeil sur nos travaux," *Revue des spécialités et innovations médicales et chirurgicales* 3 (1841), 9, suggested that his own confidence in a new surgical procedure to correct strabism had been called into question by a discussion of the subject in the Academy of Medicine. The great popularity of salicylic soda as a specific for rheumatic fever by the 1880s was attributed by one medical dictionary to the strong case which Germain Sée made for the medication in the course of a discussion he initiated in the academy in 1877. E. Ory, "Salicine, salicylique (Acide)," in *Nouveau Dictionnaire de médecine et de chirurgie pratique*, vol. 32 (1882), 178–79.

64. Devergie, "Lecture sur les travaux de l'Académie," 177.

65. Ann F. La Berge, *Mission and Method: The Early-Nineteenth-Century Public Health Movement* (Cambridge, 1992), p. 93, cites draconian cuts in government expenditures for sanitary establishments in the years following the academy's report.

66. E. A. Heaman, "Anticontagionism in France in the Nineteenth Century," M.A. thesis, McGill University, 1990, pp. 70–84.

67. The standard account of French public health during this period is La Berge, *Mission and Method*.

68. Tardieu, speech as incoming president, *BAM* 32 (1866–67), 344.

69. A good example is Barth, "Compte rendu 1872." On the larger issue of "medicalization" of social problems see Robert A. Nye, *Crime, Madness and Politics in Modern France: The Medical Concept of National Decline* (Princeton, N.J., 1984).

70. The report and discussion are scattered through *BAM* 17 (1887) and *BAM* 18 (1888).

71. The final vote is in *BAM* 20 (1888), 49. I am grateful to Harry Paul for sharing with me his considerable knowledge of wine production and consumption.

72. The discussion is in *BAM* 19 (1888), 155–470.

73. G. Hayem, *BAM* 81 (1919), 8.

74. E. Quénu, presidential address, *BAM* 103 (1930), 3.

75. See, for instance, the remarks by P. Cazaneuve, *BAM,* 93 (1925), 564.

76. A. Doléris, "Installation du Bureau, 1925," *BAM* 93 (1925), 3.

77. *BAM* 4 (1875), 256–57.

78. J. Rochard, "Comte rendu des travaux de l' Académie en 1894," *BAM* 32 (1894), 605.

79. Jaccoud, "Un adieu à la rue des Saints-Pères," 10, 6.

80. L. Labbé in *BAM* 63 (1910), 2.

81. A. Chauffard, "Un siècle de médecine à l'Académie," p. 142.

4

Academic Functions and Genres: Commissions and Prizes

Not all academic functions fit neatly into a three-tier schema of development. In this chapter we examine several forms of activity exhibiting more complex patterns of evolution. We begin with the academy's permanent public health commissions, which carried out much of the academy's day-to-day activity. We then go on to the elaborate system of prizes, which expanded substantially as the nineteenth century advanced.

Permanent Commissions

One of the chief functions of the Academy of Medicine was to serve the public health needs of the national government. Occasionally the government would submit a major policy question to the academy, which would then appoint a special commission to prepare a report. More often than not, however, the demands placed on the academy by the government followed a number of routine paths and were dealt with by permanent commissions. There were four commissions which functioned without interruption from the 1820s into the twentieth century: secret remedies, mineral waters, epidemics, and vaccination. During the 1870s an infant hygiene commission began its long existence, and at the end of the century tuberculosis and serotherapy commissions were created. (The former did not produce much material.) Several commissions meant to be permanent, like the cholera commission in the early decades of the nineteenth century and alcoholism and paludism (malaria) commissions at the beginning of the twentieth, disappeared after several years without leaving much trace.

Characteristically, a permanent commission had six members named for three-year terms that were staggered so that each year a third of the members were replaced. Two roles were associated with permanent commissions: (1) performing practical administrative and technical tasks on behalf of the national government; and (2) collecting information on specific subjects from networks of informants. The information collected in the latter case was meant to be both practically useful to the state and a contribution to medical science. All commissions played either one or the other of these roles and several combined the two. Technical administrative tasks could be fulfilled by presenting periodic short reports to the academy. The second more intellectual function involved the production of a long annual report read to the academy before being sent to the government.[1]

At the technical and administrative end of this spectrum were two commissions: one with deep roots in the ancien régime was responsible for secret and new remedies; the other, established only at the end of the nineteenth century, had jurisdiction over the production of vaccine sera and organic extracts. Both came regularly before the academy to announce their verdicts on remedies, sera, or extracts that had recently been examined. The entire academy then voted on and usually confirmed the conclusions.

The academy followed a long line of commissions and institutions, most notably the Société Royale de Médecine and the Society of the Faculty of Medicine, in evaluating secret or proprietary remedies.[2] During the first half of the century its secret remedies commission judged various patent remedies sent by the Ministry of Commerce with a view to deciding which should be purchased from the inventor by the state so that the formula could be published. Occasionally, in the absence of real approval, the commission granted the inventor the right to sell innocuous remedies (*libre disposition*). Like its institutional predecessors, the academy proved extremely reluctant to hand out authorizations. During the first three years of its existence it granted no approvals and three *libres dispositions* out of sixty submissions.[3] Most often remedies were deemed dangerous, unoriginal, or based on erroneous principles. By 1848 the commission had approved only two remedies.[4]

During the first half of the century the academy complained regularly about the legislation governing these remedies and campaigned for the eradication of secret remedies and the introduction of a new system to authorize commercial use.[5] A constant source of tension during these years was the government's unwillingness to cooperate. It showed, for instance, a proclivity for awarding inventors whose remedies were rejected as ineffective by the academy a *brevet*, or warrant, permitting unrestricted sale. Advertising frequently hinted or even claimed, much to the chagrin of academicians, that the granting of such warrants was the result of academic approval. In the three cases where the academy recommended that the government acquire remedies, no action followed except that proprietors were now able to boast of academic endorsement of their products.[6] After the reform of the laws regulating secret remedies in 1850, the task of the academy was to decide if such remedies were to be authorized for commercial use and thus added to the pharmaceutical codex. Such authorization gave the inventor the right to publicize his remedy while leaving other pharmacists free to prepare it.

Under both regimes, the commission rarely gave its approval to a remedy. The tolerance accorded to therapeutic innovations in "scientific" communications did not extend to such "commercial" submissions. On a regular basis, the commission reporter appeared before the academy with a list of remedies identified only by number and rendered negative judgments. In several cases where the commission did recommend authorization, the academy as a whole voted against the commission's proposal, so powerful was the animus against commercial exploiters of medicine.[7]

There were many reasons for this hostility. Most of those who proposed such medicines to the academy were not doctors and thus could not be taken seriously.[8] The notion of "secrecy" was deeply offensive to academicians committed to scientific openness. Most important, the law's liberality on this issue left the academy to examine "an enormous mass of formulae, which are absurd and ridiculous, and often dangerous."[9] Expectations therefore were low. They were not raised by the fact that many of the medications were submitted only because local authorities policing the remedies trade had discovered them being sold illegally.

Why then did this commission continue its work? A simple answer is that the jurisprudence regulating such matters required some sort of gatekeeping apparatus. But if academicians continued to accept the role, it was because it provided a means of combating "with firmness and without laxity, this odious charlatanism which trifles with the health and credulity of the public."[10] The commission could deny authorization and frequently heap ridicule on countless quack remedies since, in the vast majority of cases, "to examine them is to reject them."[11] According to one account, the academy did not authorize a single remedy between 1858 and 1902; not surprisingly, the number of remedies submitted declined substantially.[12]

The refusal to authorize most secret remedies had serious repercussions because courts came to interpret the notion of secret remedies very broadly. They increasingly defined as illegal secret remedies all medicines, whether secret or not, that had not been formulated according to a physician's prescription, did not appear in the pharmaceutical codex, and had not been acquired or authorized by the government.[13] This definition included most proprietary medicines. If such a broad definition of illegal drugs was almost impossible to enforce, it has been argued that it inhibited the development of the pharmaceuticals industry until legislation in 1926 allowed virtually all drugs to be sold so long as an exact list of ingredients appeared on the package.[14] Even before this reform made the secret remedies commission redundant, the academy seems to have lost interest in this task. In the early twentieth century, the reports of this commission tended to be few in number and very short.[15]

This does not mean that new remedies were no longer being evaluated by the academy. The secret remedies commission was joined at the end of the nineteenth century by another permanent commission established in response to legislation of 1895 requiring that the academy be consulted about the introduction of new sera and antitoxins.[16] This commission also examined and authorized the injectable organic animal extracts that were becoming so therapeutically fashionable.[17] Unlike the increasingly moribund secret remedies commission, this serum commission was extremely active. It typically presented brief reports every few months announcing decisions about a half dozen or so applications for the right to manufacture and distribute sera or organic extracts. It shared this responsibility with another serum commission within the Ministry of the Interior which rendered an initial verdict that was ordinarily upheld by the academy's commission. Agreement was routine because the two commissions had overlapping memberships. Furthermore, the ministerial

commission usually sent a representative to inspect and evaluate the production facilities and it was this report which determined the conclusions of both commissions.

Unlike the judgments of the secret remedies commission, those of the serum
commission were invariably positive. The reason for the difference is that the academy accepted the fundamental reasonableness of therapeutics based on the principles
of immunology and bacteriology, on one hand, and on what was to become endocrinology, on the other. (One should not forget that the development of insulin as well
as of reproductive endocrinology grew out of the mania for organic animal extracts.)[18]
Nor was there anything secret about such preparations manufactured by relatively sophisticated laboratories. The authorization of sera and extracts ordinarily depended
on a nontherapeutic criterion: that the production facilities meet accepted hygienic
and pharmaceutical norms. Whether sera or extracts actually worked was an empirical question to be settled by clinical testing. Any new product thus had to be made
available to doctors so that testing could occur.

The law regulating this rapidly expanding field caused the academy a variety of
problems. The academy initially saw its role as authorizing the public sale and distribution of sera; it did not intend to regulate doctors' use of these products for
experimental purposes. Without such experimentation, after all, how could data about
clinical effects be obtained? Consequently, a court decision in 1911 which interpreted the law of 1895 as making it illegal for doctors to ever use a nonauthorized
remedy caused quite a stir in the academy, as in other medical societies.[19] The academy appointed a special commission, which proposed new legislation that
specifically exempted from the provisions of the law of 1895 any doctor making use
of substances "as an experiment and under his responsibility"; doctors would require
authorization only when they wished to introduce a substance "into current practice."[20] The academy in secret session approved the revision after first changing the
wording to insist that the therapeutic experimentation excluded from the law had to
be justified by the results of animal experiments and that the substances being tested
had to be provided free to patients.

No revised legislation seems to have been introduced at this point. But by the
1920s the commission was getting around the problem by providing two types of
authorization. The more common was a temporary one-year authorization. The individual or laboratory receiving this was supposed to use the time to come up with
clinical data; if necessary, another temporary authorization might be awarded. Once
data were collected and published, and if they showed that a substance was not harmful, permanent authorization was usually granted.

Despite the limited terms of its legal mandate, and despite its concern to make
new substances available to doctors, the academy nevertheless claimed the right to
refuse authorization based on its judgment of probable therapeutic benefits. In 1923,
for instance, it refused authorization to a proposal for the production and distribution
of an oral vaccine on the grounds that vaccines and sera had not been shown to be
effective when taken orally. It was informed by the Ministry of Health that the Conseil d'État, which had been asked to rule on the duties of the serum commissions,[21]
had decided that it was *not* the task of either the academy's or the ministry's serum
commission to judge efficacy and utility of remedies; it had only to decide if these
remedies were potentially harmful. The academy rejected this definition of its role

and voted to ask the minister to request the Conseil d'État to reconsider its interpretation and, if that failed, to submit a new law to the legislature.[22]

The ministry submitted a proposed revision of the law to the academy in 1930 and this was introduced in the legislature in 1934.[23] But by 1940 the academy's secretary, Charles Achard, was still complaining about the commission's inability to judge anything but the chemical composition and toxicity of substances. As a result, he argued, the plethora of authorized medications posed the danger that doctors would not utilize the truly effective medications that might be available for given conditions. Achard in fact went beyond sera and organic substances and suggested that some way of evaluating the by now enormous output of the pharmaceutical industry needed to be put into effect. Although he was skeptical that it was financially feasible to set up a public testing agency, he did offer the academy's cooperation in any such endeavor.[24]

By this time there existed another precedent for academic evaluation of pharmaceutical substances. In 1926 the Ministry of Labor and Hygiene added another task to the academy's crowded agenda: inspection on behalf of hospitals and public dispensaries of the many new and occasionally dangerous antisyphilitic medications developed in the wake of Ehrlich's discoveries. A special service combining chemical and physiological testing was organized for this purpose. Although it was eventually transferred to the physical premises of the newly created Alfred Fournier Institute, it remained officially a service of the academy. It received large consignments of medications sent by manufacturers, experimented with them chemically and tested their physiological effects on mice and rats, and then sent them directly to hospitals which requested them.[25]

Two permanent commissions attending to smallpox vaccination and mineral waters combined practical administrative tasks with scientific information gathering. The vaccination commission, which replaced the Central Committee of Vaccine in 1823, organized regular vaccinations in the academy[26] and encouraged vaccination throughout the country by awarding medals to the most zealous vaccinators. The vaccination service also provided vaccine to doctors and local authorities on request and received the annual vaccination statistics, which local authorities were required to transmit to the academy. Individual doctors frequently submitted reports of their own vaccination results, the many practical difficulties they encountered, their attempts at solutions, and more general medical opinions. They occasionally submitted the results of more rigorous clinical or laboratory research.

The commission took such scientific work with great seriousness. In the second half of the century the annual sum of 1,500 francs originally used to reward particularly zealous vaccinators was diverted to provide prizes for the best written works received. The commission also reprinted in its annual report lengthy extracts from the most noteworthy submissions. The high level of interest in vaccination meant that a very substantial number of works were received. One reporter for the commission claimed that during 1893 the commission had received seventy "serious" works with at least twenty deserving of prizes.[27] Other permanent commissions almost never reported this level of activity from correspondents. The vaccination commission reported on all this material in a lengthy annual report that was published as a separate pamphlet until the 1920s. The annual report consistently publicized the benefits of vaccination and argued vigorously on behalf of the practice. From 1847 it was a firm advocate of compulsory vaccination, which was finally voted by the legislature in 1902.

The need to discuss the works it received, as well as functional imperatives, involved the commission in a certain amount of practical research: finding the best mode of preserving the vaccine being sent out, distinguishing true and false vaccines, and, later, ensuring vaccine production in sufficient quantities. The commission also became involved quite frequently in scientific controversies that were discussed in the commission's annual reports. These spilled over regularly into general academic debates, so great was interest in vaccination among academicians. Some questions under debate—whether the disease source of vaccine was smallpox transmitted to animals or a distinct animal disease—had practical implications but did not threaten the fundamental commitment to vaccination. Others might conflict with the task of encouraging the spread of vaccination.

One of the earliest controversies of this sort had to do with whether the protection afforded by vaccination was permanent or temporary; if the latter, was the problem gradual weakening of the bacterial strain spread arm-to-arm or was there a natural time limit on the immunity produced? In either case, were periodic revaccinations necessary? In the early nineteenth century, the correspondence and reports of local vaccinators mentioned occasional cases of smallpox among vaccinated individuals. By and large, leading academic vaccinators played down these reports, so committed were they to the practice and so fearful that confidence in the vaccine would evaporate. It was not until statistics in the 1840s clearly demonstrated revaccinated individuals' superior resistance to the disease that the commission, and the academy as a whole, began to enthusiastically encourage revaccination.[28]

Similarly, academicians involved with vaccination during the first half of the century discounted reports suggesting that infectious diseases, particularly syphilis, could be transmitted by Jennerian arm-to-arm vaccination. It was not until 1864, and after considerable discussion, that the academy admitted that a threat existed—albeit one that was insignificant in comparison with that from smallpox.[29] One solution to the problem, the use of animal vaccination, was not applied in the academy's vaccination service until quite late in the century (1888), partly because of serious doubts about the effectiveness of the animal vaccine and partly because the academy lacked the resources to switch over completely to the relatively expensive animal vaccine.[30]

In the twentieth century the functions of this commission changed. The introduction of obligatory vaccination in 1902 created a need for vaccine on a massive scale. Following the promulgation of a governmental decree in July 1903, the academy's vaccine service in 1907 withdrew from the actual preparation of vaccine. Under the direction of Louis Kelsch, the service became the Institute of Vaccine, which served as an organ of supervision and quality control over the institutions allowed by law to produce vaccine. It also conducted research, experimenting with new production techniques. The annual reports of the vaccination commission attempted to provide a quantitative portrait of vaccinations in France as a whole, which meant that, like other commissions, it was at the mercy of local officials required to send in annual statistics.[31]

In the first years of the twentieth century this commission continued to receive and to discuss clinical and scientific work sent in by individual doctors. By the 1920s, however, it was no longer doing so. Commission reports (now published in the *Bulletin*), all written by the director of the vaccination service, were almost exclusively concerned with administrative and policy issues. They made use of administrative documents to present an exhaustive survey of vaccination in France and its colonies. The collection of information by the vaccination commission had become an exclusively administrative task with no connection to medical science. Research was now carried out at the academy's Institute of Vaccine under the supervision of a full-time researcher.

The mineral waters commission, to which Chapter 6 is devoted, also had a gate-keeping function; it was responsible for the chemical analysis of new mineral waters and determined which could be officially developed and exploited for therapeutic purposes. The number of analyses and reports presented to the academy (which routinely followed the recommendation of the commission) became quite substantial by the end of the nineteenth century. As we shall see in the next chapter, the commission also tried to advance the scientific knowledge of mineral waters; a network of informants sent administrative and clinical statistics and various sorts of research results, which were then discussed in the commission's annual reports. Like the other commissions that played an information-gathering role, it found the collection of complete and accurate statistics impossible. But unlike the others, we shall see, it had both clinical and chemical models of scientific work to fall back on.

As the preceding account suggests, the academy's various administrative commissions became increasingly prominent and busy in the twentieth century. This placed considerable strain on laboratory resources. In the 1930s the academy's laboratories were expanded and consolidated in new premises on the rue Lacretelle. In addition to the vaccination service, three newly established specialized laboratories—one for chemistry, another for microbiology, and a third for experimental physiology—were collectively responsible for the analysis of mineral waters, drinking water, sera, and organic therapies. This expansion was made possible by the decision of the Ministry of Health to consolidate the chemical laboratory of the Superior Council of Hygiene with that of the academy under the latter institution's control.[32]

So much technical responsibility was a source of pride for representatives of the academy. But they were also aware that routine administrative work was far removed from the pursuit of science. Consequently, they emphasized the research that went on amid the routine analyses. Here is how Charles Achard described the tensions in the role of the academy's laboratories:

> The laboratories of the academy do not have as their sole object a supervision which is in a way automatic, in the manner of factory work where the hand plays the principal or even exclusive role. Numerous and interesting works have already emerged from them and it is extremely desirable that the scientific spirit continue to animate the manual work.[33]

Such tension was in many ways a sign of success. Together with the increasingly frequent public health debates which took place in the academy, these permanent technical-administrative tasks were the chief symbols of the academy's increased social and administrative influence in the twentieth century. And new responsibilities were on the horizon as the state's health needs relentlessly expanded. On the eve of World War II, the Ministry of Colonies was negotiating to get more help from the academy in colonial medical affairs.[34] But if the performance of technical tasks flourished, the other routine task of special commissions—the collection of scientific information—was languishing.

Whether they had other technical duties or not, all the information-gathering commissions had difficulties collecting materials from their networks of correspondents. These commissions all responded in very similar ways: they tried to improve the questionnaires on which reports were supposed to be based; they requested that the government put pressure on administrative personnel to send the academy the data it required; and they sought to publicly embarrass the uncooperative by listing those that had failed to submit reports. They offered more positive incentives as well: prizes for the best submissions were introduced in the 1850s; extensive discussions of better submissions were included in annual reports; the possibility of election as a corresponding member of the academy was dangled before informants. In the 1890s the Ministry of the Interior even granted the academy the right to propose names for membership in the National Legion of Honor for those provincial doctors who had already obtained all the honors which the academy itself distributed.[35] But none of these measures proved notable.

The epidemics and infant hygiene commissions both had as their primary task the gathering of data from networks of public doctors and administrators. These data were then presented and discussed in annual reports. The reports were characteristically seen as having both medicoscientific and administrative utility. While advancing scientific knowledge, they provided a glimpse of the health situation in the country that was useful to the administration. Frequently reports were used to advocate specific public health measures; occasionally these commissions produced instructions in a popular form for doctors, nursing mothers, or wet nurses. But these commissions had no routine administrative or technical tasks comparable to vaccination or to the authorization of mineral waters and secret remedies. This made the inadequacies of the information which they received all the more devastating.

The epidemics commission was in some ways the most problematic and futile of the permanent commissions throughout the nineteenth century. Modeled after the health surveys conducted by the Société Royale de Médecine in the late eighteenth century, it was charged with preparing an annual report on the epidemics and local endemic illnesses which had erupted throughout the country during the previous year. It collected this information from a network of epidemic doctors who were paid (badly) to treat local outbreaks. These doctors were supposed to present statistics about the numbers of disease outbreaks and their mortality. They were also supposed to provide all relevant information about the outbreak and the local physical environment so that the commission could determine causes and suggest public action to prevent recurrences. Later in the century, departmental hygiene councils served as intermediaries between the academy and epidemic doctors, further complicating matters.

Many epidemic doctors, however, did not submit reports regularly. The introduction in the 1850s of prizes for the best reports and essays helped somewhat, as did the occasional ministerial circular prodding local public health authorities; but these doctors did not provide the academy with anything like national statistics. Furthermore, even the reports sent in were usually incomplete. If an epidemic physician had not been called in to treat or observe an epidemic, as was frequently the case, he was not likely to have basic data, let alone detailed information. Even detailed personal observations were frequently inadequate from the point of view of the academy. It was not just that some were hastily compiled and lacking in the most elementary information; the nature of the task guaranteed failure. For, according to prevailing medical theories, virtually anything might be the cause of an epidemic under particular conditions. The range of possible factors was immense: the physical environment, climate, economic and social conditions, nutrition, human transmission. Usually a particular and highly localized constellation of circumstances was blamed for an epidemic. By the same token, virtually anything might prolong an epidemic or make it more virulent. Consequently, an adequate report had to contain almost exhaustive information about the social and physical environment as well as about the outbreak and progress of the disease. And a more general understanding of particular epidemic diseases was possible only if many such exhaustive accounts could be collected and compared.

In the absence of complete accounts, epidemics commission reports summarized descriptions of local outbreaks. They noted the possible causes, discussed curious local features, and often repeated suggested prophylactic measures. They pointed to the warning signs to which local authorities should be attentive. Reports were filled with statistical tables based on administrative documents sent in; these rarely had much connection with the rest of the narrative and were acknowledged to be incomplete. One could only hope, as one reporter put it in discussing the confusing etiology of typhoid fever, that "one day, perhaps, the rapprochement, the comparison of so many scattered facts, will spark an unexpected light."[36] But this rapprochement never arrived. One reporter commented in 1865 on the work of the commission in the following terms:"When . . . one looks for scientific or practical truths that have come to the surface, one is painfully surprised to find them so rare, and one notes with regret the enormous disproportion that exists between the length of time, the energy of the effort and the limited scope of its results."[37]

Each reporter had his own views about the most critical causes of epidemic and endemic diseases and the most useful prophylactic measures; these went into the final conclusions of the report. Such conclusions varied considerably from one report to the next, some focusing on poverty, others on environmental conditions, yet others on sanitation. But most reporters agreed on the need to improve and reform public health services in the provinces, which would, in the process, also improve the quality of the statistics sent to the academy.

The bacteriological revolution initially changed the situation little. Ideas about the importance of miasmas and climate continued to be rehearsed into the 1890s. Nor did the germ theory lessen the commission's dependence on local data. In the 1920s and 1930s the reports of the epidemics commission were still complaining about the quality of statistics received.[38] They continued to be somewhat impressionistic overviews of the most common and serious epidemic and endemic diseases of the past year. In 1931 the commission's mandate was broadened to include the prevention of all infectious disease rather than just epidemics. (Its name was changed accordingly.) Its annual report of 1934 contained a long section on the problems of hospital hygiene.[39]

The infant hygiene commission was a relative latecomer to the academic scene. Infant mortality, a traditional source of societal concern, had played a significant role in the development of public health since the eighteenth century.[40] During the 1860s concern with high infant mortality, especially among children sent out to wet-nurse, intensified considerably.[41] In 1866 a submission describing high infant mortality among infants placed with wet nurses in the Morvan sparked a debate lasting thirty-four sessions over the next four years. While this was going on, the Ministry of the Interior initiated an investigation of infant mortality; this revealed that Parisian infants placed out to nurse in ten departments had a mortality rate two-and-a-half times that of infants born and raised in those departments. The minister in 1869 appointed an extraparliamentary commission, including four members of the academy, to prepare a legislative bill to protect infants. This was the basis of the Roussel law of 1874 organizing the surveillance and protection of wet-nursing infants. Meanwhile, the academy in 1870 formally voted a series of recommendations to curb infant mortality; these included regulation of wet-nursing, general improvements in social conditions, and the creation of a permanent infant hygiene commission within the academy.

This latter commission was considerably larger than other permanent commissions. Like smallpox vaccination, infant protection was an issue that provoked great interest among academicians even outside the context of the commission; it was frequently the subject of more general discussions. The infant hygiene commission did not have routine technical and administrative chores but the Ministry of the Interior furnished an annual subvention (first 2,000, then 4,000 francs) enabling the commission to award medals to the most zealous correspondents and sponsor a prize competition. Its mandate was to encourage, collect, and discuss information and documents sent in by correspondents. In the annual reports discussing these submissions, many policy recommendations were made and maternal breast-feeding was vigorously encouraged. But its mandate became somewhat murky when, from 1880, an official network of inspectors for the administration of the Roussel law was put into place; these inspectors were obligated to send reports only to the government's Superior Council for the Protection of Infants, which, like the academy's own commission, prepared an annual report and rewarded service. There was no formal requirement to send anything to the academy.

Like other academic commissions, the infant hygiene commission began with hopes of combining submissions into accurate statistical series on infant mortality throughout the country. It heard regularly from the different sorts of inspectors now regulating the various provincial programs (public health, foundlings, wet-nursing) as well as from local practitioners. In the first report, published in 1875, the reporter, Pierre de Villiers, could point out that data on nineteen departments indicated that the leading causes of infant mortality were gastric and respiratory ailments and suggest some obvious remedies. But by 1877 de Villiers was no longer providing overall statistics but simply discussing the different materials received. One assumes that the reason—as in all the other commissions—was the difficulty of obtaining accurate and representative statistics.

From 1878 reports on the commission's prize competition constituted the bulk of its annual report, at least until 1895 when the minister withdrew funding. These competitions judged responses submitted to specific questions, which were generally quite practical, for instance, asking about ways of preventing the transmission of syphilis in wet-nursing or how best to prepare animal milk for infants. Once the prize competition was eliminated in 1895 for lack of funds, the commission resumed its unsuccessful efforts to collect statistics.[42] In 1920 the commission publicly refused to produce a report because so few of the local councils had submitted information.[43]

After gradual improvements by the mid-1920s the main complaint of reports was that methods of keeping official statistics were inadequate. Individuals were counted anew each year in the absence of individual dossiers. The academy's repeated calls for the introduction of individual dossiers induced the Ministry of Hygiene to adopt a new system of record-keeping and data-gathering in 1929. By the 1930s the reports of this commission had become more statistically oriented.

The work of this commission tended to have, as Foucault might say, a rather low epistemological status. There was more common sense than hard science involved in its activities. There was none of the sophisticated chemistry beloved by the mineral waters commission and little of the experimental science needed to resolve thorny problems of vaccination. Some academicians in fact believed that there were few scientific questions in this area needing to be resolved.[44] After the demise of the prize competition, the commission pretty much abandoned any pretense that its information-gathering had scientific significance. And its administrative significance had to do primarily with monitoring the results of and suggesting reforms to the Roussel law. In 1885, in the midst of an academic debate on depopulation in France, Roussel himself had appealed for suggestions on how to reform what he recognized was an incomplete law.[45] Henceforth the reports of the infant hygiene commission characteristically concluded with proposals for ameliorating and extending the Roussel law.

Aside from the many administrative measures it advocated, the overarching theme of the commission was the encouragement of maternal breast-feeding, *la loi naturelle*.[46] This reflected the high mortality rates of bottle-fed infants but also expressed a moral vision of the sacredness of mother-child relations. In order to encourage mothers (even unwed) to keep their nursing infants, the academy advocated the granting of temporary financial subsidies. If maternal breast-feeding was impossible, the commission preferred recourse to properly supervised wet nurses rather than bottle-feeding. In fact, the academy as a whole was quite hostile to efforts to develop safe artificial formulas, fearing that it would discourage breast-feeding. In 1877, when it was consulted about a proposal being prepared by the Paris Municipal Council to fund an experimental bottle-feeding program in a hospital, the academy firmly advised against the undertaking on the grounds that bottle-feeding was always dubious and would prove fatal in hospitals, which were death traps at the best of times. The money, it was concluded, would be better spent encouraging maternal nursing.[47] In subsequent years, bottle-feeding became less dangerous and increasingly acceptable but the commission continued to express its preference for breast-feeding.

Only two of the permanent commissions—vaccination and mineral waters—were the subjects of celebratory essays in the volume marking the centenary of the academy. Both combined routine technical-administrative tasks with information-gathering functions and both also utilized scientific modalities located in the laboratory, which made them somewhat independent of administrative chores. Nevertheless, in these commissions as well, one finds a growing separation of administrative from scientific tasks; annual reports became concerned exclusively with the former as data collection came to be seen as a purely administrative responsibility. Only the mineral waters commission, we will see in a later chapter, jettisoned its statistics-gathering role.

Prizes

By 1820 the organization of prize competitions was a traditional activity in European academies. The Montyon legacy left to the Academy of Sciences in that year permitted that institution to introduce cash prizes, which gradually replaced honorific medals.[48] Starting so much later, the Academy of Medicine had no heritage of honorific prizes to overcome and began immediately to dispense monetary rewards. Only the prizes awarded by permanent commissions lacking budgets were distributed in the form of medals.

The academy began with four prizes sponsored by the government. All but one disappeared as private donations to support prizes gradually trickled in. The first of these, devoted to pathological anatomy, was contributed by the academy's permanent president, Antoine Portal, and others soon followed. Many of the donors were doctors, including a good number of academicians, who bestowed bequests on the academy "in the absence of direct heirs" or to support a particular domain of practice and research. Some, however, were laymen responding to family illness or tragedy.[49] Since many prizes were awarded biannually, triannually, or at even longer intervals, the number available in any given year grew slowly. In 1853 there were five prize competitions worth a total of 6,000 francs. In contrast, the Academy of Sciences during that year distributed nearly 27,000 francs for its prizes in medicine, surgery, experimental physiology, and public health. (Because of the size of the Montyon legacy, this constituted a disproportionately large share of the roughly 40,000 francs the Academy of Sciences awarded for all its prizes.)[50] By the 1860s the Academy of Medicine had eleven permanent and four temporary prize foundations in operation. In most years of this decade, six or seven were in competition offering from 11,000 to 13,000 francs in prizes.[51]

The academy sought to point researchers in certain directions by posing specific scientific questions to which contestants responded with unpublished and frequently lengthy manuscripts. The original regulations establishing the academy in 1820 specified that the academy would each year propose prize questions "as likely as possible [to produce] positive experiments, observations, and research."[52] Sometimes a question provoked little or no response, in which case it could be renewed for another year or dropped. At other times, a very topical subject like the contagiousness of typhoid fever could attract nearly twenty submissions. In competitions of this sort, a commission of three or four academicians was appointed to judge responses, whose authors remained anonymous. Each prize commission produced a detailed report to be discussed and voted by the entire academy. Prize-winning submissions of particularly high quality might be published in the academy's annual *Mémoires*. Frequently a prize was not awarded and smaller sums were distributed in the form of *encourage-ments* or *récompenses* to individuals whose work was judged meritorious but not up to prize standards. The executors of the Argenteuil bequest took the academy to court in 1851 on the grounds that the Argenteuil Prize established in 1836 and offered every six years had yet to be awarded. With the scientific autonomy of the academy apparently at stake, the matter was resolved by the court in the academy's favor.[53]

The subjects of questions were frequently determined by the conditions of the be-quest. The Portal Prize always asked questions related to pathological anatomy while the Capuron Prize was divided in two, with one question relating to mineral waters and another to obstetrics. The Lefevre Prize was more narrowly devoted to melan-cholia. Within such limits, it was possible for the academy to shape questions to fit current topics of medical interest. Prize questions might follow from debates in the academy, as occurred in 1852 when the Academy Prize was devoted to the physio-logical, obstetrical, and public health aspects of rye ergot. Similarly, the Portal Prize of 1853 asked about the pathology and treatment of goiter following the publication of work on the subject in the *Bulletin*. Others responded to more general medical controversies; thus the Academy Prize of 1849 asked about the contagiousness of ty-phoid fever[54] and that of 1862 asked about the value of expectant treatment in pneumonia. Questions could also be obscure, like the one posed by the Portal Prize committee in 1849 on the pathological anatomy of cirrhosis of the liver, which drew a single submission.

Whatever the question, the evaluating committees demanded substance rather than opinions or speculation in the responses. In a word, said a prize reporter in 1850, "the academy demands demonstrations and not conjectures. . . ."[55] Extensive case materials treated quantitatively and qualitatively were encouraged, as was the use of microscopes for pathological studies.[56] In 1869 the academy's permanent secretary, Dubois d'Amiens, admitted in a prize report that, without rejecting old traditions, commissions preferred "new procedures of investigation."[57] Usually this meant focus-ing on the pathology of specific organs around which symptoms could be grouped. Prizes might be granted to a work even if the judges disagreed with many of its con-clusions, so long as it was a serious research effort.[58]

Not all prize foundations lent themselves to questions. The Itard Prize, estab-lished in 1840, offered a triennial prize for the best work, whether published or not, on practical therapeutic medicine. But such retrospective prizes were judged pretty much in the same way as the more numerous question prizes (except for the fact that anonymity was not usually required) and coexisted easily with them. More problem-atic were those in which the question was set in advance by the donor. This left the academy with little room to adjust to the evolving conditions of science or its own changing preoccupations. The worst offender, ironically, was the academician Mateo Orfila, whose bequest in 1853 established a prize in legal medicine and toxicology. The terms specified a list of questions long enough to take the academy into the twentieth century.[59] More characteristic and less obtrusive was the requirement of the Argenteuil Prize to reward improvements in the surgical procedures dealing with ob-structions of the urethra; in cases where no such improvements were to be found, the bequest allowed the academy to consider all work relating to urinary maladies.

All things considered, the prize system of the academy seems to have worked reasonably well before 1870. The small number of competitions attracted modest but respectable numbers of candidates and made academicians feel that they were influencing the direction of medical research. It is difficult to judge the quality of the work produced in this way, though many academicians of the late nineteenth and twentieth centuries were quite convinced of its inadequacies, as we shall see. But it is worth noting that winners of prizes or *encouragements* included the likes of Armand Trousseau (1836), Paul Broca (1850), and Jean-Martin Charcot (1860, 1862). The criteria were flexible enough that a substantial number of provincial medical practitioners were also prizewinners.

During the early Third Republic, the scope and nature of the academy's prize system were dramatically altered. From the 1870s the number of bequests and donations to the academy, as to other scientific institutions, increased substantially and expanded the prize system. Whereas there had been six competitions annually during the 1860s, there were in 1881 seventeen competitions worth 62,000 francs, considerably more than the medically oriented prizes of the Academy of Sciences. By 1898 the academy was offering forty-two prizes worth over 100,000 francs and attracting 230 competitors. This put it in a category not far removed from the Academy of Sciences, which at that time ran, in all fields of science, fifty-eight monetary competitions worth close to 150,000 francs as well as twelve medal competitions. Donations continued to arrive at the Academy of Medicine in the twentieth century. In 1924 the academy offered fifty-five prizes worth 130,000 francs, now seriously devalued by galloping inflation. In 1935, sixty-eight (out of a total of 116 functioning prizes) were in competition. From the late nineteenth century, the yearly report on the prize competitions read by the annual secretary and the list of prizewinners read by the president took up most of the academy's annual public meeting.

Some of these bequests and donations were very large. The Audiffred bequest of 1896 was worth 800,000 francs and generated annual interest of 24,000 francs. In 1923, Albert I, prince of Monaco, left a 1,000,000–franc bequest to the academy to support a biennial prize worth 100,000 francs. Most bequests, of course, were more modest, generating interest of anywhere from a few hundred to several thousand francs a year, which, when awarded every two, three, or five years, could constitute a fairly substantial sum. Even the more usual 1,000–2,000 francs reward represented from one-quarter to one-half the annual salary for a junior faculty post.

During the 1870s some academicians worried that the growing number of prizes would come to absorb too much of the academy's time and effort.[60] But a more immediate problem was that submissions did not keep up with the rising number of competitions. Commissions for some prizes experimented by forgoing detailed questions and opening up the competition to any unpublished work in the field;[61] but this strategy did not necessarily attract more applicants. More successful in 1875 was an effort not to limit judgment of the Barbier Prize to submissions but "to search out real merit wherever it is to be found, and to reward it, even if it requests nothing. . . ."[62]

By the late 1870s the lack of competitors assumed critical proportions. In his prize report for 1878, Bergeron reported that of thirteen prize competitions that year, six had attracted no competitors while the other seven had attracted a total of only twenty-five. A year later he told the academy that the number of submissions was up but that quality remained low. There had been some discussion within the administrative council about this state of affairs, said Bergeron, with some members laying the blame on the excessive severity of the prize commissions. But Bergeron himself had no doubt that the problem derived from the narrow conditions attached to most prizes. The best research simply did not grow out of academic programs of research but from individual initiative. The academy needed to find ways to award prizes "to the works that are most interesting or most original. . . ."[63] Not for the first or last time, the prize reporter asked potential donors to pose fewer conditions and allow the academy more latitude and flexibility in awarding prizes.

Academicians became increasingly critical of competitions based on questions. "Most often they result only in good student exercises," said one prize reporter in 1898. Nor did they attract many competitors, he claimed. "It would thus be a good thing to suppress posed questions, in every case that the expressed wishes of the testator are not opposed to it."[64] Retrospective prizes rewarding the best work in any given field were to be preferred because they "leave the field open to progress in all areas." Despite such sentiments, older prizes continued to be based on the elaboration of annual questions, either because of the terms of bequests or because some academicians remained attached to tradition. But few of the prizes established after 1870 followed this pattern. Consequently, by 1930 only 13 out of 102 prizes were built around annual questions.

The number of competitors rose substantially at the turn of the century, when the total number was well over two hundred annually. But after World War I, the problem reemerged. It was a frequent occurrence for ten or more of the prize competitions each year to be without candidates, and the total number of competitors in any given year was usually well under two hundred.[65] If prizes based on questions seldom attracted more than one or two responses, many of the retrospective prizes did not do any better.

The celebration of the centenary of the academy in 1920 included a review of private donations which should have been a celebratory exercise in keeping with the spirit of the occasion. But the talk by the academy's treasurer, Adrien-Maurice Hanriot, turned out to be unexpectedly analytical and critical of the prize system. Hanriot welcomed the shift from prize questions to retrospective rewards. Under the system of questions the winning responses were "veritable dissertations from which medical science had little to gain. Serious workers abstained from competing. . . ."[66] But even the newer system of retrospective prizes "leaving to the author the choice of research subjects to be pursued . . . no longer responds to the exigencies of modern science."[67] The problem was that even in this latter case, the subject areas chosen by donors frequently lost their scientific relevance after several years. Despite the fact that 120,000–130,000 francs was distributed annually, it proved difficult to reward the most important and original work since it often did not fit established criteria. Hanriot gave as an example the lack of prizes for research in bacteriology or radiation. Works in these fields had to be rewarded with one or another of the small number of more general prizes.[68]

It is difficult to determine whether Hanriot's criticisms, which were designed to alter the behavior of donors, were justified. Certainly there were prize subjects that had been out of date in the late nineteenth century let alone the twentieth. For in-

stance, a Dr. Stanski who had been a follower of the anticontagionist Nicholas Chervin offered a prize in the late 1870s to anyone who could show the existence or
nonexistence of *infection miasmatique*, or contagion at a distance. The Saint-Léger
Prize offered 1,500 francs to anyone who could produce tumors in the thyroids of
animals by administering extracts from the water or terrain of regions where goiter
was endemic. And the Rufz de Lavison Prize was available to anyone who could
demonstrate how movement from one climate to another provoked organic lesions
and functional disturbances.

It is also true that many, and certainly the largest of the prizes were supposed to
be rewards for finding a cure for one or more incurable diseases. The most generous
ones were offered to anyone with a cure for tuberculosis (the Audiffred Prize, 24,000
francs), improvements in surgery for urinary blockages (the Argenteuil Prize, 6,800
francs at the end of the century), or, more generally, for any cure of diseases thought
to be incurable (the Buisson Prize, 10,500 francs at the end of the century). In the
1930s, the Marmottan Prize offered 100,000 francs to anyone who could discover a
cure for cancer. Many of the responses to such general requests for cures were pre-
dictably silly. But since real cures were very rare indeed, the commission had in
many cases the right to award the prize or at least *encouragements* to more modest
scientific advances. When the Saint-Paul Prize, offering the large sum of 25,000
francs for a cure for diphtheria, was introduced in the late 1870s, the prize reporter
discouraged candidates from competing for the main prize and encouraged them to
focus on the epidemiology of the disease so that they could win a much smaller prize
based on the annual interest.

And if there were many prizes that focused on a specific disease, these did not
stipulate the scientific approaches that should be followed. Prizes in such fields as
psychiatry, obstetrics, electrotherapy, stomatology, and ophthalmology, to name but
a few specialties represented by prizes, gave academicians considerable freedom to
choose winners from fairly broad domains of medical knowledge.

Hanriot himself admitted in 1920 that eleven of the nearly one hundred prizes
then in existence were virtually without conditions. And the number increased in subsequent years. The most prestigious of the general prizes was the Albert I of Monaco
Prize, founded in 1923 (following the prince's death the year before), which gave the
academy virtually complete freedom to reward work in medical science with a bian-
nual 100,000 franc monetary reward. The academy took this prize very seriously
indeed. It met six months before the distribution of prizes to elect in secret session a
large and representative commission of fifteen members to propose candidates.
Academicians were not themselves eligible for the prize. The commission's proposals were discussed by the entire academy at a meeting held in secret session and
no decisions could be taken unless more than half the total number of titular members and *associés libres* were in attendance. No winner could be elected without
winning two-thirds of the votes cast.[69] This bequest furnished a powerful model to
future donors, a point emphasized when the academy's secretary devoted his *éloge*
of 1933 to the late prince of Monaco.[70]

All this being said, the fall in the number of competitors during the 1920s and
1930s remains unexplained. The irrelevance of certain subjects of competition and
the loss of monetary value of prizes due to inflation may well have combined to

make many of the academy's competitions uninteresting to potential candidates. And although the point cannot be demonstrated conclusively, the academy's less than central place in French medical and scientific life during the interwar period may have been another factor in the smaller number of prize candidacies.

Thus far the history of the prize system of the Academy of Medicine as described here is not dissimilar to that of the Academy of Sciences as depicted by other historians.[71] In the second half of the nineteenth century the Academy of Sciences also saw a rapid expansion of prizes thanks to private donations and bequests; there was, moreover, similar tension between donors who wanted to impose conditions and academicians who desired the fewest possible constraints on their use of monies. One also finds a comparable shift in the Academy of Sciences away from prizes based on the elaboration of specific questions and toward the retrospective rewarding of work in a specific domain. The winning of multiple prizes by certain individuals facilitated research by making funds available at irregular intervals and advanced careers by singling out the most outstanding researchers. In fact, the two academies were complementary resources for researchers like Fernand Bezançon, Stéphane-Martin Delépine, or Charles Dopter, who might accumulate four, five, or even six prizes from the two institutions during the course of a career.

The two prize systems in the middle of the nineteenth century rewarded very similar sorts of candidates in spite of the greater prestige enjoyed by the Academy of Sciences among the most ambitious members of the medical elite. Among winners of prizes or cash awards in the two institutions during the 1860s, the proportion of members or future members of the Academy of Medicine was almost identical: 38 percent in the case of the medical prizewinners of the Academy of Sciences and 37 percent for those of the Academy of Medicine.[72] The only difference one finds is that among Academy of Medicine prizewinners a slightly larger proportion were provincial doctors who were elected corresponding rather than full members of that academy.[73]

By the early twentieth century, however, the profiles of medical prizewinners had diverged in the two institutions. Its vastly expanded prize system meant that there were about three times as many winners of prizes or cash awards in the Academy of Medicine as there were of *medical* prizes or awards in Academy of Sciences.[74] The latter prizes were primarily geared to the Parisian elite. Over 30 percent of medical prizewinners of the Academy of Sciences went on to become (or in a few cases already were) Parisian members of the Academy of Medicine; another 10 percent of the winners were provincial doctors who would achieve corresponding member status. In contrast, the vastly expanded prize system of the Academy of Medicine was much more open to provincial doctors. Only 25 percent of the winners of prizes or cash awards went on to membership in that institution and nearly half of these were provincial doctors who achieved corresponding or associate status. Altogether, approximately 40 percent of the winners did not live in Paris.

The prize systems of the two institutions were thus complementary. For an elite, they provided alternative resources for research. To a large extent, however, they catered and made resources available to different populations. There is one area, however, in which the two institutions followed clearly diverging paths. The Academy of Sciences seems to have expanded its prize system to include the awarding of research grants to subsidize ongoing research programs. The process was already well under way in the mid-nineteenth century and accelerated during the Third Republic. Without abandoning its traditional questions or retrospective awards, that academy responded to a perceived lack of science funding by collaborating with donors in setting up foundations to provide research grants to French scientists. One of the most important was founded in 1907 by Prince Roland Bonaparte; it handed out 260,000 francs in grants from 1908 to 1914.[75] In 1921 seven functioning grant foundations together awarded a total of 132,000 francs in research subsidies.[76]

I have uncovered no evidence to suggest that the Academy of Medicine showed similar concerns to replace or supplement prizes with research grants. One should certainly not exaggerate the differences between retrospective prizes and research subsidies. In cases a prize was awarded not just for the quality of a work submitted but because the prize commission wished to encourage an individual to continue a promising line of research. Similarly, grants to finance research projects also depended on the previous accomplishments of beneficiaries. Nor is it very significant that prizes, unlike grants, did not have to be spent on research. Where self-financing of research was the rule, increasing individual income was tantamount to increasing research funds.[77] Still, even if we concede that the difference between the prizes and grants was essentially one of form rather than content, it is nonetheless striking that, at a time of widespread concern to increase subsidies to scientific researchers, the Academy of Medicine made no effort to introduce direct grants. At the very least, it provides striking confirmation of that growing distance between medical and scientific elites that we have encountered in the case of the academy's associés libres.[78]

It is not that medical academicians did not recognize the need for research funding. They were both beneficiaries and distributors of funds through the Caisse des Recherches Scientifiques, which later evolved into the Centre National de la Recherche Scientifique, and which devoted the lion's share of its funds to biological research.[79] But most did not see the academy's prize system as any sort of substitute for or supplement to such research funding. Achard's characterization of the Prince Albert I Prize in 1933 stands as a good description of the traditional nineteenth-century view of prizes that persisted in the Academy of Medicine well into the twentieth century. This prize, stated Achard, "provides savants with a reward for their efforts, encouragement to persevere in research, a means of action for the discovery of new truths."[80] It was a reward for past work, and it provided both moral encouragement and the financial means to pursue whatever further research the winner chose to do.

Everyone certainly recognized that research cost money. But if funding from other sources was not available, the implicit assumption seems to have been that medical researchers should bear their own research costs, at least in the first instance. Hanriot in 1920 cited as a model of enlightened philanthropy the recent bequest by Blondel, who left his entire fortune to the academy. The goal, in the deceased's own words, was not to favor "these academic dissertations which do nothing to advance science, and it is my intention to compensate financially, as much as it is in my power, those who have done experiments that are more or less costly. . . ."[81] Reimbursement of already incurred costs was the financial rationale of the traditional prize systems of the Parisian academies.[82]

There were certainly individuals in the Academy of Medicine who would have liked to use prize monies in other ways. The gigantic bequest left by Prince Albert I of Monaco provoked a small debate within the academy. There were those who wished to divide the prize monies into smaller sums, "destined to facilitate scientific research and to subsidize savants and laboratories whose great pitifulness is well known."[83] But on the grounds that the testament said nothing about dividing the prize money and that academic regulations stated that prize funds could be divided or given as *encouragements* only when the conditions of the donation actually specified that this was possible, the matter was dropped. We have seen that regulations could be overturned when academic opinion demanded. The appeal to regulations in this case probably indicated that support for the proposal was not widespread.[84]

Considering that nearly one-third of the academicians were either experimentalists or working in scientific institutions at the time, this lack of support is surprising and demands some explanation. Since the academy never openly discussed the options available to it, determining why it did not follow the example of the Academy of Sciences must be an exercise in retrospective speculation.

One possible explanation has to do with the conditions posed by donors, which most often were so specific as to preclude the use of prizes as subsidies. It is true that medicine, in comparison with, say, high-energy physics, touches everyone, including philanthropists, in very personal ways, explaining all the prizes available to anyone with a cure for cancer or tuberculosis. Indeed, some of the medical prizes of the Academy of Sciences were every bit as bizarre as those of the Academy of Medicine.[85] But the argument is not persuasive since the Academy of Medicine regularly found ways around constraining conditions. If it did not get around them so as to permit the use of prize funds as research grants and, more pertinently, if it did not actively solicit new funds specifically for this purpose, it is because academicians did not wish to do so. The best demonstration of this statement is provided by the few bequests which specifically allowed funds to be disbursed as research grants. For instance, the Monbinne Prize was designed to be used for foreign "missions" and, if no suitable candidates applied, could be used to fund ongoing research. The academy did occasionally fund travel missions but more usually rewarded a manuscript that had been submitted. Likewise, the biennial François Helme Prize was founded specifically to fund medical research. But throughout the 1930s it was awarded to the best submitted manuscripts.

To fully understand why the Academy of Medicine continued to have so little interest in research subsidies as late as the 1930s, three lines of reasoning strike me as pertinent. The first has to do with the size of the medical domain and the consequent ethos of competition which it produced. The worlds of French chemistry, physics, and astronomy were quite small because each was dependent on the existence of a small number of teaching and research institutions. It is hard to imagine that there were throughout France as many as two hundred specialists in any one of these fields in the late nineteenth century, no matter how liberally one defines the term specialist.[86] In spite of considerable expansion in the early twentieth century, one suspects that only a few disciplines in the 1920s had as many as three hundred French practitioners.[87] Within such a small universe, identifying promising individuals and research projects and providing them with financial support made eminent sense.

The world of French medicine was, in comparison, huge. Elite Parisian medicine with its hundreds of hospital physicians surrounded by their many hundreds of aco-lytes and protégés was itself comparatively large. Provincial medical elites, which also competed for prizes, brought numbers into the thousands. Elite medicine was highly competitive as well. Whatever the patronage that went on at all levels of the system, advancement required public demonstrations of proficiency.[88] The awarding of a prize in formal competition was such a demonstration and conformed to the values of elite medicine in a way that funding ongoing research did not.

A second factor that must be taken into account is the overwhelmingly clinical character of most of the prizes. There were, it is true, a handful of prizes in medical chemistry, physiology, and, by the 1930s, bacteriology, as well as some general prizes which could be used to reward experimental laboratory work. But most of the prizes, like the papers read at academic meetings, had a predominantly clinical orientation. This does not mean that experimental work was not valued or even expected. But it was an adjunct to clinical work and could usually be taken care of by gaining access to someone's laboratory and spending a bit of money on materials. The essential in-gredients of medical research—clinical case materials, corpses for postmortem analysis, junior colleagues to do much of the scut work—were available in abundant quantities to clinical researchers. In fact, the real costs of this type of research in-volved time and money lost by not practicing medicine.

And here we come to the final and probably most significant line of argument that I wish to pursue: the relative economic autonomy available to medical researchers through the practice of medicine. The sums involved were small early in a career but became progressively larger as one advanced through the hierarchy. Just as private medical practice partly financed the medical care of the poor in hospitals (since hos-pital salaries were token), so too did it support research. In fact, hospital care and research were closely related since hospitals were the major source of clinical and pathological material.

Not all medical researchers, of course, were doing work of this clinical nature. The system had its experimentalists pressing for changes to the medical education system and pressure was beginning to build for full-time hospital and faculty careers. The Caisse des Recherches Scientifiques was beginning to respond to the needs of experimental biological science. Academicians like Henri Roger and Charles Achard were active in and indeed leaders of these reform activities. It is thus significant that—aside from the debate about the legacy of Albert I—one sees no evidence of efforts to move beyond the system of prizes. My suspicion is that this silence pro-vides yet another indication that the twentieth-century academy, with its geriatric membership and its inflation-ravaged prize system, was quite simply no longer seen to be significant to the scientific concerns of the medical elite.

The different activities and genres described in this chapter evolved in rather differ-ent ways. Permanent commissions, which represented the essence of the academy's limited public health role in the early nineteenth century, became relatively less im-portant in the twentieth century as presentations and especially debates devoted to these subjects assumed increasing significance. Most commissions lost their scien-tific functions and became almost entirely oriented to technical-administrative tasks.

Those commissions either committed to technical tasks that had lost their relevance (secret remedies) or centered on the collection of information (epidemics and infant hygiene) declined into insignificance. Those with a well-defined technical task (vaccination, mineral waters, sera) flourished.

The prize system expanded throughout the academy's first century of existence. In the twentieth century it represented virtually all that remained of the institution's traditional evaluative functions and absorbed enormous time and resources. But it clearly was not at the forefront of French medical research and the many prize competitions often had difficulty attracting competitors. Prizes were a significant source of research funding for clinicians and, occasionally, laboratory scientists. But the fact that members of the Academy of Medicine did not follow their colleagues in the Academy of Sciences in seeking to transform prizes into research grants is indicative of the marginality of the twentieth-century medical elite to some of the central concerns of the scientific community.

The histories of these two forms of activity largely confirm the conclusions of the previous chapters. During the second decade of the twentieth century the academy lost many of its scientific functions and abandoned most of its evaluative scientific activities. This resulted in large part from changing institutional conditions: the establishment of state research funding agencies, the multiplication of specialized journals and societies which left little scope for traditional academies, the aging of the academic population. The Academy of Sciences, which had abandoned most of its evaluative functions a half century earlier and which was doing little in the way of providing utilitarian technological expertise to the government,[89] was, during these years, almost exclusively devoted to promoting scientific research. Yet it is doubtful whether it proved any more successful in retaining its central place in French science.[90]

In contrast to the Academy of Sciences, the Academy of Medicine took on a very active role in applying science to state needs. It performed routine technical-administrative tasks and debated public health and professional issues. The academy became an institution of elderly sages representing the collective wisdom of medicine on public issues. It is not clear that this role brought much new power to the institution. The interwar years were characterized by political paralysis and saw few professional or public health issues definitively resolved. Many of the subjects which the academy discussed were controversial and it was only one among many institutions and groups clamoring to make their voices heard. None of this is necessarily a sign of institutional failure. It merely indicates that the academy was now part of a new, more democratic, and infinitely more complex political, social, and medical order.

NOTES

1. In the nineteenth century, long reports were published in *MEM* while short administrative reports appeared in *BAM*. With the cessation of publication of the former in 1913, all reports were printed in *BAM*. Reports of the vaccination commission were exceptionally published as separate monographs until the 1920s, when they also began to appear in *BAM*.

2. Matthew Ramsey, "Traditional Medicine and Medical Enlightenment: The Regulation of Secret Remedies in the Ancien Régime," *Historical Reflections* 9 (1982), 215–32; Ramsey, "Property Rights and the Rights to Health: The Regulation of Secret Remedies in France, 1789–1815," in *Medical Fringe and Medical Orthodoxy, 1750–1850*, ed. W. F. Bynum and Roy Porter (London, 1987), pp. 79–105; Caroline Hannaway, "Medicine, Public Welfare and the State in Eighteenth-Century France: The Société Royale de Médecine of Paris (1776–1793)," Ph.D. diss., Johns Hopkins University, 1974, pp. 278–317.

3. Itard, "Rapport général sur les remèdes secrets," *MEM* 2 (1833), 24–31.

4. Matthew Ramsey, "Academic Medicine and Medical Industrialism: The Regulation of Secret Remedies in France," in *French Medical Culture in the Nineteenth Century*, ed. Ann F. La Berge and Mordechai Feingold (Amsterdam, 1994), pp. 25–78.

5. Meeting of January 25, 1834, in *AGM*, 2e sér. 4 (1834), 349–53; report by Double read to the academy on July 4, 1826, ibid., 4 (1826), 632–34.

6. Ramsey, "Academic Medicine."

7. *BAM* 17 (1852), 686–92; *BAM* 18 (1853), 450–67; *BAM* 6 (1877), 866–72.

8. See, for instance, A. Devergie, "Lecture sur les travaux de l'Académie impériale de médecine," *BAM* 25 (1859–60), 174.

9. Ibid., 175

10. Ibid.

11. A. Riche, "Le Rôle administratif de l'Académie de Médecine," *BAM* 48 (1902), 463.

12. Riche reported about sixty submissions annually in 1830 and about thirty annually since 1892. Ibid.

13. Ramsey, "Academic Medicine."

14. Ibid.

15. Ramsey reports seeing submissions in the archives whose seals were unbroken, indicating that they were never read. Ibid.

16. Riche, "Le Role administratif," 463.

17. On early responses to this type of therapy see Merriley Borell, "Origins of the Hormone Concept: Internal Secretions and Physiological Research," Ph.D. diss., Yale University, 1976, pp. 24–57.

18. On the first development see Michael Bliss, *The Discovery of Insulin* (Chicago, 1982); on the second, Merriley Borell, "Organotherapy and the Emergence of Reproductive Endocrinology," *Journal of the History of Biology* 18 (1985), 1–30.

19. A. Netter, "Sur une proposition d'addition au texte de la loi du 25 avril 1895 visant à la préparation, la vente et le débit des sérums thérapeutiques. . . ," *BAM* 67 (1912), 300.

20. Ibid., 304.

21. The Conseil d'État was the judicial authority for all matters pertaining to state administration.

22. *BAM* 92 (1924), 1205–10.

23. Jules Renault, "Sur la révision de la loi du 25 avril 1905 sur les sérums thérapeutiques de divers produits médicamenteux," *BAM* 104 (1930), 294–96; *Revue d'hygiène et de médecine préventive*, 56 (1936), 778–79.

24. Charles Achard, "La Part de l'Académie de Médecine dans la protection de la santé publique," *BAM* 123 (1940), 886–88.

25. Ibid., 885. It was felt that allowing manufacturers to directly furnish drugs to hospitals would open the door to fraudulent practices.

26. Vaccinations were usually performed twice weekly. The number varied wildly from nearly 15,000 vaccinations in 1858 to a little over 1,800 in 1872. Devergie, "Lecture sur les travaux"; J.-B.Barth, "Compte rendu des actes de l'Académie pendant 1872," *BAM* 2 (1873), viii; and S. Tarnier's outgoing presidential address, *BAM* 27 (1892), 14.

27. E. Hervieux, *Rapport général présenté à M. le Ministre de l'Intérieur par l'Académie de Médecine sur les vaccinations et revaccinations pratiquées en France et dans les colonies françaises pendant l'année 1893* (Melun, 1895).

28. L. Camus, "La Vaccine à l'Académie de Médecine," *Centenaire de l'Académie de Médecine, 1820–1920* (1921), p. 243, and Pierre Darmon, *La Longue traque de la variole: les pionniers de la médecine préventive* (1986), pp. 304–17.

29. Camus, "La Vaccine," pp. 247–48; Darmon, *La Longue traque*, pp. 340–41.

30. Darmon, *La Longue traque*, pp. 249–50. On the introduction of animal vaccination more generally see ibid., pp. 366–71.

31. L. F. A. Kelsch, *Rapport général sur les vaccinations et revaccinations pratiquées en France et dans les colonies françaises pendant l'année 1905* (1908), p. 7.

32. Achard, "La Part de l'Académie," 883.

33. Ibid., 886.

34. In response, the academy decided in 1937 to set up a new special commission for colonial medicine. *BAM* 118 (1937), 654–56.

35. *BAM* 27 (1892), 6, 63.

36. E. Gaultier de Claubry, "Rapport sur les épidémies de 1851," *MEM* 17 (1853), clii.

37. Bergeron, "Rapport général sur les épidémies pendant l'année 1865," *MEM* 28 (1867–68), liii.

38. See, for instance, Georges Brouardel, "Rapport sur les épidémies de 1929," *BAM* 104 (1930), 315–26.

39. Louis Martin, "Sur l'hygiène hospitalière et la prophylaxie des maladies contagieuses pour l'année 1933," *BAM* 112 (1934), 564.

40. On the eighteenth century see Caroline Hannaway, "From Private Hygiene to Public Health," in *Public Health*, ed. T. Ogawa (Osaka, 1981). For the late nineteenth and early twentieth centuries in comparative perspective, see Alisa Claus, *Every Child a Lion: The Origins of Maternal and Infant Health Policy in the United States and France, 1890–1920* (Ithaca, N.Y., 1993).

41. On wet-nursing see George D. Sussman, *Selling Mother's Milk: The Wet-Nursing Business in France, 1715–1914* (Urbana, Ill., 1982); and Fanny Fay-Sallois, *Les Nourrices à Paris au XIXe siècle* (1980).

42. J. A. Doléris, "Rapport sur les mémoires et ouvrages envoyés en 1911 à la Commission permanente de l'hygiène de l'enfance," *BAM* 67 (1912), 51.

43. A. Marfan, "Sur un proposition de la Commission d'hygiène de l'enfance," *BAM* 84 (1920), 250.

44. See E. Vallin, "Rapport sur le concours du prix de l'hygiène de l'enfance," *BAM* 20 (1888), 596. Depaul commented that money, not words, was needed to improve infant health. *BAM* 6 (1877), 678.

45. Th. Roussel, "De l'exécution de la loi du 23 dec., 1874," *BAM* 14 (1885), 349–62.

46. Doléris, "Rapport sur les mémoires," 53.

47. *BAM* 6 (1877), 1124–32, 1192–96.

48. Maurice Crosland and Antonio Gálvez, "The Emergence of Research Grants within the Prize System of the Academy of Sciences, 1795–1914," *Social Studies of Science* 19 (1989), 71–100.

49. E. Vallin, "Rapport sur le concours," 623.

50. Crosland and Gálvez, "The Emergence of Research Grants."

51. I am calculating the official value of prizes rather than the sums actually given away. These are based on the annual announcements in *BAM*.

52. Maurice Hanriot, "Les Bienfaiteurs de l'Académie," *Centenaire de l'Académie de Médecine, 1820–1920* (1921), p. 210. "Ordonnances relatives à l'Académie Royale de Médecine," *MEM* 1 (1828), 4.

53. *BAM* 17 (1851–52), 447. There had been two competitions, one for the period 1838–44 and a second for the period 1844–50.

54. Thirteen of seventeen works received affirmed its contagiousness.

55. C. Gibert, "Rapport sur les prix de 1849," *BAM* 15 (1849–50), 258.

56. In 1851 the question for the Portal Prize specified that microscopic observations be utilized to study the liver. Several other prizewinners in that year used microscopic research in tracing the pathological anatomy of certain conditions.

57. F. Dubois d'Amiens, "Rapport sur les prix de 1869," *MEM* 29 (1869–70), cxciii.

58. See, for instance, Gibert's comments on Lereboullet's winning essay on the microscopic analysis of the liver in *BAM,* 18 (1854), xxxv.

59. Devergie, "Lecture sur les travaux," 136. In addition to the predetermined questions, the academy was also prevented by the terms of the bequest from giving partial prizes (*encouragements* and *récompenses*) if it felt that no competitor merited a prize.

60. Barth, "Compte rendu 1872," xiii.

61. They included the Portal Prize in 1872 and 1874, the Orfila Prize in 1872, the Capuron Prize in 1873–74, the Academy Prize in 1874 and 1875.

62. J. Béclard, "Rapport général sur les prix décernés en 1872," *BAM* 2 (1873), 722.

63. E. J. Bergeron, "Rapport général sur les prix décernés en 1879," *BAM* 9 (1880), 702.

64. E. Vallin, "Rapport général sur les prix décernés en 1898," *BAM* 40 (1898), 625.

65. In 1924 there were 130 submitted works, a little over one-half the total number in 1910. In 1935 there were 166.

66. Hanriot, "Les Bienfaiteurs de l'Académie," p. 210.

67. Ibid., p. 214.

68. Ibid., p. 215. Both lacunae would be filled in subsequent years.

69. A. Souques, "Rapport général sur les prix décernés en 1923," *BAM* 90 (1923), 498–500.

70. Charles Achard, "Éloge de S.A.S., Le Prince Albert I de Monaco," *BAM* 110 (1933), 658.

71. Elisabeth Crawford, "The Prize System of the Academy of Sciences, 1850–1914," in *The Organization of Science and Technology in France, 1808–1914*, ed. Robert Fox and George Weisz (Cambridge, 1980), pp. 283–307, and Crosland and Gálvez, "The Emergence of Research Grants."

72. These figures are calculated from lists of winners of prizes and cash awards at the two institutions during the years 1860–64. (In the case of the Academy of Sciences only the winners of medical and physiological prizes have been considered.) Those for the Academy of Medicine are taken from annual prize reports in *BAM* and those for the Academy of Sciences from lists of prizewinners in Ernest Maindron, *Les Fondations des prix à l'Académie des Sciences; les lauréats de l'Académie, 1714–1880* (1881).

73. The proportion in the Academy of Medicine was 9 percent and in the Academy of Sciences 5 percent.

74. These figures and those that follow are based on the winners of prizes or cash awards in both institutions in 1900 and 1901. During these two years, there were 41 winners of medically related prizes or awards in the Academy of Sciences and 130 in the Academy of Medicine. Figures for the latter are calculated from the annual reports in *BAM*; those for the former are calculated from the lists of prizewinners in Pierre Gauja, *Les Fondations de l'Académie des Sciences (1881–1915)* (1917).

75. Crosland and Gálvez, "The Emergence of Research Grants," 190.

76. Georges Lemoine's presidential speech, December 12, 1921, *CRAS* 173 (1921), 1213–14.

77. On the use of such prize monies for research expenses see the discussions in Crawford, "The Prize System of the Academy of Sciences," 297–98, and Paul Forman, John L.

Heilbron, and Spencer Weart, "Physics *circa* 1900: Personal Funding and Productivity of the Academic Establishment," *Historical Studies in the Physical Sciences* 5 (1975), 74.

78. See Chapter 2.

79. Frédéric Blancpain, "La Création du CNRS: histoire d'une décision, 1901–1939," *Bulletin de l'Institut International de l'Administration Publique* 32 (1974), 93–143.

80. Achard, "Éloge de S.A.S. Le Prince Albert I," 658.

81. Hanriot, "Les Bienfaiteurs de l'Académie," p. 215.

82. In 1831 the Academy of Sciences decided to increase the award of one of its prizes "in order to indemnify authors for the expenses which their research might occasion." Maindron, *Les Fondations des prix à l'Académie des Sciences*, p. 87.

83. Souques, "Rapport de 1923," 498. Since this discussion occurred in secret session there was no direct record of it.

84. In fact the academy did somewhat transform the terms of the bequest, which specified that the prize be awarded for the best "work" (*travail*) in any branch of medicine. It amended the awarding formula to "the best work or ensemble of works." Ibid., 490.

85. For instance, the Bréant Prize, which offered 100,000 francs to anyone who could come up with a cure for cholera, the Argut Prize for a "medical" cure of an illness that was then treatable only by surgery, and the Mège Prize to anyone who could explain the factors favoring or retarding the progress of medicine since antiquity. These are from the Academy of Sciences's list of prizes in *CRAS* 153 (1911), 1408–10.

86. One study of physics at the turn of the century found 105 physicists (excluding applied industrial and medical physics) throughout France in higher teaching and research institutions. This includes junior staff and assistants. The number reaches 145 if one includes those with research affiliations. Forman, Heilbron, and Weart, "Physics *circa* 1900," 6–12.

87. The vast majority of scientists would have been working in the science faculty system. In 1888 there were only 256 individuals at all levels of the system; by 1919 there were 625 but many were low-level laboratory technicians. George Weisz, *The Emergence of Modern Universities in France, 1863–1914* (Princeton, N.J., 1983), p. 318.

88. The nature of advancement within the elite medical institutions of Paris is analyzed in Chapter 10.

89. Maurice Crosland, *Science under Control: The French Academy of Sciences, 1795–1914* (Cambridge, 1992), pp. 327–28, 399–402.

90. Crosland does not fully evaluate the role of Academy of Sciences during this period but suggests in his conclusions that it was, by the turn of the century, in clear decline. Ibid., pp. 436–40.

5

Representation and Memory in the Academy

When the medical journalist Louis Peisse called the academy's new building on the rue des Saints-Pères a "monument" in the 1850s, he was not just referring to the building's classical architecture. The rooms and corridors were cluttered with works of art donated by the state (in whose storage rooms they had frequently languished) and by academicians or their loved ones. The new premises, said Peisse, were like a museum whose very walls communicated to those able to comprehend:

> The walls speak. Everywhere the eyes rest within the confines of the academy, they meet only paintings, gilding, inscriptions, busts, statues, back to back, attached to, encrusted on the walls. The outsider who enters this sanctuary of science for the first time believes himself to be in a museum and is tempted to request the catalogue.[1]

In filling itself with art, much of which was recognized to be relatively mediocre, the Academy of Medicine was following a pattern common to public institutions generally in France and abroad. The portraits of the Royal Institution in London are justly famous,[2] while the magnificent art in French court buildings has recently received attention from art historians. Nevertheless, though we know a great deal about how state patronage influenced the development of art in France,[3] we know relatively little about what this art meant for the institutions that displayed it. The following comments are thus somewhat speculative.

It seems fairly obvious that in a country like France where official institutions routinely exhibited their official art, a relatively new institution like the Academy of Medicine would inevitably follow the prevailing fashion. It was to some extent a matter of aesthetics. Empty spaces seem literally to have been insupportable, demanding to be filled.[4] At the same time, the imperative was social. Art was part of the very definition of a public institution. Deploying it thus consecrated the academy's status as an official institution. It did so in a number of ways. Most art was donated by the state or by individuals. Possessing it thus demonstrated visibly an institution's ability to command public support. One suspects as well that, in a country where presidents routinely express literary aspirations, public art in the academy reflected the cultural pretensions of the medical elite. Doctors, it proclaimed, were as cultivated as any other sector of the bourgeoisie. And medicine was as worthy a subject for great art as any other human endeavor.

Perhaps most significantly, such art provided the academy with a visible history filled with heroic figures and great actions. It linked the present to the past, confirming the centrality of the academy to the progress of medicine and the centrality of medicine to the progress of the nation. It affirmed and reinforced collective values and group identity in much the same way as did academic eulogies. Both described a sphere of scientific progress in which the academy was actively participating and within which the illustrious dead continued to exist as exemplars of medical and scientific virtues. The premises of the academy, through the arrangement of institutional space, became the *physical* embodiment of this transcendent world. Simultaneously, academic eulogies (*éloges*) constituted the *oratorical* evocation of this sphere.

These two forms of representation—artistic space and eulogies—will be described in this chapter. They were of course very different. In the case of the first, academicians had little control over the fundamental elements with which they had to work since almost everything was donated. Nor was meaning necessarily very precise. *Éloges*, on the other hand, constituted a major academic genre through which collective representation of a very detailed sort was carried out. But this representation was constrained by another one of the *éloge*'s functions: serious and lengthy scientific evaluation. This combination of elements in the *éloges* proved unstable and gradually unraveled as the nineteenth century came to a close.

Art and the Academic Environment

Upon entering the academy, individuals penetrated a world of embodied collective memory in which past and present, dead and living, intersected. All memory is selective, and more successful works of art did not just represent the physical likeness of the dead but also served a pedagogical function, representing and affirming collective professional ideals.[5]

The difficulty faced by academicians in constructing this space was their lack of control over most of its elements. There was, for instance, little that could be done about the inadequate layout of the rue des Saints-Pères. Viewed objectively, moreover, the artistic elements filling this space were, to put it bluntly, rather motley. Works donated were of uneven quality and came to the academy in haphazard fashion. The challenge was to organize and display these ramshackle elements in such a way as to transform the former chapel and teaching amphitheater into a locus of memory and representation for the medical elite.[6]

We possess a remarkable evocation of the way this physical space was organized in the mid-nineteenth century thanks to an essay by the medical journalist and occasional art critic Louis Peisse (himself elected an *associé libre* of the academy in 1866), written soon after the move to the rue des Saints-Pères. Fancying himself

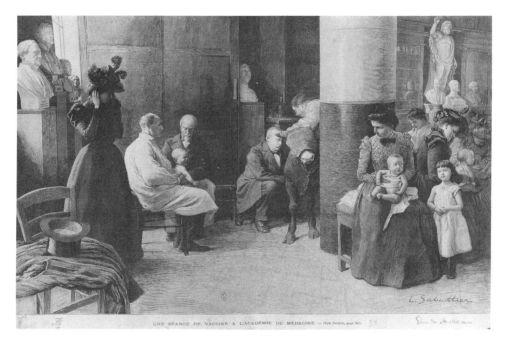

FIGURE 5.1. Vaccination session in the Salle des Pas Perdus of the academy. Engraving by
L. Sabatier, 1898. (Bibliothèque des Arts Décoratifs)

something of a connoisseur, Peisse took it upon himself to review and evaluate the
artwork in the academy.

On entering the building one passed through a small vestibule into a larger atri-
umlike antechamber, the Salle des Pas Perdus, which was the sight of many activities
including the weekly public vaccinations which the academy conducted. It also held
all of the institution's very considerable statuary. Immediately upon entering, the visitor was confronted by a large statue of the Greek healing god, Asclepius, which
identified the medical character of the building and represented medicine: "His de-
meanour" said Peisse, "is affable but proud. The posture of his body is simple, grave,
and full of dignity. What traits could more felicitously personify medicine?"[7]

Busts and statues filled nearly all the available space in the academy. But if
quantity could not be increased, Peisse suggested, quality could be much improved.
Of the many busts of academicians in the vestibule, a good number were, to Peisse's
chagrin, not of marble but of a plaster that was impossible to clean of dust. Others
busts were mediocre and even grotesque. Among the better pieces were two particularly large and grand marble statues dominating the rest and representing two glories
of military surgery, René Desgenettes and Dominique Larrey.[8] The finest busts and
statues did not merely reproduce accurately the features of the academician being
celebrated but personified the best features of the physician. One captured the "grave

and virile head" of Béclard. A portrait of Double reproduced "this tone of refined politeness, of effortless dignity, of persuasive authority and elegant finesse." Before leaving the antechamber and entering the meeting room, academicians passed marble busts of the academy's founder, Louis XVIII, and of the current emperor, Napoleon III. Both expressed the academy's links to the ruling powers. Both were of "colossal" dimensions but Peisse felt that they lacked grandiosity; "they are only gross, and too gross." Behind and above these three figures was a marble wall plaque listing in gold letters the financial benefactors of the academy.

One then entered the main meeting hall, which was, by all accounts, an architectural triumph over lack of space. Its courtroomlike look, whether intended or not, proclaimed it to be a tribunal of medical science. It was, like the antechamber, cluttered with works of art, here attached to the walls. Following the example of the Academy of Sciences, an effort had been made to display the names of especially illustrious academicians.[9] In the front and back near each corner of the room was a box listing nine names (inscribed in gold on a blue background) of deceased academicians. Each list represented a particular medical or scientific category. To the left of the speaker's podium (from the audience) was a list headed by the name of

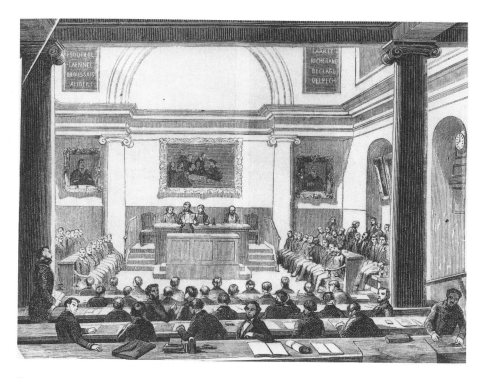

FIGURE 5.2. The meeting hall of the academy in 1852. From E.-A. Texier, *Tableau de Paris* (Paris, 1852). (Bibliothèque des Arts Décoratifs)

Jean Corvisart and representing internal medicine. To the right of the podium was a roll of prominent surgeon-academicians. At the back of the room was a second listing devoted to internal medicine and another headed by Cuvier grouping prominent figures in the natural sciences. Peisse remarked that it was possible to quibble about the omission of specific individuals. He did not, however, note the placement of the lists, probably because he found it perfectly natural for internal medicine and surgery to be at the front of the room behind the speaker's podium while lesser internists and natural scientists languished at the back.[10]

The most "brilliant part of the ornamentation" (in Peisse's words) was the academy's paintings. Most had been donated, making them difficult to evaluate since "one does not look a gift horse in the mouth."[11] Among them, the most prominent was a copy of Rembrandt's *Anatomy Lesson* at the very front of the meeting room above the president's desk. This copy had been painted by Pierre-Félix Cottrau in 1845 and had been donated to the academy by the government. One might be tempted to consider the visibility of this painting as a reflection of the importance of anatomy for medical science. But Peisse emphasized artistic merit. This, he said, was a first-rate copy of one of the three major works of the master.[12] In discussing it he devoted nearly a page to identifying the personalities represented but did not discuss its medical significance.

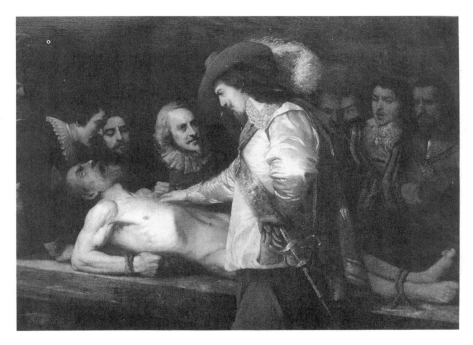

FIGURE 5.3. *Harvey Demonstrating the Circulation of the Blood*, by Eugène-Benjamin Fichel. (Académie de Médecine)

Surrounding the Rembrandt copy were four portraits. One depicted J.-M.-F. Lassone, founder of the eighteenth-century Société Royale de Médecine, which had in many ways served as a model for the Academy of Medicine.[13] The three other portraits were of the deceased academicians Corvisart, Antoine Dubois, and N.-L. Vauquelin, representing respectively internal medicine, surgery, and experimental science.

On the opposite wall hung an original painting by the well-known academic artist, Eugène-Benjamin Fichel, depicting William Harvey demonstrating the circulation of the blood on a living man before the young King Charles I. Despite his desire not to look gift horses in the mouth, Peisse was incensed by this work. It was historically inaccurate, Peisse insisted, because Harvey had never performed human vivisection. Furthermore, the chest incision being shown could not possibly have demonstrated the circulation of the blood. "There is thus nothing of interest from the scientific point of view."[14] Artistically it was equally insignificant. But most problematic of all was the image of suffering and death conveyed in the picture. Did the academy want to prove true the old saying that medicine is nothing but a meditation on death? "Would it not be better, for the honor of the profession and for the consolation of humanity, to present medicine to people from its attractive side, in its smiling images of life, of health, of which it is the guardian and protector?"[15]

The rest of the collection was made up of portraits. There was one of Vesalius that the academy's first president, Baron Portal, had donated to the academy and that was attributed to Titian. Peisse thought it was probably a copy of an original portrait by Jan van Calcar. Many other portraits, most of which Peisse thought mediocre, were displayed wherever there was room, not infrequently in poor circumstances. (The alienist Esquirol seems to have hung over a door.) Peisse suggested with apparent seriousness that these were regularly moved so that each could have a turn in the light.

There was, in addition, a very large painting on each of the side walls of the meeting room. These stood out not merely because of their size but because the academy had specially commissioned them from the young academic artist Charles Müller, who was a disciple of Thomas Couture. One depicted the military surgeon Larrey on the battlefield; the other showed Philippe Pinel causing the chains to be removed from the insane at the Bicêtre. (This mythic event never in fact took place.)[16] Since they had been expressly conceived for the academy, Peisse had no qualms about judging whether they were successful artistically. Although they were pleasing to the eye, the journalist felt that the decorative predominated over the intellectual and moral. It left dissatisfied "those . . . who would prefer in these works the elevation of sentiments and of thoughts, grave teachings, strong and noble emotions, and the poetic ideal of great historical painting."[17] More fundamentally, Peisse disagreed with the idea of seeking living personifications of medicine represented in acts "best able to place in relief the grandeur and the beauty of the scientific and professional character."[18] This reduced medicine to anecdote. It was preferable to apprehend and render the symbolic or emblematic form for the "idea," as Raphael had done in the chambers of the Vatican where he depicted the domains of knowledge.

Peisse's sense that the two scenes did not somehow do full justice to medicine may have been due to the fact that they constituted an incomplete set. Originally the

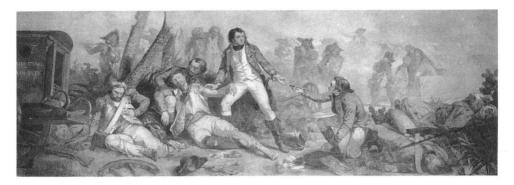

FIGURE 5.4. *Larrey on the Battlefield*, by Charles Müller, c. 1849. (Académie de Médecine)

academy had hoped to commission Müller to paint four tableaux, one for each wall of the meeting hall.[19] Two smaller paintings for the front and back walls were to depict Jenner discovering smallpox vaccination and Laënnec inventing auscultation. Both subjects celebrated medicoscientific innovations, the first central to public health and the second to clinical medicine. Larrey on the battlefield represented surgery and military medicine as well. (It may have also constituted a subtle tribute to the new ruler, Louis Napoleon, in whose uncle's army Larrey had distinguished himself.) Pinel at the Bicêtre gave recognition to internal medicine and, secondarily, to the field of psychiatry that had recently emerged.[20] But both of the latter paintings also celebrated aspects of medicine quite distinct from the intellectual and scientific genius to be personified by Jenner and Laënnec. Larrey, for instance, is not yet in the process of operating, in

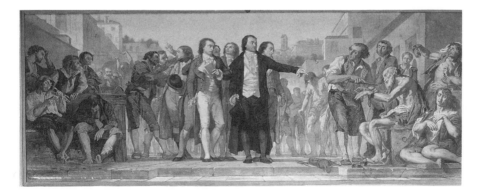

FIGURE 5.5. *Pinel Freeing the Insane from Their Chains at the Bicêtre Hospital*, by Charles Müller, c. 1849. (Académie de Médecine)

Müller's rendition, though an instrument is being handed to him. He is, however, standing tall while the battle rages around him. Here he exudes not surgical skill but physical courage and sangfroid.[21] These are characteristics that were frequently associated with surgeons in the early nineteenth century; but they had wider reverberations in the medical world, as we shall see in Chapter 9 when we examine the theme of political courage in the academic eulogies of the early nineteenth century.

The representation of Pinel is in some ways even more striking. He is not touching a patient but is rather giving an order. In response to this order, someone is actually removing chains from an inmate while someone else (Esquirol) is recording Pinel's words or the scene for posterity. The attempt to do without restraints was of course part of a medical effort to cure madness through moral therapy. But it can also be seen as an essentially humanitarian and even political act whose symbolism extends beyond the mad to all those who suffer from superstition and ignorance. Even as medical activities, the elimination of restraints and moral therapy are efforts to effect cure through the rational organization of the environment. It is not too hard to see Pinel in this painting as the personification of professional aspirations to utilize medical knowledge in order to effect a rational ordering of social reality. The effect is heightened by the fact that the courtyard of the hospital in which the action takes place resembles a public square. In contrast, a rendition of the equally fictitious liberation of the madwomen of the Salpêtrière by Pinel, painted by Tony Robert-Fleury in 1878 (and which now hangs in the library of that hospital), situates events in a cramped hospital courtyard. It looks inward toward the hospital, whereas Müller's painting looks outward.

Taken together, the four tableaux covered a fairly wide range of medical ideals and virtues. But the government provided only enough money to commission the two large tableaux.[22] The officers of the academy reminded the government on several occasions about the two smaller paintings but were rebuffed. By 1852 they seem to have been willing to settle for a single one to fill the empty space at the front of the meeting hall. And rather than choose between Laënnec and Jenner, they seem to have abandoned historical personages, as Peisse had advised. in favor of symbolic abstraction. The academy's permanent secretary, Dubois d'Amiens, told the ministry that Müller had made a sketch for a third tableau whose theme was the "value for medicine of the accessory sciences like hygiene, physics, chemistry, etc."[23] One would have liked to see his rendering of this abstract notion. But in the face of a major financial crisis for public art in the early 1850s, money never became available and the academy's third Müller painting did not materialize.

One does not want to go too far in using the choice of subjects as an indicator of the medical ideals and virtues which had priority in the 1850s. That the academy ended up with two paintings that appear to us so "unmedical" is probably a result of historical accident. It is not at all clear that these would have been chosen had academicians known that no others would be added. The dissatisfaction of certain journalists with the paintings would furthermore suggest that there was no unanimity within the medical profession about the ideal characteristics of medicine that should be rendered. Still, any combination of themes to represent medicine that included the two that were finally completed suggests just how different the medical world of the mid-nineteenth century was from that of the late twentieth.

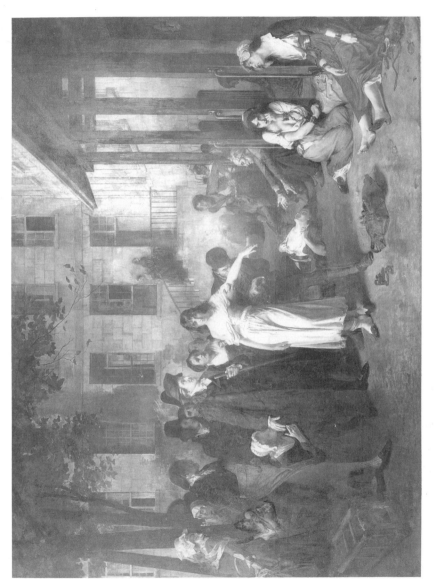

FIGURE 5.6. *Pinel Freeing the Insane Women of the Salpêtrière*, by Tony Robert-Fleury, 1878. (Salpêtrière Hospital, Photographie Bulloz)

The deposition of the academy's art seems to have changed little in the late nineteenth century. One journalist noted in 1893 that "artistic riches are crammed together in a confused jumble, and one begins to deplore that a permanent refuge has not yet been found in which to gather together all these marvels."[24] The vestibule area outside the meeting hall, the "salle des pas perdus," remained teeming with statuary increasingly made from bronze or marble. With the coming of the Third Republic, the statue of Napoleon III disappeared but Louis XVIII's political presence remained. A good many new pieces had been donated since Peisse's tour in the early 1850s. The meeting hall was not much changed, though Fichel's *Harvey* had been moved from the meeting hall to the "salle des pas perdus," no doubt because of its lack of authentic detail. In its place was a new painting donated by the state depicting Dutch savants discussing the discovery of quinine.[25] In 1870 Baron Hippolyte Larrey donated a large canvas called *Spanish Plague* (or *Yellow Fever*) by the Spanish painter José Aparicio, who had been a student of David. It took up the top part of the front wall behind the speaker's podium and president's desk (just above the Rembrandt copy).[26] The need to fill an empty space with an artistically respectable painting seems to have taken precedence over thematic considerations since there are no doctors in the picture; several priests, helpless to aid the sick and dying, are in fact

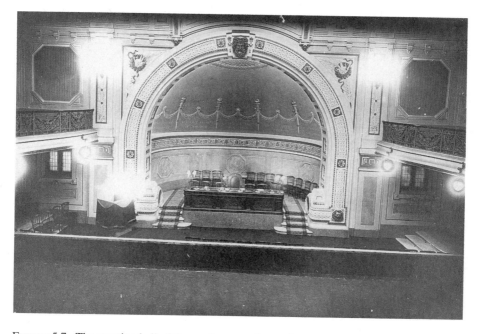

FIGURE 5.7. The meeting hall of the academy on the rue Bonaparte in the early twentieth century. (Collection Roger-Viollet)

gazing toward heaven. The meeting hall now held many more portraits as well as
several busts that did not fit into the "salle des pas perdus." Other areas also held artwork; the room where the administrative council met featured an Ingres portrait of
the hygienist François Mélier.

In 1902 the academy finally moved into its new premises on the rue Bonaparte,
adjoining the École des Beaux-Arts. Unlike its predecessor, the new building had
been designed and constructed especially for the academy and space was organized
in a more precise way, with specific rooms for specific functions. These rooms were
also full of art but disposed rather differently.[27] The building's classical facade proclaimed its medical orientation with decorative sculpture of medical flora and a head
of Asclepius at the top of the principal bay. Consequently, there was no longer need
for the massive Asclepius in the vestibule where one encountered only the large
marble Desgenettes facing the equally substantial Larrey; there were as well five
busts and a list of financial benefactors on the wall facing the entrance.

The main meeting hall, in the form of a large semicircle, was in a modernized
Empire style meant to evoke, in a more spacious way, the old meeting hall on the rue
des Saints-Pères. However, it differed in one significant respect. It seems to have initially been without paintings or sculpture. A possible reason is that its design
incorporated a great many decorative flourishes and much ornamention in the walls
and ceilings; it thus may have had no aesthetic need for the ramshackle collection of

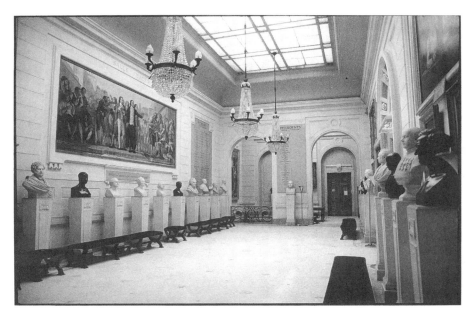

FIGURE 5.8. The Salle des Pas Perdus of the academy as it appears today. (Académie de
Médecine)

artwork that had cluttered its predecessor. The emptiness was noted by several journalists, who remarked that prominent empty spaces could easily be filled with frescoes.[28] Still it is tempting to attribute this spareness to a new hardheadedness that separated the space in which medical science took place (or at least was discussed), which had little need of art, from the spaces of memory where the history of the academy and of French medicine was enshrined.

The "salle des pas perdus," just outside the main hall, in fact seems to have been quite deliberately chosen to be the chief repository of this history.[29] At the inauguration of the new building in 1902 this area contained thirty busts (many still apparently made from plaster). On the walls hung Müller's *Pinel*—now in a position of particular prominence—the copy of *The Anatomy Lesson*, and Fichel's *Harvey*. It is probably indicative of the changing concerns of the medical elite that Müller's second tableau, *Larrey on the Battlefield*, was even further removed for the main meeting hall, hung as it was in the small library reading room. The courage of the battlefield surgeon was not very relevant to the career-driven Parisian medical elite of the early twentieth century; nor were the heaven-gazing priests of *Spanish Plague,* who were also relegated to the library.

In the twentieth century, works of art continued to find their way into the academy. In the mid-1930s the glaring absence of any representation of Hippocrates was remedied when a francophile Greek physician donated a large marble statue of the "father of medicine" that was placed in the main assembly hall amid much fanfare. It served as a reminder of the filiation between Hippocrates and the academy, "his spiritual child and heir," and as a symbol of interwar Franco-Greek friendship.[30] As of this moment, busts still predominate but several more recently acquired paintings have gradually satisfied the need for scientific and clinical themes. Jenner's achievement is finally celebrated in the academy on a landing of the main staircase. Painted in 1879 by Gaston Mélingue, it depicts the great man vaccinating a child. The often reproduced painting by Léon Lhermitte (1889) of Claude Bernard in his laboratory has been moved from its long-time home at the Sorbonne and now hangs in one of the academy's corridors. Clinical devotion is now represented in a 1921 painting by Vuillard hanging in the elegant salon and depicting a paternal doctor (Henri Vaquez) treating a patient at the Pitié hospital.[31] The themes of the newer paintings are familiar to our own sensibilities; they are an indication of how much elite medical self-images have changed since the mid-nineteenth century.

The representational role of art in the academy was relatively straightforward. That of academic eulogies was more complex. These sought to combine the representation of collective memory and values with elaborate scientific evaluation.

Eulogies

One of the permanent secretary's primary tasks was the presentation at annual public meetings of *éloges* devoted to the achievements of a deceased academician—a tradition that had become established in nearly all academies during the eighteenth century. The academic *éloge* was itself part of a more general tendency in the France of the eighteenth and early nineteenth centuries to celebrate great men in literature,

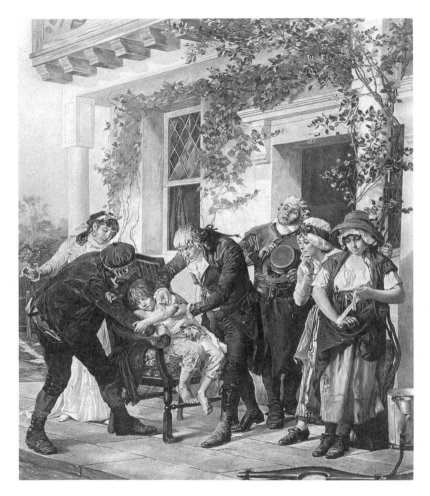

FIGURE 5.9. *Jenner Performing the First Vaccine Innoculation*. Engraving based on the painting in the academy by Gaston Mélingue, 1879. (Photographie Jean Loup Charmet)

art, public architecture, and even popular almanacs. This cult of great men reflected a new faith in progress and in individuals as vehicles of this progress. It expressed as well more traditional beliefs in the pedagogical efficacy of exemplary lives to stimulate virtuous behavior. It exemplified the bourgeoisie's identification with a celebration of merit (usually its own) rather than noble birth or military heroism. Finally, it expressed a secular displacement of the desire for immortality away from religious afterlife to posthumous presence in this world as a result of special achievement.[32]

The academic *éloge* in medicine and science was a strange genre;[33] it was at once an oral presentation of a particularly ritualistic kind and, when subsequently published, a literary text full of careful evaluation of specialized scientific work. The *éloge* had three explicit purposes. First, it was a form of instant history which located the work of individuals within an interpretation of recent medicoscientific developments. This is how the Academy of Medicine's first secretary, Etienne Pariset, defined his task:

> Gentlemen, when my task requires me to speak before you in order to honor the memory of a colleague, this colleague appears to me on the spot, surrounded by his writings and by the writings of his predecessors. I cannot then prevent myself from connecting the present to the past; I see there something like a treasure of science; I attempt to comprehend its origins, follow its progress, call attention to its importance, scope, variations, difficulties; and in this revue of so many excellent minds, I seek to measure the merit of each one of them, and to mark the rank which he ought to occupy in men's esteem.[34]

An *éloge* was, in the second instance, a reward which the academy accorded illustrious members and that assured the deceased a certain degree of immortality. The public *éloge* was thus a ritual act of initiation celebrating the transition from the impermanent world of the living to the timeless pantheon of medical heroes that was physically embodied in the statues, busts, and paintings which cluttered the academy.

Finally, and this was the traditional function of the classical encomium out of which it developed, the *éloge* had an explicitly moralistic purpose. The lives of the deceased were presented to academicians as exemplars of professional and personal behavior. As Pariset put it, death leaves a memory of virtue "that becomes both the consolation of our pain and the model that we must imitate."[35] Emulation of the subject was the surest route to both professional achievement and peer approval.

A fourth function was never explicitly acknowledged. *Éloges* allowed the secretary to project an idealized image for public consumption of medicine and the medical elite. Numerous tangents and asides, moreover, allowed the secretary to press the sovereign or government for favorable treatment of savants.

Such diverse purposes sometimes came into conflict. The presentation of models of virtue or scientific excellence required some degree of idealization of subjects, whereas scientific evaluation demanded historical accuracy. Consequently, there were sporadic attempts to introduce more veracity into biographies. Despite a great deal of theoretical justification for such practices,[36] there were practical limits to what could be said. Presenting an individual in the best possible light was indispensable to the moralizing purpose of the *éloge* since models of behavior had necessarily to be positive. At the same time, it was argued, such idealization permitted the eulogist to more nearly approach the truth by transcending the rivalries, prejudices, and weaknesses of character which obscured an individual's achievement.[37] In this way, contemporaries could view the deceased as he would be seen by future and more objective observers. Finally, there was the outside world to consider. Eulogists were not unaware of their power to disseminate a particular view of the medical elite. Pariset, for instance, explained his practice of presenting subjects in historical perspective:

[S]upposing that this recapitulation is an hors-d'oeuvre for you, it will at least have
the advantage of giving notice to the outside world that, in the mold of the one
whose memory you are glorifying, you belong to an elite class of men who, scattered in time and space, labor in silence for the well-being of their fellows.[38]

Excessive criticism of subjects was not the way to achieve such ends.

Pariset presented his first *éloge*—devoted to Corvisart—in 1824. From then on,
an *éloge* was usually read each year at the academy's annual public meeting. These
éloges were subsequently published in the academy's *Mémoires*, which appeared
from 1828 to 1911.[39] Such panegyrics were substantial literary efforts ranging from
ten to forty pages in length and required the collection of biographical materials and
close reading of the subject's publications. The permanent secretary ordinarily presented all major *éloges* but he could in special cases delegate responsibility, as most
secretaries did at least once or twice during their tenures.

It was the secretary who ordinarily decided which academicians were to be honored. Although he was sometimes subject to peer pressures, he enjoyed considerable
freedom in his choices.[40] Occasionally, however, pressure was irresistible. A ceremony organized by the academy's section of pathological anatomy to honor
Laënnec, the inventor of auscultation, forced Pariset to respond with an *éloge* of
Laënnec a year later.[41] Near the end of Pariset's tenure, the academy's administrative
council moved to curb some of the permanent secretary's powers. In response to
Pariset's decision in 1846 to eulogize a corresponding member rather than one of
many deceased Parisian members, the council decided that the permanent secretary
was obligated to inform it in advance of the subject of his *éloge*. And when Pariset,
soon after, refused to prepare an *éloge* for the recently deceased academician
François Broussais, the administrative council intervened and asked Louis Bégin,
then serving as annual president of the academy, to eulogize Broussais at the next
public meeting.[42]

Pariset's successor, Dubois d'Amiens, began his career by successfully reasserting the prerogatives of the secretary; at his insistence, Bégin agreed to leave the
forthcoming *éloge* of Broussais to the new secretary.[43] However, in his quest for objectivity and scientific honesty, Dubois d'Amiens soon managed to alienate his
colleagues with panegyrics that were considered excessively critical. As a result of
the controversies which he ignited, he chose not to present any *éloges* during his last
decade as permanent secretary.[44] His successors avoided such altercations and retained considerable freedom to choose subjects.

All usually honored titular members of the academy, although occasional *associés libres* of particularly high stature like Cuvier, Pasteur, and Émile Littré could be
the subjects of tribute. Clinicians were most frequently *éloge* subjects but efforts
were sometimes made to satisfy other constituencies so that the occasional pharmacist, veterinarian, or laboratory scientist was honored. Each secretary had special
interests which determined his choice of subjects. Some of Jules Béclard's selections
between 1863 and 1887 reflected his commitment to the scientific reform of medical
education. E. J. Bergeron (1887–1900) had a lifelong career interest in public health,
devoting three of his panegyrics to public health figures. The clinician Sigismond
Jaccoud (1900–1913) also devoted three *éloges* to prominent public health figures
and several others to teachers and close friends.

Since only a very small number of individuals could be the subjects of *éloges* at public meetings, another form of eulogistic practice was introduced in the academy. Many deceased academicians were honored at their funerals by an oration presented by a representative of the academy. Starting in 1837 these shorter orations, presented at graveside by the permanent secretary or, more frequently, by another academician, were repeated at one of the academy's regular meetings and then published in the recently established *Bulletin*. This practice was justified on the grounds that all academicians deserved some posthumous recognition. "There are the illustrious [*des gloires*] who aspire to the honor of an academic *éloge*; there are those who are more modest and who would be content with a simple notice; but one can refuse it to them all the less since it is a right of ours acquired when we are admitted within these walls."[45]

In actual fact, many full members of the academy in the nineteenth century were not the subjects of any sort of panegyric.[46] The reasons for the lack of an appreciation in these cases remain obscure, but in many cases it resulted from the death of academicians far from Paris; it was thus impossible for the academy to send a representative to the funeral in time to present an oration. In other cases individuals specified that no orations be presented at their funerals.

Unlike the academic *éloge*, a funeral oration at graveside was not the appropriate place for a detailed evaluation of the deceased's scientific work. It tended rather toward platitudes and moral lessons. This may well be the reason that funeral orations lost popularity in the last decades of the nineteenth century. Increasingly, from 1870 on the *Bulletin* of the academy reports cases of academicians specifically requesting that no speeches be made at their funeral. In 1873 the annual president of the academy suggested that since so many academicians refused funeral orations, perhaps newly elected academicians should present a scientific appreciation of their predecessor, as was the practice at the Académie Française.[47] This suggestion was never implemented but another solution was eventually found.

Funeral orations continued to appear in the *Bulletin*, albeit in ever-shrinking numbers, until World War I.[48] They were gradually replaced by brief biographical notices read by the annual president at the moment when he announced the death to the academy. These notices imperceptibly expanded as time went on from a few paragraphs to about two pages, but they were never very elaborate. On rare occasions, however, another academician might present a more substantial necrological notice. After World War I, funeral orations completely disappeared. Longer and more elaborate notices by academicians other than the president became more frequent until by the late 1920s they were as important as the presidential necrologies. Frequently a student or colleague of the deceased might present the notice. But increasingly a number of more "literary" academicians tended to specialize in these notices, which gave them an opportunity to exercise literary skills and perhaps establish their credentials should the post of general secretary fall vacant.[49]

All such notices tended to be rather dry and more preoccupied with careers and publications than funeral orations had been. Their spread eliminated a variety of technical impediments to appreciations of deceased academicians. No longer was it necessary to actually attend a funeral. Virtually all full members who died in the twentieth century could thus expect some form of necrological notice. Similarly, it now became possible to honor corresponding and foreign members in fairly large numbers. This wider coverage in necrologies was also part of a more significant broadening of horizons that made the Parisian elite at the turn of the century increasingly aware of events occurring outside the capital. Non-Parisian French members were first recognized in significant numbers during Bergeron's tenure as secretary. Foreign members began to be eulogized during Jaccoud's tenure because the new secretary was eager to open the academy and French medicine more generally to international medical science.[50] The fact that so much important medical science was taking place outside the capital, indeed outside France, undoubtedly contributed to this more cosmopolitan perspective. Nonetheless, corresponding and foreign members were seldom the subjects of full academic *éloges*.[51]

Outwardly the traditional academic *éloge* did not change as dramatically as the funeral oration. It became somewhat shorter as tangential discussions were eliminated.[52] More significantly, it became increasingly retrospective. In its initial phase, the *éloge* served to distinguish the true heroes of medicine from other academicians. If every deceased academician was owed a funeral oration immediately following his death, only a handful were singled out with an *éloge* a year or two later. But starting with Dubois d'Amiens, secretaries frequently devoted *éloges* to individuals who had died during the tenure of predecessors. By the twentieth century this practice had become the norm. Only after a period of time, explained academic spokesmen, could the true contributions of academicians be fully appreciated and placed in perspective.[53] Thus orations and necrological notices presented immediately after the deaths of virtually all Parisian members came to represent the initial evaluation of an academician; the academic *éloge* became a second, more elaborate treatment of special individuals whose extraordinary achievement had become clearer with time.

More significantly, perhaps, *éloges* were gradually stripped of metaphorical content and social vision. The genre was from its origins a compromise between scientific and more literary forms of writing, between evaluation and representation. Pariset's immensely long presentations provided space to describe the work of subjects, pursue his own hobbyhorses (the importance of clinical and scientific observation and the need to temper anatomical localism with vitalist insights, for instance), develop an extensive repertoire of social and moral themes (to be discussed in Chapter 9), and explore a variety of exotic tangents. By the twentieth century, little remained of this rich literary potpourri but the details of elite medical careers and the publications which they generated.

Among the reasons this occurred was the desire to make *éloges* more "scientific." There emerged a consensus among Pariset's successors that, as brilliant as his *éloges* were as literature, they were weak as scientific documents.[54] Dubois d'Amiens carried, to a particular extreme the desire to redress the balance and created enormous controversy. With greater moderation, his successors showed equal concern to produce more scientifically respectable documents. Scientific aspirations did not completely eliminate literary figures and moral concerns from *éloges*; but these became increasingly marginal to the main scientific and career narratives.[55] The increasing brevity of the form, as well as the tendency to write about individuals who had died many years before and who were therefore dimly remembered, also discouraged efforts to go much beyond accounts of careers and scientific achievement.

In 1921 the recently elected secretary, Charles Achard, presented not a standard *éloge* but a historical review of the genre in the academy. His views about the functions of *éloges* were in some ways conventional. They were useful, he suggested, in three ways. First, they established historical truth, tracing the role of an individual in the evolution of a science. Second, they served science by surveying the state of particular questions and suggesting new directions. Last, the *éloge*—"like the fable"—provided a moral and educational service through the examples of goodness and virtue leavened by inevitable human imperfections.[56] The main difference between Achard's views and those of Etienne Pariset a century earlier is the disappearance of the belief that *éloges*, by promising immortality, stimulated academic zeal; on the contrary, Achard emphasized that a revue of *éloges* made it clear that many academicians had produced nothing memorable, demonstrating that "immortality is not among the privileges of our academy."[57] Instead, Achard suggested that academic eulogies could point medical science in new directions. This small shift produced a rather unbalanced list. The first two tasks—reconstructing scientific history and surveying the state of scientific questions—are enormous and complex tasks. The last—providing examples of virtue—seems in comparison both slight and simplistic in the context of the "fable" analogy.

If one finds in Achard's *éloge* little of the social imagery that made Pariset's depiction of the medical elite so vibrant, and if evaluation seems in these works to dominate over representation, the reality is that evaluation had become a form of representation. His scientific histories turned frequently on the defense of the recent achievements of French medical science at a time when leadership in international science had manifestly passed to other nations. The most ubiquitous topos in his work is that the achievements of subjects, usually Frenchmen, had not been fully recognized.

In a few cases the neglect was temporary. The military physician Alphonse Laveran faced and ignored widespread skepticism regarding his findings about the parasitic origins of paludism.[58] More often than not Achard's subjects had been treated unfairly by posterity and it was one of the eulogist's self-declared tasks to remedy this situation posthumously. Raphael Lépine, for instance, was in Achard's account the unsung precursor of the modern conception of diabetes.[59] The eulogy of Henri Dutrochet discussed the subject's discovery of osmosis but also argued that he and not Schwann was the real discoverer of the cellular structure of tissue.[60] The eulogist tried to set the record straight in the case of Casimir Davaine whose pioneering discovery of the first illness-causing microbe (anthrax) and more general role in explaining the role of microbes had, it was argued, been largely ignored.[61] Elsewhere, Achard emphasized that Joseph Grancher had demonstrated the clinical unity of tuberculosis even before Koch's discovery of the causative microorganism confirmed what French pathological anatomy had already demonstrated.[62]

Achard did not just argue for the contribution of academicians to such medically relevant fields as bacteriology or the conceptualization of diabetes. In his *éloges* of Dutrochet and Adolphe Wurtz, Achard demonstrated the contribution of medical men to such more general discoveries as osmosis and atomic notation in chemistry. This was the same impulse which led the academy to spend a number of sessions in early 1924 trying to win official recognition for the view that E. J. Marey (1830–1904) was the inventor of cinematography.[63] What was at stake was the role of French medicine and of the academy in the mainstream of scientific developments at a time when France was desperately seeking to reaffirm its international scientific role.[64] We shall return to this theme in another chapter when we examine the evolution of Laënnec's reputation in the twentieth century.

Despite or perhaps because of his nationalist agenda, Achard's *éloges* during the interwar years continued to be substantial, well-researched, and full of more or less original judgments. And yet, during his tenure, the academic *éloge* was already in decline. In certain years Achard preferred to present historical or topical essays rather than *éloges*. In 1921 he reviewed the history of the *éloge* at the academy and in 1937 he discussed the historical forms of charitable health assistance.[65] At the first public meeting after the French defeat at the hands of Nazi Germany, he discussed the role of the Academy of Medicine in the protection of public health.[66] Whether under the pressure of other tasks or due to advancing age, Achard was also increasingly likely to delegate *éloges* to other academicians. From 1931 to 1940 the general secretary presented just three *éloges*.

Under Achard's successors, *éloges* became short and rather perfunctory, ritual rehearsals of accepted views of medical heroes; the ritualistic celebratory function seems in fact to have altogether replaced serious evaluation of any sort.[67] Little by now remained of the remarkable vitality and richness of the nineteenth-century academic *éloge*. It had been gradually stripped of its function of representing the social and moral reality of the medical elite so that it might be devoted to scientific evaluation. This was not unlike the attempt in the new building on the rue Bonaparte to separate the academy's locus of scientific activity, its meeting hall, from its locus of memory, the *salle des pas perdus* where its art collection was displayed. But just as art never completely disappeared from the main hall, representation did not vanish from the *éloge*. The evaluation of current or almost current science gave way to a retrospective historical evaluation which proclaimed the excellence of French medical science. Even this seems to have been abandoned as a serious activity after 1940.

We have now completed our survey of academic structures and activities. In the following section we will return to special commissions, debates, *éloges*, membership. But rather than describing the institution we will be using them as historical sources in order to examine issues that go well beyond the Academy of Medicine.

NOTES

1. Louis Peisse, *La Médecine et les médecins; philosophie, doctrines, institutions, critiques, moeurs et biographies médicales*, 2 vols. (1857), vol. 2, p. 307.

2. Katherine Fisher Taylor, *In the Theater of Criminal Justice: The Palais de Justice in Second Empire Paris* (Princeton, N.J., 1993); Association française pour l'histoire de la justice, *La Justice en ses temples: regards sur l'architecture judiciare en France* (Poitiers, 1992); Sophie Forgan, "Context, Image and Function: A Preliminary Enquiry into the Architecture of Scientific Societies," *British Journal of the History of Science* 19 (1986), 111.

3. Among the many relevant works on this subject, see Albert Boime, *The Academy and French Painting in the Nineteenth Century*, 2nd ed. (New Haven, Conn., 1986), and *Hollow Icons: The Politics of Sculpture in Nineteenth-Century France* (Kent, Ohio, 1987); Michael Marrinan, *Painting Politics for Louis Philippe: Art and Ideology in Orleanist France* (New Haven, Conn., 1988).

4. In a speech describing the premises, the academy's president commented: "There were large spaces to fill around the cupola; two tableaux by a distinguished painter . . . now occupy them." I. Bricheteau, "Inauguration de la nouvelle salle," *BAM* 25 (1849–50), 1088.

5. The most important work on spaces of memory is to be found in Pierre Nora, ed., *Les Lieux de mémoire*, 3 vols. (1984–93). For the Anglo-American literature on memory see the extensive footnotes in Pnina Abir-Am, "A Historical Ethnography of a Scientific Anniversary in Molecular Biology: The First Protein X-Ray Photograph," *Social Epistemology* 6 (1992), 323–54.

6. According to Charles Achard, the placing of portraits and busts, at least in the twentieth century, had to be voted on by the entire academy in secret session. But Achard made it clear that this procedure was not always followed. *BAM* 118 (1937), 394. Under normal circumstances, one suspects, it was the permanent secretary who made decisions about such matters.

7. Peisse, *La Médecine et les médecins*, p. 316.

8. The first was by Jacques-Louis David (d'Angers); the second was commissioned by the academy from Pierre Robinet.

9. The example of the Academy of Sciences was explicitly acknowledged in Bricheteau, "Inauguration de la nouvelle salle," 1088.

10. My reconstruction of their placement is based on pictures of the meeting hall from the period.

11. Peisse, *La Médecine et les médecins*, p. 325.

12. Ibid., p. 329.

13. This was a gift to the academy from Portal. Dr. A. Cabanès, "Notice historique sur l'Académie de médecine," *Gazette des Hôpitaux* 66 (1893), 25.

14. Peisse, *La Médecine et les médecins*, p. 331.

15. Ibid.

16. "Introductory Essay," in Philippe Pinel, *The Clinical Training of Doctors: An Essay of 1773*, ed. Dora B. Weiner (Baltimore, Md., 1980), pp. 16–17; Jacques Postel, "Philippe Pinel et le mythe fondateur de la psychiatrie française," *Psychoanalyse à l'Université* 4 (1979), 197–244.

17. Peisse, *La Médecine et les médecins*, p. 327. A later journalist also found that Müller's tableaux lacked "a teaching or an emotion." Cabanès, "Notice historique," 25.

18. Peisse, *La Médecine et les médecins*, p. 327.

19. My understanding of the origins of these paintings is based on unpublished material kindly placed at my disposal by Nancy Davenport and on Isabelle Violet, "Le Mythe de la libération des aliénés de Bicêtre par Philippe Pinel pendant la Révolution Française," Travail d'Étude et de Recherches, Université de Paris IV-Sorbonne, U.E.R. d'Histoire.

20. That the two paintings were primarily intended to honor surgery and internal medicine is suggested by the comments of the academy's president, Bricheteau, "Inauguration de la nouvelle salle: discours de M. Bricheteau," *BAM* 25 (1849–50), 1088.

21. This is not just my opinion. F. Roubaud's discussion of the painting in *Gazette des Hôpitaux*, 3e sér. 2 (1850), 464, emphasizes the contrast between the carnage all around and Larrey, who is "sublime with calm and serenity."

22. Even so it was slow to pay Müller, who complained to the academy in February and March 1849. AM Liasse 13.

23. Letter of February 3, 1851, in Violet, "Le Mythe de la libération," p. 109.

24. Cabanès, "Notice historique," 24.

25. All that one journalist could say about it is that it succeeded in covering the nudity of the wall. Ibid., 25.

26. Cabanès judged it as "not of the first order" but nonetheless "estimable." He compared it unfavorably, however, with the "ideal frescoes" of Puvis de Chavannes. Ibid., 26–27.

27. My discussion is based on E. De Lavarenne, "La Nouvelle Académie de Médicine." *Presse médicale* 10 (1902), 1131–34, and J. Noir, "La Nouvelle Installation de l' Académie de Médicine," *Progres médical*, 3e sér., 161 (1902), 425–27.

28. *Gazette des hôpitaux* 133 (1902), 1318. L.-C. Boileau, "La Nouvelle Académie de Médicine," *L Architecture* 15 (1902), 84. The architect's drawings suggest that at least one was envisaged at the front of the hall. The ceiling vault was eventually filled in with a fresco.

29. Boileau, "La Nouvelle Académie," 83, reprints a press release stating that this room "will receive the portraits, tableaux, and busts which the academy possesses."

30. Both points were made in the speeches celebrating the installation. *BAM* 118 (1937), 390, 393.

31. I am grateful to the director of the academy's library, Mme Michèle Lenoir, for a guided tour of the academy's rich artistic heritage in April 1992.

32. On the cult of great men during the eighteenth century see Jean-Claude Bonnet, "Naissance du Panthéon," *Poétique* 33 (1978), 46–55; Mona Ozouf, "Le Panthéon: l'École normale des morts," in *Les Lieux de mémoire: I, La République*, ed. Pierre Nora (1984). On its manifestation in popular culture, Jean-Jacques Tatin, "L'Homme du peuple au Panthéon," *Revue d'histoire moderne et contemporaine* 32 (1985), 537–60, and "Relation de l'actualité, politique et culte des grandes hommes dans les almanachs de 1760 à 1793," *Annales historiques de la Révolution française* 57 (1985), 307–16.

33. On Academic *éloges* see Daniel Roche, "Talents, raison et sacrifice: les médecins vus par eux-mêmes," *Annales ESC*, 32 (1977), 866–86, and *Le Siècle des lumières en province: académies et académiciens provinciaux, 1680–1789* (1978), pp. 166–80; Dorinda Outram, "The Language of Natural Power: The *Éloges* of Georges Cuvier and the Public Language of Nineteenth Century Science," *History of Science*, 16 (1978), 153–78; Charles B. Paul, *Science and Immortality: The Éloges of the Paris Academy of Sciences (1699–1791)* (Berkeley, Calif., 1980). On *éloges* in the context of the development of biography see Daniel Madelinat, *La Biographie* (1984), pp. 32–63.

34. E. Pariset, *Membres de l'Académie Royale de Médecine*, 2 vols. (1850), vol. 2, p. 316.

35. *Éloge* of Alibert, *BAM* 2 (1837), 164.

36. The best summary of such justifications of *éloges* as historical notices rather than panegyrics is F. Dubois d'Amiens's introduction to his *Éloges académiques* (1872), pp. iii–lxiv, which develops the ideas of earlier writers like Thomas and D'Alembert.

37. F. Vicq d'Azyr, "Éloges historiques; considérations générales," in *Oeuvres de Vicq d'Azyr, recueillis et publiés avec des notes et un discours sur sa vie et ses ouvrages*, 6 vols., ed. Moreau de la Sarthe, vol. 5 (1805), p. 1.

38. Pariset, *Membres de l'ARM*, vol. 2, p. 317.

39. In the following years they appeared in *BAM*.

40. In 1835 an academician, Gilbert Breschet, suggested that two recently deceased provincial associates (Lobstein and Fodoré) be eulogized at the next public meeting and his motion was adopted. But Pariset devoted his *éloge* four months later to the physiologist F. Chaussier.

41. This will be discussed in detail in Chapter 8.

42. Minutes of the administrative council, January 11, 1847, in AM Liasse 13.

43. Ibid.

44. He continued, however, to present the annual prize reports while his eventual successor as secretary, J. Béclard, took charge of *éloges*.

45. *BAM* 1 (1837), 387.

46. At mid-century nearly one-half of the full members were without orations; in subsequent decades the figure was slightly higher than one-quarter.

47. Barth, "Compte rendu des actes de l' Académie pendant 1872," *BAM* 2 (1873), xvii.

48. By the late 1890s there were no more than one or two a year.

49. E. Rist, for instance, published a collection of his necrological notices, *Vingt-cinq portraits de médecins français, 1900–1955* (1955).

50. P. Ménétrier, "Éloges de François-Sigismond Jaccoud (1830–1913)," *BAM* 104 (1930), 589.

51. In his *éloge* of one corresponding member, Raphael Lépine, Charles Achard could cite only two other corresponding members who had been the subjects of academic *éloges*. He attributed this neglect to the lack of regular contacts between members and correspondents. Charles Achard, "Raphael Lépine (1840–1919)," *BAM* 94 (1925), 1127–28.

52. *Éloges* gradually become shorter throughout the nineteenth century but it is in the early years of the twentieth century, starting with Debove's tenure as permanent secretary (1913–20), that they shrank significantly. One suspects that aside from changing rhetorical conventions, the main reason for the decreasing length of *éloges* was the expansion of the program of prizes, which was also reported on at the annual public meeting.

53. See, for instance, Pierre Marie, "Éloge de Charcot," *BAM* 93 (1925), 576.

54. His eulogist, Dubois d'Amiens, referred explicitly to the lack of scientific understanding in Pariset's *éloges* ("Éloge de Pariset," in Pariset, *Membres de l'ARM*, vol. 1, p. 17); this judgment was echoed in Charles Achard, "Cent ans d'éloges à l'Académie de Médecine," *BAM* 86 (1921), 360. This attitude may have reflected Pariset's low stature as a medical scientist rather than the quality of his analyses.

55. By the twentieth century one tended to find them isolated in the introductory and concluding paragraphs.

56. Achard, "Cent ans d'éloges," 358–59.

57. Ibid., 375.

58. Charles Achard, "Alphonse Laveran (1845–1922)," *BAM* 102 (1929), 602.

59. Achard, "Lépine," 1138.

60. Charles Achard, "Henri Dutrochet (1776–1847)," *BAM* 114 (1935), 586–87. This continues to be a burning issue for Frenchmen. See Émile Aron, *Henri Dutrochet: médecin et biologiste, honneur de la Touraine, 1776–1847* (Chambrey, 1990), pp. 53–62; J. Schiller and T. Schiller, *Henri Dutrochet: le matérialisme mécaniste et la physiologie générale* (1975), pp. 35–40.

61. Charles Achard, "Casimir Davaine (1812–1882)," *BAM* 100 (1928), 1343–56.

62. "Joseph Grancher," *BAM* 90 (1923), 537.

63. *BAM* 91 (1924), 306–10, 335–47, 395–98. Six years later the centenary celebration of Marey's birth gave the academy another opportunity to insist on his role as inventor of cinematography. Charles Richet, "Le Centenaire de Marey," *BAM* 103 (1930), 706–14.

64. On this matter see George Weisz, *The Emergence of Modern Universities in France, 1863–1914* (Princeton, N.J., 1983) pp. 252–68.

65. Charles Achard, "Cent ans d'éloges," 358–75, and "Coup d'oeil historique sur l'assistance aux malades," *BAM* 118 (1937), 499–510.

66. Charles Achard, "La Part de l'Académie de Médecine dans la protection de la santé publique," *BAM* 123 (1940), 878–90.

67. For instance, those eulogized in the 1940s were Esquirol (1940, d. 1840), 2 pages; Claude Bernard (1944, d. 1878), 9 pages; Charles Richet (1945, d. 1935), 6 pages; A. Beclère (1948, d. 1939), 5 pages; Félix Terrier (1949, d. 1908), 5 pages; Charles Bouchard (1950, d. 1915), 7 pages.

II

ACADEMIC PERSPECTIVES ON CLINICAL SCIENCE

6

Water Cures and Science:
The Academy and Mineral Waters

During the nineteenth century the Academy of Medicine played a predominant role in the regulation and scientific study of spas and mineral waters. No one, I think, would argue that this represented the most important work done in the academy. There were, when all is said, few fundamental scientific discoveries in this domain. Nor were there many obvious repercussions for public health. Using the criterion of national mortality statistics, one discovers that the institutional activities of the nineteenth century which contributed most to saving lives were unquestionably those related to smallpox vaccination. And yet there was a special status attached to the academy's mineral waters activity which made it one of the subjects of a celebratory essay at the institution's centenary celebration in 1920. There is thus much to be learned about the academy from a chapter devoted exclusively to this aspect of its endeavors.

But if I examine the academy's role in this sector at an intensified level of magnification, I do so, first of all, because the academy provides a privileged perspective on the sizable and largely unexplored world of spas and mineral waters. Second, the academy's activity in the elaboration of a science of hydrology has much to tell us about the nature of clinical medical science in the nineteenth century. It thus allows us to make a small contribution to the sociology of medical knowledge. Third, this subject permits us to bring to the fore the specificity of the French medical tradition and, more generally, the profound divergences between European and North American medical traditions.[1]

There is a particularly striking contrast between the medicine of Europe and that of North America in the therapeutic use of mineral waters. The eminent historian Henry Sigerist remarked on this fact fifty years ago while criticizing North Americans for ignoring their considerable hydrological resources.[2] Distinctions in this respect between the two continents continue to be remarkable. Unlike Americans, Europeans in large numbers drink, bathe, shower, inhale, and introduce into various orifices waters of different types and at a variety of temperatures. In France, Italy, and Germany several million people spend time each year at a spa.[3] Approximately 600,000 French people annually take full cures (usually lasting three weeks) under strict medical supervision. The French government funds more than 85 percent of these through the national health insurance system. Since 1970 the number of medically supervised cures in France has risen by more than 40 percent.[4]

The European outlook is not completely rosy. The spas of England have declined to virtual insignificance.[5] Everywhere, it is claimed that water therapy is badly represented in medical curricula and that it does not attract the best young doctors. Certain spas specializing in diseases now treated easily and effectively by chemotherapies face serious economic difficulties. French observers complain—unjustifiably according to Christian Jamot—that French spas are underutilized in comparison with those of European competitors. They are probably on firmer ground when they observe that the identification of spas in that country with the health insurance system has led both wealthy French and foreign curists to the more luxurious spas of central Europe and has, more generally, severely constrained the expansion of the waters industry. Such complaints notwithstanding, water cures remain firmly entrenched as part of French and European medicine.

Differing medical attitudes to mineral waters on the two continents are to some extent due to cultural traditions. European doctors, in comparison to those of North America, tend to be relatively more attracted to therapeutics that are natural and holistic. There is also a greater tolerance for medical traditions and experience that do not meet the rigorous standards of demonstration characteristic of physiological and clinical testing.[6] This European attitude was wonderfully expressed by Sigerist:

> It is very unscientific to deny the experience of 2000 years merely because we have no ready-made theory that explains all phenomena in every detail. It would have been foolish to deny the existence of lightning because electricity was not yet known. Experience has preceded science in medicine more than once.[7]

Whatever the cultural differences at work, structural factors also come into play. Mineral cures in North America represented an essentially entrepreneurial activity with few links to public health agencies or academic medicine. In certain parts of Europe, however, mineral waters constituted a quasi-public form of healing from whose exploitation the state profited directly and in which the academic medical elite was directly involved in both regulatory and scientific capacities. It is this connection, I would argue, that has kept water cures within the frontiers of clinical medicine in some parts of Europe.

In making this last statement, I am not suggesting that European medicine is less scientific because the water cure (or "thermalism," as it is known in France) has not disappeared. I am arguing rather that in each national context, the survival or disappearance of the water cure as part of medicine depended on the number and power of institutions committed to its survival and development. It is relatively easy to demonstrate how the economic importance of European spas, which became a major sector of the tourist industry, required that these be protected and promoted by governments. In this chapter, however, I hope to show that in France, at least, important groups *within* the medical elite were committed for historical reasons to thermalism as a medical and scientific enterprise.

Demonstrating this point does not of course prove that the link between spas and elite medicine was a major factor in the survival of French thermalism in the twentieth century. A demonstration of this sort would have to center on medical developments in the period following World War II, particularly the setting up of a comprehensive health insurance system. This chapter proposes somewhat more modestly to lay the groundwork for such a demonstration by investigating the connection between the Parisian medical elite and mineral waters in France through the work of the Academy of Medicine. It will argue that during the first half of the nineteenth century the emerging science of hydrology, which served as the chief link between the medical elite and the waters industry, was shaped by the academy's need to combine scientific and administrative functions. After mid-century, a partial and gradual separation of scientific from administrative roles created a variety of difficulties and new opportunities. The academy's mineral waters commission, unlike most of the institution's other permanent commissions, did not abandon its scientific role for more purely administrative functions, primarily, I argue, because of its traditional close links to clinical medical practice and the chemical laboratory. More briefly, this chapter will also suggest that besides lending scientific credibility to the water cure, the academic hydrology that emerged at the end of the nineteenth century came eventually to shape French thermalism in its own "biomedical" image.

The Role of the Academy of Medicine

As popular works on the subject invariably point out, the medicinal use of mineral waters goes back at least to Antiquity. In France, however, the water cure was, until the nineteenth century, a predominantly local therapy since few provisions for travelers existed. If a handful of prerevolutionary spas like Vichy were patronized by the rich and famous, they do not for the most part seem to have achieved the fashionable status or level of conspicuous consumption attained by watering holes like Bath and Baden-Baden. On the other hand, as early as the seventeenth century, French spas could boast a degree of medical supervision and control that was unusual.[8] This provided the framework for the major expansion of installations and clienteles that occurred in the mid-nineteenth century. The number of French curists in 1822 was estimated at about 30,000.[9] By the end of the century there were well over 300,000 at 160 or so major springs.[10] Many other French men and women were drinking bottled water from over 1,100 authorized springs.

The links between spas, the French state, and elite medicine have been particularly close since the early seventeenth century when Henry IV appointed his First Physician as Superintendent of Baths and Mineral Fountains. In the nineteenth and twentieth centuries, the major instrument of this intersection was the Academy of Medicine, which in 1823 took over tasks previously fulfilled by a succession of committees and institutions like the eighteenth-century Royal Society of Medicine.[11] The academy was during the course of the nineteenth century joined in this task by other institutions and agencies, most notably the state corps of mining engineers, responsible for underground installations and channeling, and the national Consultative Committee of Public Hygiene. But to the extent that there existed a French science of balneology or hydrology, it is the Academy of Medicine that played a predominant role in its development.

Most of the academy's activity in this area occurred within its permanent commission for mineral waters. Unlike the sister vaccination commission, whose controversial debates regularly spilled over into the discussions of the entire academy, the mineral waters commission ordinarily functioned on unproblematic terrain and only occasionally required the active intervention of the entire academy. In all its tasks related to mineral waters, the academy tried to combine the technical and administrative functions that made it useful to the government with its mandate to advance hydrological science.

One of the academy's major functions was to authorize the use of new mineral waters. Authorization was based on chemical analyses carried out in the academy's laboratory. The commission did not ordinarily make judgments about therapeutic efficacy. It simply determined whether a specific water contained significant amounts of mineral elements and whether its chemical composition bore similarity to that of one of the known waters with recognized therapeutic properties. While less than 60 percent of the requests received a positive verdict during the early 1860s, over 70 percent were approved during the early 1880s, with the approval rate approaching 90 percent at the end of the decade. The academy did not become more lenient in its judgments. Rather, as mineral waters turned into big business, those seeking authorization became increasingly proficient in strictly following the administrative procedures for submitting waters for analysis.

Authorizations were requested in increasing numbers, stretching the capacities of the academy's laboratory to its limits. From 1820 to 1870 the academy authorized the exploitation of a little over 400 sources. During the next thirty years, powerfully stimulated by Franco-German political, commercial, and scientific competition, as well as by changing patterns of bourgeois leisure and sociability, nearly 1,200 French sources were granted authorizations. Only a small minority of course became real spas. Many others provided bottled water for home cures or normal drinking. The academy, for its part, was continually trying to make this "gatekeeping" function more effective. By the end of the nineteenth century, it had added bacteriological analyses to the authorization procedure.

During the first half of the century authorization was usually restricted to French waters. Foreign waters were only approved if they possessed properties absent from any French sources (like the original Seltzer water). Academicians were keenly aware of economic realities and tried to protect from foreign competition French waters which they believed to be inherently superior to those available elsewhere. By the end of the nineteenth century, however, international commercial realities forced the academy to be relatively liberal about authorizing bottled foreign waters.[12]

The chemical analyses performed by the academy were also viewed as one of the primary means of advancing hydrological science. Hydrology was modestly represented among the various types of communications presented before the academy but it was not a subject about which many doctors had much expertise. There were no teaching positions in the field and few physicians resided in or near spas until the last third of the nineteenth century. The academy itself relied on a small number of members who took turns serving on its mineral waters commission. This commission, in turn, based its work largely on the corps of inspectors appointed by the government to be its representatives in the larger spa towns.

The 100–125 inspectors in this corps were the successors of the intendants of mineral waters brought into existence in the early seventeenth century. They were, by the nineteenth century, expected to study scientifically the properties of local waters, supervise the medical functioning of spas, suggest improvements to the appropriate authorities, and provide free medical care to indigents. Although they were supposed to receive salaries from the spa establishment to which they were attached, most of their income came from private practice. They were also required to submit to the academy annual reports about the waters under their jurisdiction; these reports were to provide information about such matters as the numbers of patients and their illnesses, treatments, and outcomes, needed improvements, weather conditions, and estimates of the monies spas added to the regional economy. These reports served in turn as the basis for an annual survey of the nation's mineral waters, which the academy's mineral waters commission prepared for the government.

One rationale for these reports was administrative. The government sought detailed knowledge about the workings of spas, institutions with both medical and economic significance. At the same time these reports were an integral part of the academy's scientific work. The reasoning was seldom made explicit, but the model for this, as for the reports of the other permanent commissions, clearly came from public health statistics; the aim was to set down information in a logical manner so that correlations among what we would call variables could be made visible.[13] The key question in this case was the extent to which a particular water could be shown to be especially effective against particular diseases or conditions. The goal was to determine each water's therapeutic specificity (understood as a range of therapeutic effects from the very to the less strong). Crucial to this task were the elaboration and constant improvement of questionnaires whether in the form of synoptic tables (*tableaux*) or more detailed case notebooks (*cahiers*) that forced inspectors to note information in the most logical and complete form possible and which "filled out scrupulously and with discernment [are] finally capable of leading to positive results."[14]

The inspectors were not merely passive purveyors of information; they were encouraged to supplement their tables with manuscripts reporting on their personal research whether clinical, physiological, or chemical. But it was the task of the academy which received and processed all their information to synthesize hydrological knowledge so that the nuances of every water (and every form of its utilization) could be correlated on a national scale to the nuances of every physical condition and disease. This centralized vision of hydrological knowledge (understood primarily as therapeutic knowledge) thus depended on "a well-organized inspectorate which constitutes the best means of coordinating into a unit [*un faisceau*] all the progressive acquisitions of hydrology."[15]

However, in reality, many inspectors, like the correspondents of other permanent commissions, stubbornly resisted the data-gathering and research roles assigned to them. In any given year a majority of the inspectors were likely to have neglected to submit reports. Many of those sent were of poor quality, made up of speculative claims for the miraculous powers of the local waters. Diagnostic categories were imprecise and administrative statistics about the use of waters incomplete. The commission used pretty much the same tactics as other permanent commissions to improve numbers and quality, relying on both the carrot and the stick. Its annual survey published in the journal of the academy contained long summaries of the inspectors' views, including their complaints against spa proprietors. The names of sources for which reports were lacking were prominently displayed. In response to complaints from inspectors, attempts were made in 1837 and 1848 to improve the tables that had to be filled in. From the mid-1850s medals were presented to authors of the best reports. The outstanding hydrologists among the inspectors might expect to be elected corresponding members of the academy. Occasionally the ministry was cajoled into issuing warnings that almost always led to a temporary rise in the number of reports received. But none of these tactics resolved the problem.

The inadequacies of these reports as administrative documents, together with inspectors' failures to fulfill other supervisory tasks, were more disturbing to the government than any scientific weaknesses. At the end of the 1850s the government appears to have considered abolishing the inspectorate, which led to a substantial but unfortunately temporary rise in the numbers of inspectors' reports received. In 1862, following a recommendation by the academician François Mélier, inspector-general of mineral waters, the ministry ordered local inspectors to send the administrative segment of their report to the Consultative Committee of Public Hygiene (the main advisory body to the national government on public health matters) rather than to the academy. Initial reaction in the academy was relief that an administrative burden had been lifted; energy could now be devoted exclusively to scientific activity. In reality, however, the annual surveys of the mineral waters commission changed hardly at all. They continued to include administrative information and to feature demands for local improvement made by the inspectors. Hydrologists in the academy saw themselves as the true defenders of the interests of mineral waters and could not resist becoming involved in local details as well as large policy issues. They used the annual survey of the mineral waters commission to regularly defend a number of general positions.

First, the academy stood for the development of adequate facilities around mineral waters; these included comfortable living premises for guests, improved transportation, and above all thoroughly hygienic circumstances for the complete panoply of therapeutic facilities. Academicians were well aware and regularly reminded ministers of the economic importance of mineral waters for specific regions and for the country as a whole. It was clear to the hydrologists in the academy that France could compete with central European spas only if it was willing to make significant capital investments in facilities.

Second, the academy stood for maintaining the purity of sources; purity was synonymous with therapeutic efficacy. Any adulteration or change in the composition of waters was vigorously condemned. The academy in fact eventually concluded and convinced the government that authorization should be temporally limited since waters might be transformed deliberately or accidentally during the course of commercial exploitation.[16] Since any transportation of waters might lead to chemical change, hydrologists insisted that only on-site cures were effective. Later in the century when bottling waters became a large-scale industry, hydrologists insisted for similar reasons that all bottling be done at the source.[17] The academy and other regulatory bodies like the Committee for Public Hygiene also became increasingly opposed to the manufacture of synthetic mineral waters.[18] It seemed clearly impossible to reproduce the complexity of even the simplest water.[19]

Third, the academy stood for medical authority over waters. During the first half of the nineteenth century its annual survey scrupulously recorded the complaints of inspectors about their lack of control over cures and insisted regularly on the need to subject the utilization of waters to a doctor's supervision. The properties of certain waters were too powerful, they argued, the modalities of treatment too complex, subtle, and individualized to allow curists to proceed without medical direction. And some spas actually implemented rules to this effect. However, no French government in the nineteenth century would accept the identification of waters with dangerous medicines. In 1860, in fact, the government of the Second Empire officially proclaimed the principle of unrestricted use of waters forcing certain spas to abandon the medical controls that had been introduced.[20] This situation was a continuing source of discontent for hydrologists in the academy, who regularly reminded the ministry of the dangers presented by the lack of regulation. Most wanted all therapies at an establishment to be under the direction of the local inspector. At the very least, patients should be required to show a prescription from a licensed doctor.

The academy also stood for medical authority in the face of commercial interests. Owners and administrators of spa establishments were perceived as fundamentally unscrupulous in pursuit of profit. The only counterbalance to commercial greed was medical authority. One of the reasons the academy consistently campaigned for the expansion of the powers of local inspectors, despite its own unhappiness with their performance, was that these were the only possible instruments of medical authority. They seemed the sole barrier to an unbridled commercialism that would tarnish the reputation of French water. However, if the academy's annual survey of mineral waters is to be believed, the diminution of inspectors' power over patients in the nineteenth century went hand in hand with growing impotence with respect to proprietors.

Hydrological Science in the Academy

The academy's influence on government policy regarding mineral waters was, as we have seen, rather meager. The academy, however, was predominant when it came to the scientific study of waters. No other institution competed with it in this domain. Nevertheless, the academy's scientific activity was severely constrained by circumstances and by hydrologists' perceptions of the waters industry.

Hydrologists viewed their science as vital to the economic prosperity of spas, which were themselves a source of national wealth. Few members of the academy doubted that the therapeutic effectiveness of water cures for chronic ailments had been proven by centuries of practical experience.[21] But most believed that a great deal of irrational and sometimes harmful activity took place in spas because of the widespread lack of knowledge of the actual properties of each water. This made it easy to discredit water cures, especially in view of widespread medical skepticism that was frequently alluded to in hydrological writing.[22]

The prosperity of the spa industry would be ensured if water cures were made rational, so that physicians fully understood the range of conditions for which each water was useful. Explaining the mechanisms through which waters acted on the body might be part of this task but was secondary to the precise determination of therapeutic efficacy. Debates in the academy on matters of hydrology almost always centered on whether a particular water or new mode of treatment was indeed effective against a particular condition.

A second constraint had to do with scientific personnel. The public health model of collecting information from informants for processing by a central authority did not just reflect a certain style of knowledge. It was dictated by administrative necessity. For much of the nineteenth century inspectors were the only doctors in a position to do research on mineral waters. With limited time at their disposal, they were required to provide basic statistics about waters for administrative purposes. It was sensible to try to use scientifically the administrative information they were required to provide.

Inspectors were encouraged by the academy to pursue research in addition to collecting information. In 1828 the mineral waters commission drew up two sets of instructions to orient the research efforts of inspectors. The first listed five topics for individualized research including studies of the chemical composition of waters and the effects of specific waters on animals of different types and on humans of different age, race, and sex. A second set of instructions explained the procedures for the proper chemical analysis of waters.[23] Similar encouragement was offered regularly in subsequent years, and some inspectors made an effort to comply but most lacked both time and training for serious research.[24] Consequently, the collection of clinical statistics necessarily predominated among them.

By and large the quality of the hydrological knowledge produced in this way was recognized to be poor.[25] It was not just that many inspectors did not submit reports or that their data were incomplete if not worthless. The whole enterprise was fraught with difficulties. Diagnostic categories, the basis for any classification, were highly imprecise. Waters could more easily be typed but sophisticated methods of chemical analysis uncovered an increasing complexity of composition that called into question the whole effort to classify waters into a manageable number of basic categories. How, moreover, could an inspector rigorously determine the effect of a particular cure if his observation of the patient inevitably came to an end when the latter went home? (This was especially problematic since it was widely believed that full relief from a chronic condition could be expected only several months after completion of the cure.) How in fact did one judge improvement or cure in cases of chronic disease, which predominated at spas? Furthermore, the growing tendency to submit patients to a wide array of thermal procedures, including showers and inhalation as well as the more traditional drinking and bathing; the utilization of waters at various temperatures and potencies; and the fact that other types of medications were imbibed along with waters made it virtually impossible to attribute cures to any specific factor.[26] It is hardly surprising that the few efforts to make serious statistical correlations of spas and disease showed that most of the large spas handled a similarly wide variety of ailments and had very similar rates of success for each.[27] One could attribute such results to the general tonic properties of all waters and to the fact that all provided patients with a rest in the country. But this interpretation called into question the drive for therapeutic specificity that seemed necessary to make hydrology fully "modern."

Many of these difficulties were hardly unique to mineral waters. Therapeutic evaluation of all kinds was problematic in the absence of widely accepted methods of clinical testing. But even the rough and ready efforts at increasing the rigor of evaluations so characteristic of Parisian hospital medicine were beyond the capacities of hydrologists coping with especially fluid diagnostic categories, multiple modes of therapy, and, most significantly, patients who were far less tractable than the patients of modest means who peopled the Parisian hospitals.

Consequently, while more rigorous procedures for clinical testing of waters were frequently proposed, they were never carried out. One suggestion made was to establish near waters more hospitals in which doctors "could make more complete observations."[28] But in the few hospitals that did exist, hospital physicians were not notably more rigorous than their colleagues in reporting to the academy.[29] The annual survey for 1834–36 proposed that patients be given no medication other than waters in order to better evaluate the effects of waters.[30] In 1842 the academy decided to test the disputed effects on scrofula of the waters of Forges-sur-Brie by inviting the Paris hospital administration to send, at its own expense, its scrofula patients to that village. Half would take the waters while the other half would benefit only from the location.[31] Not surprisingly, the test was never carried out.

Physiological science did not provide an alternative model for academic hydrology partly because it was not well suited to explain which waters were most effective for each illness and, perhaps more pertinently, because there was little institutional contact between academic physiology and mineral waters. (When hydrologists referred to physiological testing during the early nineteenth century, they usually meant the study of symptomatic effects.) Unlike chemistry, physiology had no role to play in the administration or authorization of mineral waters. Only in the late nineteenth century, when the number of medical physiologists began to assume sufficient critical mass, could the methods of laboratory physiology become widely utilized in hydrological research.

Hydrological chemistry, as well, despite its very visible role in academic hydrology, could not suggest a new intellectual direction. Chemistry was in certain respects hydrology's main claim to rigorous scientific status. Chemical methods of analysis were becoming highly sophisticated and increasingly capable of identifying trace elements in waters. However, chemistry could not offer a model to hydrologists because so many were ignorant of its procedures and skeptical of its usefulness. Tension between chemistry and clinical therapeutics was frequently expressed in the academy.[32] Even the authorization of waters, ordinarily no more than chemical analysis, could be problematic if the results of chemical analysis contradicted clinical experience. This occurred in 1862 when, after lengthy discussion, the weakly mineralized waters of Forges-les-Bains were authorized on the basis of their history of therapeutic efficacy. The primacy of therapeutic effects over chemical analysis was explicitly affirmed.[33]

The view that chemical composition was totally irrelevant to the therapeutic efficacy of waters (since all waters had pretty much the same effects) gradually declined during the course of the nineteenth century. But even the hydrologists sympathetic to chemistry had to admit that chemical composition could not fully account for their action since chemically similar waters frequently had very different therapeutic effects while chemically different waters sometimes behaved similarly.[34] Even if one admitted that specific mineral properties that could be analyzed chemically gave waters their therapeutic powers, chemical analysis still brought little knowledge of therapeutic effects beyond provoking speculation about how certain waters worked. Therapeutics, the primary concern of most academic hydrologists, could be based only on some form of *clinical* science.[35] Collecting data on the model of public health statistics seemed in fact one of the few ways to bridge the gap between chemistry and therapeutics. It was supposed to permit the academy to mine inspectors' reports in order to process these two types of knowledge into data which might show clear correlations between chemical composition and the capacity to heal particular diseases.[36]

Inspectors' reports rarely permitted such correlations. Instead the academy usually received "under the name clinical studies, views that are more or less ingenious, more or less exact, about the curative properties of the waters of the station in this or that illness, the whole thing demonstrated with the help of some well-chosen observations."[37] The weaknesses of the public health statistics model did not become immediately apparent because in the academy's early years, the annual survey of the mineral waters commission appeared infrequently. It was easy to blame its inadequacies on the failure of inspectors to submit proper reports. The problem was also masked by the fact that the man who wrote most of the early annual surveys knew pretty much what the inspectors' data were supposed to demonstrate.

Philibert Patissier,[38] who was the most influential hydrologist of the early nineteenth century, had a well-developed theory of the action of medical waters loosely based on the neogalenic theories of the eighteenth-century physician Théophile de Bordeu. Like many of those who studied mineral waters, Patissier believed in both the general tonic effects of waters and their chemical specificity. In his view, the general effects observable for all waters were due to their capacity to stimulate secretions and excretions, along with the benefits of resting in the country. The specific effects stemmed from the different chemical compositions of waters, which, along with their temperature, determined the particular degree of stimulation. More important, their chemical composition allowed waters absorbed by the circulatory system to transform the constitution of body solids and humors. The mode of taking waters also made a difference since drink allowed water to come into contact with the gastrointestinal mucous membranes, whereas baths stimulated the integumentary membrane.

Consequently, each type of water was most, though not exclusively effective for particular kinds of maladies. Sulfurous waters, for instance, were especially efficacious for skin diseases, waters with bicarbonate of soda were highly effective for digestive problems, and the alkaline waters of Mont-Dore were particularly good for chronic chest ailments. But the therapeutic use of waters was no simple matter. The physician had also to take account of the intensity of the malady and the age, condition, and even income of the patient in recommending a complex and highly individualized water regimen.[39]

Having as he did his own elaborate account of the operation of different waters on diseases (and his reports contained detailed tables correlating maladies with the most appropriate waters), Patissier did not really require complete reports from all inspectors, although he regularly demanded them. In every survey he wrote, he reformulated his account and mined the inspectors' reports for data and opinions which supported, qualified, or extended what was already known. More often than not he merely reproduced without comment the statistical tables that had been sent to him. Under such conditions the fundamental weaknesses of the public health statistics model did not become widely apparent.

In the post-Patissier period after 1850, and in the absence of any single dominant personality, the surveys lost focus. They became critical summaries of the reports and manuscripts submitted by inspectors, followed by a list of inspectors awarded medals for their work. A semblance of scientific order was maintained by grouping the discussion of reports according to a shifting chemical classification of waters. But even this practice disappeared in the 1870s to be replaced first by an alphabetical principle of ordering according to the name of the spa and later by one based on the quality of the submitted work. Any theory of how mineral waters worked pretty much disappeared from the post-1850 surveys until the 1880s. Patissier's successors were content to repeat without much comment the views found in the works they examined.

The statistics-gathering model was widely seen to be unworkable by the 1860s though it continued to have its defenders.[40] The promulgation in the early 1860s of regulations allowing patients to take waters without medical supervision made it impossible for inspectors to accumulate complete statistics. The decision to have inspectors send the administrative portion of their report to the Committee of Public Hygiene also removed an important rationale for the academy's concern with statistics. By then the academy was in any case vigorously supporting the second traditional aspect of its hydrological activity: encouraging and rewarding individual scientific work. Increasingly, local inspectors were submitting manuscripts in addition to and usually more substantial than their formal reports. These were as likely to win medals as were the reports. The academy also began to receive submissions from and award medals to individuals who were not members of the corps of inspectors. The academy could even award cash prizes for meritorious research through the Capuron Prize competition established in 1851.[41] From the 1850s, moreover, academic hydrologists worked closely with the most ambitious of the local inspectors to promote research in the Paris Society for Medical Hydrology as well as in several scientific journals.

This model of academic intellectual activity was not new. But rather than being seen as complementary to the public health statistics model, it was increasingly being viewed as an alternative to it. It too depended primarily on local inspectors who made up the bulk of researchers in the field; but instead of providing data to be processed by the academy, these inspectors were to constitute a corps of researchers whose work was stimulated and rewarded by the academy.

This form of scientific activity was in many ways as illusory as the statistical model; inspectors were busy practitioners with heavy administrative duties and often lacked both the leisure and the scientific training to do research at a high level. But it was more in keeping with developing norms of scientific activity than was the gathering of statistical information. It was thus hoped that the work of inspectors could be improved. One remedy for low quality was thought to be a greater role for the academy in the nomination of inspectors. This would ensure more scientific competence and industriousness than the present system of recruitment, which was largely political. Training in hydrology for future inspectors also seemed to be in order. The academy took a small step in this direction by instituting the Vulfranc Gerdy Prize in 1863 in order to allow medical students to spend a year or two doing research on mineral waters. But the number of candidates for the prize was small.[42] From 1875 the academy began appealing regularly for the creation of courses and chairs of hydrology in the medical faculties.

During the 1860s and 1870s the two models of hydrological knowledge coexisted in uneasy equilibrium. The public health model of research might conceivably have disappeared gradually as a result of changing criteria of scientific practice. Similarly, the academy's reliance on inspectors would undoubtedly have lessened as more physicians and scientists working in a growing network of laboratories developed an interest in hydrology. But the fate of the academy's traditional mode of hydrological activity was sealed precipitously when the government eliminated the office of local inspector on which it was based.

Abolishing the Inspectorate

For the Academy of Medicine, we saw, the inspectorate represented medical power within the expanding spa industry and provided the personnel for hydrological science. Neither of these functions, it was widely admitted, was well performed. But the solutions envisioned by the academy were to expand the administrative powers of inspectors and to transform their scientific role through better recruitment and education. Other forces, however, were pushing in another direction.

The pressure to abolish the office of local inspector was inspired initially by the small but growing number of physicians who had begun to settle in spa villages (often on a seasonal basis). They deeply resented the existence of semiofficial competitors whose visibility attracted wealthy private patients. There were only about four hundred spa physicians in 1880 but they were highly vocal. They were supported, defenders of the inspectorate charged, by owners of establishments who wished to be freed of troublesome medical adversaries.[43]

A bill to abolish the inspectorate came before the legislature in 1872. It appears to have had the backing of the Ministry of Commerce but gained little support within the medical establishment where it was opposed by both the public health administration and the General Association of French Physicians, representing the organized medical profession.[44] Nevertheless, the Academy of Medicine took advantage of the situation to mount a vigorous defense of the inspectorate while at the same time demanding its reform. Among the recommendations made was that official reports be abolished and that inspectors be encouraged to submit original scientific manuscripts. The academy also demanded a role in the nomination of inspectors. To satisfy some of the aspirations of spa physicians, the academy suggested that these be organized in each center into a consulting committee meeting once each year to suggest needed improvements.[45]

The inspectorate was, in this instance, neither abolished nor reformed. The minister of commerce wrote to the academy in 1875 to explain why he considered the statistical reports of the inspectors vital.[46] But the forces arrayed against the inspectorate were increasing in strength. Most ominously for the academy, the public health administration was gradually coming to the conclusion that the inspectorate was an inadequate basis for the administration of mineral waters. It wished moreover to integrate the regulation and inspection of waters into a reorganized and unified public health administration which it hoped to establish.

The first steps were innocuous enough. In 1883 the legislature passed a law stating that inspectors were not to receive a public salary. The motive seems to have been a desire to save money. Regulations governing the inspectorate specified that inspectors were to receive a small salary paid by the spa establishment and guaranteed by the government. No one took either provision seriously until 1881 when two inspectors who had been dismissed from their posts sued the government for back salaries and won. Fearing that the judgment would establish a dangerous and expensive legal precedent, the government protected itself by legally eliminating salaries. In the process, it promised to review the entire administrative structure governing mineral waters.[47]

Soon after, the government kept its promise by appointing an extraparliamentary committee dominated by politicians and administrators but including three representatives of the Committee of Public Hygiene. After nearly two years of debate, the commission agreed on a plan to abolish the local inspectorate and transfer its administrative and scientific functions to four national inspectors, each responsible for an extended region of the country. Such national inspectors, it was believed, would be in a far better position to serve the national government than local inspectors dependent on the good will of proprietors. Nor could they be viewed as unfair competitors by local practitioners.[48] Nonetheless, and despite vigorous support from several academicians representing the public health administration, the academy rejected the proposal and once again affirmed its support for the inspectorate. Only inspectors, the academy argued, could ensure adequate medical control of waters.[49]

The public health administration, however, was less concerned with medical control than with effective administration. The position it took was based on a distinction between administrative and medical roles. Inspectors were simply not up to the required tasks of administrative supervision. They were too involved in the activities of the spas to effectively supervise and inspect and they lacked the required expertise. Paul Brouardel, president of the Consultative Committee of Public Hygiene, argued in the academy that the inspection of waters should be taken over by local public health councils that would be more independent of entrepreneurs and that could respond more flexibly to problems by sending chemists, engineers, or doctors, as the situation warranted. From an administrative perspective, medical expertise was only one of several types of expertise needed.[50] The Committee of Public Hygiene rallied behind the plan of its president, Brouardel, in April 1888.[51] On June 22, 1889, the government issued a decree eliminating about three-quarters of the inspectors. The surviving inspectors gradually disappeared through attrition.

In the first survey of the mineral waters commission that followed the academy's debate on the inspectorate, Albert Robin,[52] himself newly elected to the academy, issued a call for a program of experimental research into the physiological and clinical effects of mineral waters based on the premise that waters affected cell nutrition. He called as well for laboratories to be set up at each spa and faculty courses in hydrology to be introduced.[53] The abandonment of hydrological statistics by the academy's mineral waters commission occurred just at the time when other permanent commissions were moving to consolidate their statistics-gathering activity. (See Chapter 4.)

There seem to have been two reasons for this unique situation. First, the government clearly lost interest in the forms of administrative statistics which constituted the commission's stock-in-trade. Unlike statistics about epidemic outbreaks, infant mortality, or vaccinations, the dubious therapeutic statistics coming out of spas had little significance for public health. Second, the mineral waters commission was never totally committed to this form of administrative knowledge because it also utilized clinical and chemical models of medical knowledge. In contrast, the epidemics and infant hygiene commissions, which lacked alternative prototypes of knowledge production, were irrevocably tied to the public health statistics model.

The Twentieth Century

One should not exaggerate the effects of either the elimination of inspectors or the abandonment of statistics. The mineral waters commission continued to play an administrative role into the twentieth century. Without the annual reports submitted by inspectors, the commission could no longer keep in touch with the details of spa life. But its other functions remained unchanged. It continued to serve as the main body authorizing the exploitation of new springs. From the 1930s its mandate expanded to the authorization of "climatic stations" whose climate was believed to have therapeutic benefits.[54] A law passed in 1939 gave the academy the further task of distinguishing climatic stations devoted to the cure of tuberculosis from those of more general therapeutic rest (station de villégiature).[55] It continued to press for improvements in the legislation that regulated the use of mineral waters, focusing in the early twentieth century on the regulation of bottled waters.[56] It repeatedly urged that tourist facilities be upgraded, recognizing that this was the only way to compete against the spas of central Europe. Nor did it abandon efforts to bring spas under medical control; several annual surveys, for instance, discussed the need to harmonize the diet provided by hotels with the therapeutic regimen.[57] In the late 1930s the academy directly took on a powerful spa industry fearful of medical monopoly by repeatedly advising the government that the use of many waters be subject to a doctor's referral. It also suggested that prominently displayed signs in each establishment warn of the dangers of unsupervised use of facilities.[58]

As the local inspectors disappeared, the commission's scientific role failed to expand notably. Its main scientific task, in fact, became the administration of an annual prize competition for works on mineral waters submitted to the academy.[59] It used this forum to encourage more sophisticated experimental and clinical research on the effects of waters. By the 1920s the commission was mainly receiving works sent by spa physicians and based on clinical observation.[60]

As time went on, however, even these modified annual surveys of submitted publications became increasingly unrepresentative of hydrological science. The reporter for the mineral waters commission complained in 1936 that only fifteen works had been sent in that year. The following year the winner of the commission's highest prize was the organizer of a large resource book summarizing information on all the thermal and climatic centers of France. Its merits were clearly practical rather than scientific.[61] In both 1938 and 1939 the annual report of the mineral waters commission abandoned all pretence of rewarding recent work. It awarded its medals to individuals who had over the years made major contributions to mineral waters. Some of those honored in this way had advanced science; others, like Geist, who organized regular tours of French spas to familiarize French and foreign doctors with national hydrological resources, had contributed in more practical ways.[62] Clearly, the mineral waters commission was no longer at the forefront of hydrological science.

The real hydrological work of the academy was now localized in the papers read before the entire academy. During the 1920s a small number of scientific papers on mineral waters were presented and the number increased during the 1930s. Often presented by members of the academy,[63] they were usually written by nonmembers working in the network of laboratories that had recently been established in medical faculties, scientific institutions, and the largest spas.

In the early twentieth century the mineral waters industry began to devote substantial resources to hydrological science. By the 1930s most medical faculties in France were offering industry-subsidized courses in hydrology. An industry-sponsored Institute of Hydrology was created at the Collège de France, after the Paris Faculty of Medicine turned it down. Hydrology was recognized as an academic medical specialty when a special *agrégation* in this subject was established in 1933.[64] Larger watering holes like Vichy and even smaller ones like Bourbonne-les-Bains established their own institutes and research laboratories. The papers read at the Academy of Medicine thus represented only the tip of a research and publication iceberg.

Looking at the hydrological papers appearing in the *Bulletin*, one is struck by the relative absence of practical therapeutics, the subject that had dominated nineteenth-century academic writings. Most papers were resolutely laboratory-based. Characteristically, they utilized some recently developed instrument in order to analyze waters in new ways,[65] much as hydrologist-chemists of the nineteenth century had operated, or used physiological procedures to demonstrate some metabolic effect in animals or humans of imbibing or bathing in certain waters.[66]

The lack of therapeutic data is not really surprising. By the twentieth century experienced hydrologists "knew" which waters were useful for which conditions. In 1920 the leading hydrologist in the academy could point to recent research in the field and blithely remark that it would have little impact on thermal practices, which were the product of several centuries of practical experience.[67] What then was the function of all the laboratory data?

First, just as they had done during the nineteenth century, chemistry and physiology provided theories that could be used to "explain" why some waters seemed to work to ameliorate certain conditions while others did not. Evidence of increased tissue oxidation or increased elimination of uric acid could, with some leaps in logic, be used to explain perceived therapeutic effects. Second, even without making therapeutic connections, simply demonstrating that waters affected metabolism served to refute the most common criticism of water therapy: that rest in the country rather than water was responsible for any "cures" which took place. All these physiological data might not demonstrate therapeutic efficacy but they did show physiological effect, which was the next best thing. And third, such research associated hydrology with the latest and most up-to-date laboratory techniques. By producing the appropriate graphs and tables, researchers situated hydrology, and by extension water cures, within mainstream "scientific" medicine. No one seems to have doubted that sophisticated laboratory-produced knowledge would validate and facilitate the acknowledged patriotic task of augmenting the reputation and profitability of France's system of mineral waters.

By this time the Academy of Medicine was no longer the only, or even the major medical institution concerned with the science of mineral waters. It continued, however, to be the most prestigious and a visible reminder of the commitment of the nation's greatest physicians to the system of mineral waters. As it had in the past, the academy rewarded, sometimes with membership in the academy, medical scientists who pursued hydrological research and encouraged its own members to take the field seriously. One can document this latter point by referring to the sales catalogue put out in 1939 by Masson, one of the leading medical publishers in Paris. Thirteen works published between 1932 and 1936 were listed under the rubric *Hydro-Climatologie*. Fourteen individuals appeared as authors or coauthors, in several cases more than once. Of these, no fewer than nine were already or would be elected members of the academy. All four of those who authored or coauthored two or three publications were or would become academicians.[68] It would be hard to make a better case for the strong link between the science of mineral waters and the Academy of Medicine in the early twentieth century.

Hydrological knowledge in nineteenth-century France was dominated by a state institution, the Academy of Medicine, because governments required or thought they required certain kinds of information. The needs of the administration profoundly shaped the direction that hydrology took in the nineteenth century, partly explaining the emphasis on chemical analysis (a requirement for authorization of waters) and public health statistics. By appointing inspectors of mineral waters, the state also provided the academy with a cadre of researchers in hydrology whose level of knowledge and skill helped define the boundaries of the field.

If the state both made possible and shaped hydrological science, the benefits of this knowledge to state power were less evident. This undoubtedly accounts for the government's growing indifference after 1850 to the system of knowledge (and its institutional manifestations) constructed by the academy. It was the state's gradual retreat from the domain of hydrological knowledge, culminating in the elimination of inspectors, which gave the academy free rein to abandon the public health model of hydrology and move firmly in the direction of individual research.

The relationship of the academy to the private spa industry was a complex mixture of complicity and conflict. On one level, the work of the academy was self-consciously intended to increase the profitability of spa resorts. Investments by entrepreneurs were required in order to equip spas with all necessary technologies and facilities. Yet the resolutely medical orientation of academicians, their insistence on strict medical control over all water therapies, inevitably provoked friction with entrepreneurs.

The academy clearly exercised only limited administrative influence on French thermalism during the nineteenth century, though it did perform an important but technically low-level gatekeeping function based on the chemical analyses of waters. Its scientific influence was much more significant. Out of the motley collection of inspectors, it struggled to create an organized body of researchers in the field. Even by its own criteria, it was not very successful but it helped keep hydrology alive as a scientific specialty in the nineteenth century and invested it with whatever prestige it itself possessed. It also produced a body of medical writing that pretty much confirmed belief in the efficacy of water cures.

From the end of the nineteenth century, the academy in conjunction with other medical institutions pushed the waters industry firmly in the direction of therapeutic specificity. The move has been so successful that critics now view French thermalism as excessively medical to the point where the expansion of the industry is severely constrained. They look enviously at Germany and Italy where, alongside a narrow medically oriented thermalism, there exists a kind of "health tourism" which brings to spas large numbers of people who are not ill.[69] Such criticisms reflect the extent to which waters have been "biomedicalized" by virtue of their association with France's medical and scientific elite. Things may of course be changing. There is evidence to suggest that during the past two decades France's most successful thermal centers have diversified successfully into other forms of tourism.[70]

The academy in the twentieth century has with other institutions also pushed hydrology (now called crenotherapy) firmly in the direction of laboratory experimentation. In the process, it has continued to provide legitimacy to waters as a therapy by providing legitimacy to hydrology as a science. Its activities in this domain have made a clear statement about the value and validity of water cures. In so doing, it has helped keep this therapy within though far from the center of orthodox medicine in spite of its inability to conform easily to dominant models of scientific explanation and therapeutic evaluation.[71] This lack of conformity has led to growing skepticism among doctors in France as elsewhere. However, until relatively recently, the activities of the academy and other institutions of elite medicine defined such difficulties not as reasons to abandon thermalism, but as scientific problems requiring and capable of scientific solutions. That, I would suggest, has been the Academy of Medicine's chief contribution to France's system of mineral waters.

NOTES

1. See, for instance, Lynn Payer, *Medicine and Culture* (New York, 1988).

2. Henry E. Sigerist, "American Spas in Historical Perspective," *Bulletin of the History of Medicine* 11 (1942), 133–47.

3. Thomas Maretzki and Eduard Seidler, "Biomedicine and Naturopathic Healing in West Germany: A Historical and Ethnomedical View of a Stormy Relationship," *Culture,*

Medicine, and Psychiatry 9 (1985), 412, cite the figures of the Confederation of Thermal Stations to the effect that nearly 6 million West Germans take cures annually. Christian Jamot, *Thermalisme et villes thermales en France* (Clermont-Ferrand, 1988), p. 71, gives a more modest West German figure of 2.5 million, only slightly more than the number of curists in Italy and France.

4. Jamot, *Thermalisme et villes*, pp. 70–71; Guy Ebrard, *Le Thermalisme en France: situation actuelle et perspectives d'avenir. Rapport au Président de la République* (1981), p. 27.

5. William Thomson, *Spas that Heal* (London, 1978), pp. 23–31. On the effect of this decline on spa towns see J. A. Patmore, "The Spa Towns of Britain," in *Urbanization and Its Problems: Essays in Honor of E. W. Gilbert*, ed., R. P. Beckinsale and J. M. Houston (Oxford, 1970), pp. 47–69. Also see David Cantor, "The Contradictions of Specialization: Rheumatism and the Decline of the Spa in Inter-war Britain," in *The Medical History of Waters and Spas*, ed. Roy Porter, *Medical History*, Supplement No. 10 (London, 1990), 127–44.

6. This statement is almost impossible to *prove* satisfactorily. For the French case, I base it on twenty years of personal experience. The German situation is discussed by Maretzki and Seidler, "Biomedicine and Naturopathic Healing"; Thomas Maretzki, "Cultural Variation in Biomedicine: The Kur in West Germany," *Medical Anthropology Quarterly* 3(1989), 22–35, and "The *Kur* in West Germany as an Interface between Naturopathic and Allopathic Ideologies," *Social Science and Medicine* 24 (1987), 1061–68; and Paul Unschuld, "The Issue of Structured Coexistence of Scientific and Alternative Medical Systems: A Comparison of East and West German Legislation," *Social Science and Medicine* 14B (1980), 15–24. Some of the differences among European medical systems in this regard are documented by Payer, *Medicine and Culture*.

7. Sigerist, "American Spas," 140.

8. Lawrence W. B. Brockliss, "The Development of the Spa in Seventeenth-Century France," in *The Medical History of Waters and Spas*, ed. Roy Porter, *Medical History*, Supplement No. 10 (London, 1990), 26–27, 34–39. On British spas during this period see Phyllis Hembry, *The English Spa, 1560–1815: A Social History* (London, 1990).

9. E.-H. Guitard, *Le Prestigieux Passé des eaux minérales* (1951), p. 67.

10. Armand Wallon, *La Vie quotidienne dans les villes d'eaux 1850–1914* (1981), p. 118. Also see Paul Gerbod, "Les 'Fièvres thermales' en France au XIXe siècle," *Revue historique*, 277 (1987), 309–34. About a dozen establishments were owned by the state or the military while the rest were the property of private individuals or municipalities.

11. On the role of this institution see Pascale Muller, "Les Eaux minérales en France à la fin du 18e siècle," Mémoire de maîtrise, Université de Paris I 1975; Pascale Cosma-Muller, "Entre science et commerce: les eaux en France à la fin de l'Ancien Régime," *Historical Reflections*, 9 (1982), 249–63; and Caroline Hannaway, "Medicine, Public Welfare and the State in Eighteenth-Century France: The Société Royale de Médecine of Paris (1776–93)," Ph.D. diss., Johns Hopkins University, 1974, chap. 5.

12. This change of policy occurred gradually during the 1880s. In neither 1876 nor 1877 was a foreign water among those analyzed. Five foreign waters were analyzed in 1889, seven in 1892. For a brief debate about the degree of severity which foreign requests required see *BAM* 11 (1882), 82–83.

13. On this subject see William Coleman, *Death Is a Social Disease: Public Health and Political Economy in Early Industrial France* (Madison, Wisc., 1982), chap. 5, and James C. Riley, *The Eighteenth-Century Campaign to Avoid Disease* (London, 1987), esp. chaps. 3 and 4. On the epidemics inquiry of the Société Royale de Médecine, which was in many ways the prototype of academic data-gathering activity, see J. Meyer, "L'Enquête de l'Académie de Médecine sur les épidémies 1774–1794," *Médecins, climat et épidémies à la fin du XVIIIe siècle*, ed. J. P. Desaive et al (1972), pp. 9–20, and Hannaway, "Medicine, Public Welfare and the State," chap. 4.

14. G. Ferrus, "Extrait d'un rapport fait au nom de la Commission des eaux minérales," *AGM* 14 (1827), 68. On efforts to improve information forms, see the minutes of the mineral waters commission, AM Liasse 29, for 1826–30, 1833, 1834, 1837. Also *AGM* 22 (1830), 130–35, and I. Bourdin, "Rapport au nom de la Commission des eaux minérales," *BAM* 14 (1848–49), 499–530.

15. A. Bouchardat, "Rapport général sur les eaux minérales en 1861," *MEM* 26 (1863–64), cxlv. In another expression of this vision, J. Guérard, "Rapport général sur les eaux minérales en 1853," *MEM* 20 (1856), xci, compared the inspection of waters with the system of meteorological stations. "One and the other have as their object to gather carefully the facts of observation relating to the science on which they depend; the analysis of these facts and the utilization of these *units* is the task of the *scholarly corps* whose mission it is to apply them and who are able to bring out the large-scale laws which regulate therapeutics on one hand and terrestrial physics on the other."

16. In the twentieth century the academy began granting authorizations for only a limited period.

17. M. Hanriot, "Rapport général sur les eaux minérales en 1898," *BAM* 44 (1900), 666.

18. J. Regnaud, "Eaux minérales: fabriques en grands d 'eaux minérales dosées," *Recueil de travaux du Comité Consultatif d'Hygiène Publique de la France* 14 (1884), 448–94.

19. Attitudes toward mineral waters were undoubtedly linked to mythical beliefs surrounding water in general. The classic study of water in this respect is Gaston Bachelard, *L'Eau et les rêves: essai sur l'imagination de la matière*, 13th ed. (1976).

20. The academy was equally unsuccessful in winning medical control over therapeutic sea baths. In 1862 the administration abolished the few positions existing for inspectors of sea baths.

21. The author of one annual survey summed it up when he wrote: "in a manner similar to most of our therapeutic agents, natural mineral waters cure sometimes, relieve often and console always." Ph. Patissier, "Rapport général sur les eaux minérales en 1837," *BAM* 3 (1838–39), 478. This attitude is not surprising in view of the fact that hydropathy with non-mineralized waters was a staple of medical and especially hospital practice during the first half of the nineteenth century. See Jean-Pierre Goubert, *La Conquête de l'eau* (1986), pp. 130–43.

22. See, for instance, E. Verjon, "Eaux minérales: modes d'action et effets thérapeutiques," in *Nouveau Dictionnaire de médecine et de chirurgie pratique*, vol. 12 (1870), p. 253.

23. *AGM* 18 (1828), 585–87.

24. The ignorance of many inspectors about the most recent medical innovations is difficult to overstate. In the early 1840s Patissier felt compelled to urge inspectors to take account of Laënnec's diagnostic categories in diseases of the thoracic cavity. *BAM* 6 (1841), 986–87. Another hydrologist complained a decade later that most inspectors did not utilize either auscultation or percussion in establishing diagnoses. I. Bourdon, "Rapport au nom de la Commission des eaux minérales," *BAM* 14 (1848–49), 512. Later a standard complaint was that inspectors did not utilize the most modern diagnostic instruments like the thermometer and sphygmograph. A. Gubler, "Rapport général sur les eaux minérales en 1870–1871," *MEM* 30 (1871–73), 256.

25. For a critical view of hydrology, see J. Raige-Delorme in *AGM* 29 (1852), 122–28.

26. Many of these problems were inherent in the enterprise of public health or "environmental" statistics, as Riley argues in *The Eighteenth-Century Campaign* (esp. chap. 4). To this day, rigorous determination of therapeutic effects remains a problem for holistic therapies. See Manesh S. Patel, "Evaluation of Holistic Medicine," *Social Science and Medicine* 24 (1987), 164–75.

27. Ph. Patissier, "Rapport général sur les eaux minérales en 1847–48," *MEM* 15 (1852), 45–46; A. Devergie, "Rapport général sur les eaux minérales en 1867," *MEM* 29

(1869–70), cccxii; G.-S. Empis, "Rapport général sur les eaux minérales en 1875," *MEM* 32 (1879), cccv.

28. Ferrus, "Extrait d'un rapport," 73.

29. A. Devergie, "Rapport général sur les eaux minérales en 1866," *MEM* 29 (1869–70), cxlix.

30. F.-V. Mérat, "Rapport général sur les eaux minérales en 1834–1836," *MEM* 7 (1838), 49. For more modest variants of this proposal see Ph. Patissier, "Rapport général sur les eaux minérales en 1838–39, *BAM* 6 (1841), 957, and Bourdon, "Rapport au nom," 508.

31. *BAM*, 8 (1842–43), 263–97.

32. See, for example, the discussion within the mineral waters commission in AM Liasse 29, meeting of June 23, 1836, and the exchange between Hayem and Robin in *BAM* 25 (1891), 761–62.

33. *BAM* 27 (1861–62), 828–34.

34. For this reason some hydrologists eagerly seized on the discovery of electrical charges and later radioactivity in some mineral waters to explain therapeutic effects.

35. See, for instance, Devergie, "Rapport général 1866," cxlviii.

36. Philibert Patissier summarized this hope best: "if these *tableaux* are filled in with care and good faith, the academy will be able, in a few years, to make a reasoned judgment about the medicinal effects of the various mineral sources of France, to compare them one with the other, from the point of view of their action in illnesses that are more or less identical, and by comparing this action with the constituent elements of waters, substitute rational principles for the most often empirical criteria which direct doctors in their use [of waters]." "Rapport général 1837," 520. Similar views are expressed in Devergie, "Rapport général 1866," cl.

37. J. Fauvel, "Rapport général sur les eaux minérales en 1877," *MEM* 34 (1883–84), xxi–xxii.

38. Patissier (1791–1863) received his medical degree from the Paris Faculty of Medicine in 1815. He never held an official teaching or hospital position.

39. These basic points recur in most of Patissier's surveys. But for a full explication see especially Patissier, "Rapport général 1838–1839," 951–1023 and "Rapport général 1847–1848," 41–127. A more sophisticated version of this widespread view can be found in Maxime Durand-Fardel, *Traité thérapeutique des eaux minérales* (1857).

40. Opponents included A. Tardieu, "Rapport général sur les eaux minérales en 1859," *MEM* 25 (1861–62), cxxcv, cxxxv; A. Gubler, "Rapport général 1870–1871," 247.

41. This was not, however, one of the more successful prizes in the academy. It was awarded only four times after 1860.

42. There were usually three or fewer *stagiaires* chosen annually.

43. E. Vidal, "L'Inspectorat des eaux minérales doit-il être supprimé ou modifié? Rapport fait au nom de la Commission permanent des eaux minérales," *BAM* 17 (1887), 231. Fauvel, "Rapport général 1877," ix.

44. See Fauvel's comments to the academy, February 11, 1873, in *BAM* 2 (1873), 200.

45. Gubler, "Rapport général 1870–1871," 247–96. For the academy's extensive discussions of Gubler's conclusions see *BAM* 2 (1873), 200–220, 225–39, 243–69, 283–98, 301–36, 342–71.

46. *BAM* 4 (1875), 222–24. Surveys by the mineral waters commission defending the usefulness of statistical reports were A. Laboulbène, "Rapport général sur les eaux minérales en 1871–1872," *MEM* 32 (1879), lix; Fauvel, "Rapport général 1877," xii.

47. *Journal officiel; Assemblé nationale; Sénat*, January 22, 1883, 19–22.

48. Vidal, "L'inspectorat des eaux," 241–45.

49. Ibid., 228–54. For discussion of Vidal's report in the academy see *BAM* 17 (1887), 321–33, 343–57, 387–402, 416–27, 436–41, 453–74.

50. The administration's position was expressed most vigorously within the academy by J. Rochard, *BAM* 17 (1887), 321–33, and P. Brouardel, ibid., 395–401, 453–62.

51. Paul Dupré, Chabrin, and A.-J. Martin, "Réforme de l'inspectorat médical des stations d'eaux minérales," *Recueil de travaux du Comité Consultatif d'Hygiène Publique de la France* 18 (1888), 175–99.

52. Robin (1847–1928) became a member of the Academy of Medicine in 1887 and assumed the chair of clinical therapeutics at the Paris faculty in 1905.

53. Albert Robin, "Rapport général sur les eaux minérales en 1886," *MEM* 36 (1891), 1–67. Two years later he repeated his call in "Rapport général sur les eaux minérales en 1888," ibid., 2. (Each of the surveys in this volume was paginated separately.)

54. G. Pouchet, "Sur la définition d'une station climatique," *BAM* 118 (1937), 786–87. The availability of proper sanitary facilities was an important criterion for granting this classification.

55. *BAM* 122 (1939), 776.

56. See, for instance, Hanriot, "Rapport général 1898," 656–73; G. Meillère, "Rapport général sur les eaux minérales en 1909," *MEM* 42 (1909–10), 1–9.

57. For instance, Robin, "Rapport général 1886," 3.

58. P. Le Noir, "Rapport sur l'emploi des eaux minérales prises à la source et dans les établissements thermaux," *BAM* 119 (1939), 406–10.

59. Unlike most of the regular prize committees, it issued medals rather than cash prizes to winners.

60. See, for instance, A. Sireday, "Rapport sur les travaux envoyés pour le concours des eaux minérales," *BAM* 98 (1924), 268–76, and "Rapport sur les travaux envoyés pour le concours des eaux minérales," *BAM* 102 (1929), 195–207.

61. A. Sireday, "Sur les travaux envoyés à la Commission des eaux minérales," *BAM* 118 (1937), 352–60.

62. P. Carnot, "Sur les récompenses proposées par la Commission des eaux minérales," *BAM* 120 (1938), 267–68. Also Carnot, "Rapport sur les travaux concernant les eaux minérales," *BAM* 122 (1939), 355–59.

63. Having a paper presented by an academician was useful because members had priority in presenting papers and because such sponsorship might attract more serious attention.

64. Guitard, *Le Prestigieux Passé* p. 121. For an extended discussion of the role of the *agrégation* in medical careers, see Chapter 10.

65. For instance, R. Glenard, "L'Evolution des eaux alcalines au rayonnement Tyndal," *BAM* 118 (1937), 315–17; Rog. Glenard et al., "Pouvoir catalytique des eaux alcalines à l'émergence," *BAM* 122 (1939), 189–91.

66. For instance, A. Desgrez et al., "Contribution à l'étude des eaux bicarbonates calciques considérées comme éliminatrices d'acides uriques," *BAM* 96 (1926), 483–88; L. Merklen et al., "Effets immédiats du bain de Bourbonne sur la circulation artérielle," *BAM* 117 (1937), 672–76; M. Piéry et al., "Mécanisme d'action des eaux minérales ferrugineuses naturelles; activation de la respiration tissulaire," *BAM* 120 (1938), 774–78.

67. G. Meillère, "Un siècle d'hydrologie à l'Académie," *BAM* 84 (1920), 502.

68. These were B. Villaret and L. Justin-Besançon (three books each), E. Chabrol and M. Piéry (two books each). In Masson et Cie., *Ouvrages de médecine récents: extraits du Catalogue général*, May 1939, p. 27. I am grateful to Alberto Cambrosio for bringing this source to my attention.

69. P. Viceriat, "Un thermalisme à la française?" *Espaces* 67 (1984), 5–7; Jamot, *Thermalisme et villes*. It is impossible for me to evaluate the accuracy of such views of thermalism in Germany and Italy. There does, however, seem to be a naturopathic component of the German water cure (see Maretski and Seidler, "Biomedicine and Naturopathic Healing") that is only

beginning to emerge in France. For a French attempt to identify thermalism with alternative medicine see Henri Bergueran, "Eaux thermales: nous ne sommes pas celles que vous croyez," *Espaces* 67 (1984), 10–12.

70. Christian Labenne, "Stratégie thermale et fréquentation," *Espaces* 67 (1984), 8–9.

71. One wonders how a randomized clinical trial could possibly be conducted in this domain.

7

Academic Debate and Therapeutic Reasoning in the Mid-Nineteenth Century

Having examined academic debates as a scientific genre (Chapter 3), I go on in this chapter to analyze a number of therapeutic debates that occupied the Academy of Medicine in the mid-nineteenth century. By concentrating on this "golden age" of academic debate, I hope to cast some light on three aspects of medicine in nineteenth-century France. First, I am interested in the nature of therapeutic reasoning, a task which remains complex and messy in our own day.[1] Second, I will be particularly concerned with the ways in which members of the Parisian medical elite, in the multi-disciplinary setting of the academy, succeeded or failed in reaching consensus about scientific "facts" at a time when medical science was undergoing what can be described only as a medical revolution. Finally, I am interested in the influence that the Parisian medical elite, and the Academy of Medicine in particular, wielded over French medical science.

The evaluation of therapeutic innovations of one sort or another constituted the largest single category of major debates in the mid-nineteenth-century Academy of Medicine.[2] Relatively few of these therapeutic debates were about internal medications. Most had to do with surgery, major and minor. Even if doctors wished to affect the functioning of deep organs, they characteristically did so through minor surgical procedures on the surface of the body. Because debates were so often set off by works sent in for evaluation, they characteristically focused on claims of innovation by French rather than foreign doctors. The academy rarely condemned therapeutic innovations outright unless they clearly seemed harmful. Most often the final conclusion expressed polite interest and called for more research. This tactic reflected more than fear of being proven wrong. Given the limited therapeutic means at the disposal of doctors, innovations were warmly welcomed. Because of the complexity and individuality of disease processes, even apparently unpromising remedies might prove useful in specific cases that could be determined only by medical experience. One academician summed up the prevailing attitude. "What is one to conclude? that one should not accept, that one should not reject any single [therapeutic] method."[3]

If conclusions were seldom voted, there were occasionally clear winners and losers in these debates that were covered widely and in detail by the medical press. The different positions in a debate might be defended by interventions that were unequal in number and quality. Such imbalance would not be lost on listeners and readers.[4]

Conditions of Argument

During the first half of the nineteenth century, debate took place at several different levels. Many discussions began in a mode that can be characterized only as the exchange of technical information among skilled craftsmen. Successive speakers spoke about their experiences with a particular procedure or condition, seeking to account for either failures or successes. Suggestions or experiences recounted in this way might prompt an academician to experiment in turn with a new procedure. The direct experiences of speakers might be supplemented by those described in the medical literature, both recent and ancient.

If it was sustained for any length of time, discussion usually moved into another mode: that of disagreement and debate. Individual experiences might diverge significantly. An opinion might seem absurd in the light of someone's views about the nature of a particular condition. A new therapy being discussed might threaten the validity of another therapy with which someone had become closely identified. Sometimes the therapy being discussed was only the pretext for a debate about other matters that had long divided academicians.

Once such a debate broke out, discussants attempted to make a convincing case for the correctness of their views. Rhetorical skill was certainly an important element in these efforts since eloquence was much prized by the medical elite. The backhanded compliment which upon reflection turned into a devastating putdown became something of a native art form. But academicians themselves were not very impressed with rhetorical proficiency unless it was accompanied by something like data. It was not uncommon for one academician to dismiss the views of another on the grounds that no new "facts" had been introduced. While such comments were themselves rhetorical strategies, they suggest the need to take seriously the criteria of validation and demonstration which academicians used in trying to resolve medical issues.

Therapeutic "facts" were usually of two general types. Data could speak directly to the efficacy of a procedure or medication or focus on theoretical appropriateness. Ideally, both types should be present but the former was by far the more fundamental. To base therapeutics exclusively on theoretical speculation was at worst pernicious and at best a necessary evil.[5] Frequently, however, data of the first sort were unavailable, leaving academicians no alternative but to focus on theoretical appropriateness. This did not make methods of judgment "unscientific." Great methodological sophistication could sometimes be mobilized to determine whether a therapy "made sense" or not.[6]

One method for judging the appropriateness of a therapy was correspondence with accepted notions about the workings of the body and the nature of a particular illness. In a few cases, such considerations could be determinant. For instance, a discussion of homeopathy in 1835 was extremely critical of this form of practice despite an almost total lack of empirical data about its effectiveness.[7] Here the outrageousness of its central tenets from the perspective of accepted medical knowledge was sufficient to disqualify it from serious consideration. Such unanimity, however, was rare during the first half of the nineteenth century when doctrinal conflict was the rule. Even such seemingly marginal doctrines as animal magnetism and phrenology found defenders in the academy. Consequently, correspondence with theories seldom resolved disputes.

What of the kind of evidence that could be culled from the three most famous developments of early nineteenth-century Parisian clinical medicine: pathological anatomy, experimental physiology, and clinical statistics? The answer, as we shall see in considerable detail, is that all three had gained widespread acceptance by mid-century but within fairly narrow parameters. Use of one or the other method tended to be pragmatically determined by the question at hand. Each was part of a repertoire of procedures more or less available to medical men. Claims of exclusive legitimacy for one or the other, like the notion that any one superseded clinical judgment, aroused vehement objections.[8] Clinical judgment itself was perceived to be the result of an open-ended and undogmatic search for information gained from many different intellectual procedures. The attitude was not unlike the pragmatic openness to therapeutic innovations described earlier.

Reference to the structure of organs or organic growths (often by actually bringing them to the academy) was a fairly standard procedure of academic discussion. Pathological anatomy could provide authoritative evidence in such matters as diagnosis or establishing the existence of disease entities. But its uses for therapeutic evaluation were more limited. The major difficulty, of course, was that one could not ordinarily examine internal organs until after death had occurred. This might permit clinicians to determine from the state of an organ or growth whether a particular therapy had had local effect. It sometimes also permitted more accurate clinical prognosis, which in turn affected therapy.[9] But in these cases pathological anatomy served as an adjunct to clinical observation and evaluation. As Gabriel Andral put it in 1836, for the clinician "the anatomical lesion can never be anything but one of the numerous elements whose [central] idea can guide him in the determination of therapeutic measures."[10] When these bounds were overstepped, clinicians were quick to react. The claim made by certain microscopic pathologists to the effect that the cellular structure of cancerous tumors was the only sure indicator of curability or incurability provoked a vigorous reaction from surgeons in the academy who possessed their own practical knowledge of such matters.[11]

Laboratory experimentation was an increasingly common feature of French medicine of the period. Chemical analysis was beginning to make possible the preparation of pharmaceuticals that were uniform and of precise composition. But it was unable to provide direct evidence of therapeutic efficacy. Chemical processes were usually utilized either to suggest theoretical rationales for why certain remedies seemed to be effective for particular ailments or to argue for the appropriateness or rationality of specific medications or procedures.[12] Although chemists in the academy were invariably modest about their service role in medicine, clinicians at mid-century were quick to jump on and denounce what they perceived as the excessive pretensions of medical chemists.[13]

Physiological experimentation in medicine could not ordinarily be performed on humans except by such indirect means as the analysis of secretions or observation of visible symptomatic effects. For the most committed physiologists, experimentation meant animal experimentation. Here new procedures of laboratory physiology, identified most prominently with François Magendie and later Claude Bernard, blended in with an older and simpler tradition of testing surgical procedures on animals.[14] Animal testing provided analogical data which might or might not be convincing when applied to humans. Such testing was used on a number of occasions in academic debates and in some cases, as we shall see, determined the outcome. There was of course some opposition within the academy to the use of vivisection even in purely physiological matters, let alone those devoted to therapeutics. During an extended discussion in 1839 of the Bell-Magendie thesis distinguishing between sensory and motor nerves, the role of animal experimentation in medicine was called into question by several academicians.[15]

One common objection was the difficulty and unpredictability of such complex procedures. Not only did different vivisectionists come up with conflicting results; individuals might find it impossible to obtain consistent results, as Nicholas Gerdy, the most implacable opponent of the procedure, argued on the basis of personal experience.[16] One of the principal defenders of the Bell-Magendie thesis, Philippe Blandin, admitted that of the three procedures which furnished arguments for the theory—vivisection, clinical observation, and the anatomy of the nervous system— vivisections were the most complex and difficult to understand "so that, alone, they are unable to produce conviction."[17] In the view of the academician Charles Londe, it was not possible to determine precise physiological function from the destruction of parts of the brain or the severing of nerves because of the suffering and general physiological shock caused by such brutal procedures.[18]

Despite Blandin's view of animal experimentation as only one of many potential sources of knowledge, it was the perception of opponents of vivisection that physiologists had more exclusive, indeed imperialistic tendencies. "What I reproach the devoted partisans of the experimental method in physiology for," Gerdy asserted, "is in particular the extreme confidence and the superiority which they accord vivisections over other methods of study."[19] A final and in some ways most critical objection had to do with the assumption that animals were comparable to humans, particularly with respect to something so complex as the nervous system. It was precisely the nervous system which seemed to distinguish man from lower animals.[20]

Despite such statements from a handful of academicians, there was not a great deal of principled opposition to vivisection and remarkably little resistance to its use as evidence in therapeutic debates. One reason for this relative acceptance is that the problematic relationship between experiments done on animals and what might be expected from humans meant that the former could be used only in quite restricted ways. Animal experiments seemed to demonstrate very convincingly the dangers of a particular surgical or mechanical procedure, as our discussions of empyema and tracheotomy will show. Likewise, even Gerdy admitted the usefulness of animal experimentation in determining the toxic qualities of poisonous substances.[21] In both cases it seemed likely that what harmed or killed animals was bad for humans.[22]

Nevertheless, it was difficult to utilize such procedures to test therapeutic properties. One could simply not assume that animal illnesses, even when experimentally induced, were anything like human illnesses or that they responded similarly to therapeutic measures.[23] On the few occasions when animal experiments were brought up in debate for this purpose, the presenter got virtually no response from the academy. The relative lack of controversy about the utilization of animal experimentation was thus due precisely to the great distance between the physiological laboratory and the therapeutic activity of the physician. Experimental results could not be anything but one form of data among many which the physician might or might not take into account in making judgments.[24]

Unlike vivisection, the numerical method—the third great innovation of Parisian clinical medicine in the early nineteenth century—went to the heart of traditional therapeutic judgment. It offered new procedures to organize the clinical experiences of individuals, shape judgment, and resolve dispute. Because it hit so close to home, its use provoked major disagreements.

In the early nineteenth century a clinical paper would characteristically be composed of a series of detailed case histories. In French (but not in English) the word for such written case histories is *observation*. In the early nineteenth century and beyond, "observation" in its larger sense had polemical connotations and was associated with scientific induction as an alternative to both theoretical speculation and experimentation.[25] For those influenced by the sensualism of the Ideologue school, particularly as it had been developed and transmitted by the medical philosopher Cabanis, it had to do with the rigorous application of the senses (the only source of legitimate knowledge) to the objects of medicine.[26] Observation was widely perceived as the essence of clinical science. By carefully observing a case one could compare it with cases of a similar nature. By reasoning about many cases of the same type clinicians could reach generalized conclusions about illnesses and therapeutics. The use of the term *observation* for the written case history was not just fortuitous. The written history was both the result of and a precious aid to clinical induction. As a consequence, the precise composition of the written *observation* received considerable attention in early medical dictionaries.[27]

Written case observations compelled belief in much the same way as clinical experience did; a succession of good or bad therapeutic results produced opinions that varied from tentative to certain. The control for such generalizations was the level of detail that was provided. This permitted readers to judge the plausibility of the author's conclusions.[28] Above all, it seemed to do justice to the specificity of each case while permitting general conclusions.

In an age of science, the evidence provided by the accumulation of case studies left something to be desired. Systematic counting of results had long been a method utilized for the evaluation of smallpox immunization. In the realm of therapy, a number of British clinicians in the eighteenth century counted the number of successes and failures of particular treatment modes.[29] After the publication in 1814 of the popular essay on mathematical probability by Pierre-Simon Laplace,[30] the idea of utilizing the "calculus of probabilities" clinically floated around the Parisian medical world, popularized particularly by Pinel. But it became a concrete procedure defended as an alternative to the setting down of detailed case observations with the publication of Pierre Louis's book-length study of bloodletting in 1835.[31] The term "calculus of probabilities" was frequently utilized in the ensuing debate and Louis's opponents sometimes spoke as if he was advocating the probability theories of Laplace, Quetelet, or Poisson. But the actual procedures of Louis and his followers owed virtually nothing to the mathematical theorists of probability; they involved rather simple comparisons of proportions and averages.[32] Since none of the academicians of the period had real mathematical sophistication, it was not until several years later that Jules Gavarret demonstrated the mathematical inadequacies of Louis's procedures.[33]

The year 1835 saw a critique of the statistical method applied to medicine in the Academy of Sciences in a review of statistical efforts to demonstrate the superiority of lithotrity over lithotomy as a method of removing stones from the urinary tract.[34] In 1837 a dispute in the Academy of Medicine on the comparative virtues of bloodletting and purgatives in typhoid fever bloomed into a full-scale debate about the statistical method, which lasted several months. Many academicians expressed opposition to or at least reservations about this method for clinical therapeutics (though not necessarily for public health purposes).[35]

The hostility of some doctors to medical statistics was due to Louis's militant rhetorical posture. He seemed to be rejecting both traditional methods of clinical observation and traditional therapeutics whose efficacy was self-evident to many. Louis's rhetoric also gave rise to the perception that quantification, in the minds of its proponents, superseded individual clinical judgment; taken to its logical conclusion it would leave the doctor little to do but apply mechanically predetermined formulas. "Instead of facts to analyze and compare, you will have nothing more than chances to calculate; medicine will no longer be an art, but a lottery."[36]

Aside from the scope of Louis's claims, the method was unconvincing to many academicians. Chief among its practical difficulties were the contradictory results it seemed to yield, which depended on who did the counting. Much of that undoubtedly resulted from poor observation and recording, as proponents of the numerical method argued.[37] But the problem went deeper for it was not clear that the units being counted were in fact comparable. Different cases of what was labeled as the same disease might have a different symptomatology and prognosis. On what basis then could different therapies be judged statistically? It was precisely the variations in the dominant forms of puerperal fever from year to year that made academicians twenty years later skeptical about Semmelweiss's famous mortality statistics; these seemed within the range of normal variations as experienced by clinicians.[38]

This difficulty was not insurmountable for those who believed that diagnostic imprecision was being gradually overcome as medical science progressed. But to many doctors the individuality of disease states was a fundamental article of faith. One did not have to deny the reality of disease entities, as some did, to believe that each case varied because the disease principle (whatever that was) could itself change and because each individual's physical and environmental makeup was unique. Such cases were impossible to lump together for statistical purposes because they were fundamentally incommensurable. "An illness is a variable series of mobile acts, changing every day, at every instant. The pneumonia of today is not the pneumonia of yesterday, and the pneumonia of Paul is not the pneumonia of Pierre."[39] The sheer complexity and variability of conditions doomed all efforts at calculation. Only traditional observation of individual cases could do justice to the individuality, variability, and contextuality of diseases.

This led to one final objection. If diseases and therefore therapeutics were fluid and individualized, knowing that a larger number or proportion of patients were cured or relieved by one therapy as opposed to another was meaningless. The essential question was: which therapy was best for any particular patient?

> In any case, every method has reverses; every method successes; from which it follows that the problem to pose should not be the old problem: given a certain malady, find the treatment; but rather the following: given this particular case, deduce from it the treatment.[40]

Diseases in the aggregate could be treated only with multiple therapeutic modalities rather than the single best one that clinical statistics seemed to be striving for. And choice in any specific case required the experienced practitioner to utilize some barely analyzable form of judgment based on knowledge, observation, and, above all, logical induction which could take account of variability.[41] Determining the best treatment for an individual based on collective data made about as much sense as seeking to predict the sex of a fetus from statistics about the proportion of masculine to feminine births or the date of someone's death from general mortality tables.[42]

Supporters of quantification argued that rather than displacing observation and logical induction, the use of calculation brought new rigor and exactitude to them. Clinicians always judged individual cases by comparing them to other cases and made quantitative approximations. Counting was simply more rigorous comparison.[43] Louis himself was uncompromising: "without statistics, therapeutics is nothing more than a jumbled heap of banal and doubtful recipes."[44] Quantification might be difficult to do well but it was not impossible; the variations that everyone talked about—precisely what made statistics necessary—could be incorporated into calculations.[45] Counting was now possible because the progress of pathological anatomy had made it possible to identify many specific and stable disease entities.[46] Individual variations while inevitable were not necessarily significant and could frequently be safely ignored by the clinician.[47] In a considerable number of diseases, moreover, there *was* a single fundamental treatment, despite variations that might dictate individualized applications.[48]

Some of Louis's supporters saw opposition to Louis's quantification as the product of the antireductionist vitalism associated with the Montpellier School of Medicine.[49] It is true that two of the most virulent critics of the procedure, François Double and Benigno Risueño d'Amador, were representatives of this tradition. But many individuals not associated with Montpellier vitalism shared such reservations, albeit less flamboyantly, while vitalists like François Malgaigne had no problem with clinical statistics. Some opponents, like Louis Castel, were thoroughgoing intellectual conservatives; others, like Jean Cruveilhier and Gabriel Andral, were at the center of developments in Parisian medicine. Nor can one reduce the disagreement to a conflict between those like Louis who sought to make medicine a science and those defending it as a humanitarian art.[50] Many of those opposed to or expressing reservations about quantification were quite happy to utilize scientific procedures that seemed appropriate to the complexity of the medical task. At issue for them was the scientific appropriateness of counting as opposed to logical analysis based on observation.

In fact, between the extreme position taken by Louis and those of his bitterest opponents was a middle ground occupied by figures like the hospital physicians François Guéneau de Mussy and F. Martin-Solon, who accepted the value of clinical statistics but only to resolve uncomplicated issues and only as one among various clinical techniques.[51] Even as uncompromising a calculator as Jean-Baptiste Bouillaud insisted, early in the debate, that units compared and counted needed to be simple; "wanting to count the cases of successful or unsuccessful treatment in complex ailments, this is what I cannot admit."[52] Such a conditional and limited embrace of clinical counting would prove, after the dust had settled, to be the lasting legacy of the academic debates of the 1830s.

During the next few years, statistics did not loom very large in the therapeutic debates of the Academy of Medicine. It is not that they were never presented in papers or argument.[53] But they seldom became the focus of debate as physiological or anatomical questions did. This may have had more to do with the institutional conditions of statistical production than with any principled opposition to them. If an academician, for instance, disagreed with an argument couched in physiological terms, it was not inconceivable to spend several days performing counterexperiments that might be introduced into debate. But statistics could be accumulated only over a fairly lengthy period. Consequently, they could become an element of academic debate only if significant numbers of clinicians were routinely amassing them as part of their clinical practice.

This seems to have occurred by the mid-1850s when statistical argumentation began to play a significant role in certain kinds of debate. Academicians were particularly likely to resort to numbers in cases involving surgical therapeutics where the consequences of acting or not acting were survival or death. These could be quantified more or less unproblematically, whereas more subtle changes could not. It is not accidental, I think, that a number of debates over variants of traditional internal therapies relied almost exclusively on case descriptions. The therapeutic results of such procedures were too inconclusive or subtle, depending on one's perspective, to permit much quantification.

In the sections that follow I shall discuss in some detail several debates. Separated by nearly twenty years, the first two both focused on surgical procedures meant to stave off suffocation and both culminated in fairly unambiguous conclusions. Together they illustrate the limits and possibilities of animal experimentation and clinical quantification in surgical debate. The two others pertain to internal medications. They exemplify the indirect intellectual strategies common in matters of internal medicine where direct testing of efficacy was virtually impossible. Taken together, these debates give some idea of the ways in which particular scientific procedures and forms of evidence shaped academic debate and therapeutic thinking more generally.

Empyema

In 1836 an ad hoc commission presented a report written by a controversial professor of clinical medicine, Bouillaud, evaluating a submitted work that discussed empyema, a condition in which liquid collects in the pleural cavity.[54] In cases of empyema where suffocation set in, the sole remedy was surgical drainage.[55] The report expressed pessimism about this operation, citing the work's own results: of eight cases, only one resulted in cure while six patients died. For Bouillaud, the poor prognosis of surgery suggested that everything possible should be done to make the operation unnecessary. In particular, once pleurisy was diagnosed, extensive bleedings should be undertaken to prevent fluid buildup. The report provoked an extensive discussion in the academy.[56]

A close look at the published minutes of the discussion reveals that several different debates, in fact, took place as new debates were superimposed on older ones that gradually faded. The first issue to emerge directly from the report by Bouillaud had to do with the dangers of the operation.[57] No one argued that it should never be performed since it obviously brought relief from suffocation as no other procedure could. But the conviction that it was rarely successful suggested that it should be used only as a last resort. Academicians discussed their own professional experiences with the operation, mainly unsuccessful, as well as the opinions of deceased colleagues like Laënnec and Duypuytren. Eventually Bouillaud's report was adopted, which should have ended matters. But in subsequent meetings of the academy individuals continued to speak about their experiences. It soon became clear that a record of failure with this surgical procedure was by no means universal.

Two issues emerged directly from this divergence of experiences. For those who believed that surgery was both useless and dangerous, it was vital to prevent pleurisy and fluid buildup as Bouillaud had suggested. Pierre Louis elaborated on this point with statistical evidence. He reported on 150 cases of simple pleurisy—defined by the fact that patients had been healthy before they developed pleural inflammation—that were treated successfully with intensive bleeding, diuretics, and digitalis powder so that empyema did not occur. He went on to suggest that the popular belief that the condition was always fatal arose because it often occurred in tandem with more serious diseases. In such cases, surgical drainage served no useful purpose.[58] These statistics were not very believable to Louis's academic colleagues. Bouillaud, a fellow "counter," attributed Louis's results to luck since they contradicted his own and others' statistics.[59] Louis Castel denied that pleurisy was not dangerous, citing Morgagni and anonymous Greek medical authors in defense of his view. Later, in response to claims that he had introduced no "facts" into the debate, Castel offered his own statistics showing that by bleeding patients lightly he got better results with pleurisy than did Louis and Bouillaud.[60] P. A. Piorry questioned Louis's definition of "simple" pleurisy on the grounds that he had seen very few cases like those Louis described. This issue then faded from view while others took its place.

As more surgeons reported favorable results from surgical drainage, they also began to suggest reasons for their success and others' failures. One widely accepted explanation was that outcome depended on prior health. The sicker the patient and the greater the number of complications, the less the chances of successful surgery. But debate came to focus on variations of surgical technique. Two major distinctions were made. The first had to do with the speed with which evacuation took place. Some surgeons preferred to drain all liquid at one time. Others preferred to evacuate gradually over a number of days, usually leaving an opening in the interval. A second less fundamental distinction had to do with the nature of the opening made in the pleura. Some preferred an incision of fairly substantial size while others preferred tapping with small punctures. In almost all cases personal surgical experience was cited as the major reason for the preference.

Rationales for the various techniques emerged gradually, mainly from those academicians who believed in the usefulness of surgical drainage. Some academicians were simply afraid of any rapid changes in the body. One favored slow drainage in order to give the lungs time to resume their normal shape.[61] Another suggested that rapid evacuation led to a drop of pressure around the lungs, which caused vessels to fill too quickly with blood and thereby rupture.[62] Other academicians believed that air was the chief villain, although explanations of the mechanism varied. Barthélemy claimed that the primary problem was inflammation of the pleura and corruption of the liquid in the lungs through exposure to air.[63] Others suggested that when air entered the pleural cavity, air pressure caused lung collapse and made breathing impossible.[64] The two views of the dangers of air seem to have been reactions to different phenomena. "Corruption" undoubtedly referred to the problem of infection, whereas air pressure referred to the danger of lung collapse. Several academicians minimized both dangers unless other lung problems existed or the organ was damaged by surgery.[65]

Gradually the minority arguing in terms of air pressure began casting their views in the language of animal experimentation. In order to resolve the dispute about rapid as opposed to gradual evacuation, the pathological anatomist Jean Cruveilhier reported on his animal experiments to determine the effect of air on the lungs. He had opened up the sides of the chest with perforations of different sizes without causing death. He concluded that air did not collapse the lungs or inflame the pleura and that draining was acceptable if the surgeon opened wide and evacuated quickly.[66] Two other academicians, Jean Amussat and Eloi Barthélemy, reported on their own experiments showing that puncturing the pleura made inspiration impossible.[67] They suggested that results depended on the length of time air was permitted to enter the lungs; the longer the pleura remained open the greater the chances of death. Thus challenged directly, Cruveilhier repeated his experiments taking care to keep the incisions open for "several moments." The animal still survived.[68] Other experiments confirmed the views of his critics,[69] who suggested that Cruveilhier had performed the experiment incorrectly. Cruveilhier in turn suggested that his opponents had used sick animals in their experiments.[70]

After debate ended, papers and letters continued to trickle in.[71] Cruveilhier himself read a most unusual paper describing new experiments with dogs that made certain that the pleural opening was not closed by the movements of the animal. Permanent communication of air in both pleural cavities, he now conceded, led to asphyxiation; intermittent penetration or even permanent penetration on a single side did not. Whatever reservations one might have about comparative physiology, he asserted, there was no doubt that these findings, in conjunction with the human case descriptions other academicians had already provided, applied to man. Cruveilhier concluded that the operating surgeon should take care to close any pleural incision. He did not, however, admit to any change of mind regarding surgical therapy and claimed that the published proceedings which had him advocating large incisions in preference to surgical tapping were inaccurate.[72]

Several communications on this subject followed the conclusion of the debate. At least two continued to insist that air was harmless to the lungs.[73] But the tide had clearly turned. In 1841 J.-F. Reybard of Lyon published a description of his procedure, designed to keep air out of the pleural cavity.[74] Two years later, Armand Trousseau came out with the first of a series of publications in which he promoted the surgery on the basis of Reybard's technique. Disagreements about the advisability of the procedure persisted,[75] but few disputed the need to avoid the entry of air into the chest when the surgery was performed. By the 1860s Littré's *Dictionary of Medicine* emphasized the need in cases of empyema to quickly close the pleural cavity in order to prevent the penetration of air.[76] One American historian of empyema even found somewhat excessive the concern of French surgeons during the second half of the nineteenth century to keep air out of the lungs.[77]

The debate on empyema was unique for a number of reasons. It was at one level rather unfocused and wide-ranging; yet on a single narrow issue a major disputant publicly changed his mind (though he did not admit it). This result followed from the achievement of a consensus that a certain type of experiment would resolve the issue and that certain experimental conditions needed to be fulfilled. The debate was also unique insofar as animal experimentation had actual therapeutic implications: that surgeons should keep to a minimum the time during which air entered the chest. Still, the narrow issue that was decided, in comparison with the broad issues raised in the debate, is striking. Nothing was concluded about the advisability of drainage in particular circumstances, about the dangers of infection, or about how best to perform drainage. Academicians quite simply lacked the procedures around which to construct agreement about such matters.

Tracheotomy Versus Tubage

The following debate, which took place twenty years later, was considerably more focused. Tracheotomy in cases of croup (usually defined as the formation, ordinarily but not always due to diphtheria, of a false membrane in the throat hampering breathing) had been discussed in the academy in 1839.[78] The format was very much that of artisan discussion with various individuals informing the academy of their experiences. The general feeling was that the procedure was worth doing in spite of the high rate of mortality associated with it. A good deal of quantified information was cited during discussion because, I suspect, results in this case were without ambiguity. For the patient *not* to die from either suffocation or the procedure was both rare and a clear indicator of success. Isidore Bricheteau began discussion with a report on several works on the subject received by the academy. He added together clinical statistics from various published sources and was able to claim eighteen "cures" out of sixty operations performed. By 1850 the procedure was widely accepted, thanks largely to the popularizing efforts of Trousseau.[79]

It was in this context that a young physician, Eugène Bouchut, read a paper to the academy in September 1859, proposing an alternative treatment. In cases of suffocation due to croup, he inserted into the trachea a metal tube which then rested on the vocal chords and facilitated breathing.[80] In advocating the new procedure, Bouchut was critical of tracheotomy, which had by now become the treatment of choice. The most inflammatory aspect of his claim was the charge that mortality statistics had risen in recent years as a direct result of the increased use of tracheotomy. The entire paper was seen as a direct assault on Armand Trousseau, who was recognized to be the father of tracheotomy and whose student Bouchut had once in fact been. It could also be seen as an attack on the Hôpital des Enfants Malades where Trousseau had once worked and which was closely identified with the tracheotomy procedure. Significantly, Bouchut himself worked at a rival hospital for children, the Hôpital Saint-Eugénie.

Trousseau himself was chosen to prepare the report evaluating the communication of a nonmember. This appointment was a good indication of support within the academy for Trousseau and for tracheotomy, widely celebrated as a "French" medical discovery. Trousseau's report[81] was extremely critical of Bouchut's work but some academicians complained that its final conclusions—conceding an important role to tubage in croup therapy while insisting that tracheotomy remained the principal therapeutic modality—were far too mild. Among academicians, only the surgeon Malgaigne took on Trousseau and defended tubage. Given this constellation of forces, it is not surprising that the final conclusions voted by the academy not only reaffirmed tracheotomy as the treatment of choice for croup but concluded that lack of evidence about the efficacy and dangers of tubage made it impossible to encourage the procedure. Only the fear, admitted by some academicians, that a formal rejection of tubage might damage the academy if the procedure turned out to be successful kept the conclusions from being even more harsh.[82]

These conclusions were not preordained by the initial imbalance of forces arrayed on either side. Trousseau and his supporters were in fact able to mount a far more powerful case (in the judgment of participants) than their opponents. Their very ability to do so reflected the extensive institutional resources at their disposal. The dispute hinged on two questions. First, was tubage dangerous when continued for a significant length of time? Second, how successful was tracheotomy in preventing death from suffocation?

In his report Trousseau had claimed that a tube inserted into the larynx was probably safe for a day or two but that it inevitably damaged the pharynx and vocal chords if left in for an extended period. He offered no evidence for this claim—as Malgaigne was quick to point out—which rested on his understanding of human anatomy. Bouchut himself unwittingly provided the missing evidence by letting it be known that he had done experiments on dogs to resolve the issue. Although he did not respond to Trousseau's request for the results, one of his assistants in these experiments just happens to have been a former student of Trousseau. This assistant refused, according to Trousseau, to divulge Bouchut's results but he did agree to help set up a repeat experiment which was performed by Professor Henri Bouley of the Veterinary School at Alfort. Trousseau reported that after twenty-four hours of tubage the throat of a dog exhibited a swollen and inflamed mucous membrane; after forty-eight hours there was considerable tumefication and deep ulcerations sometimes as far as the cartilage; and after seventy-two hours the cartilage was totally uncovered while surrounding tissues exhibited violent inflammation. He clinched his argument by exhibiting a number of opened dog larynxes that he had conveniently brought with him. Even Malgaigne was forced to bow before this evidence.[83]

In contrast to the effects of tubage, determining the efficacy of tracheotomy depended on statistical evidence. One academician, Piorry, expressed skepticism about the validity of blanket statistics about success and failure, arguing that what doctors called croup was in fact several different conditions.[84] Nevertheless, most academicians seemed satisfied with comparing the number of successes, defined by patient survival, with the number of failures, defined by death.

Trousseau had no difficulty disposing of the argument that tracheotomy had increased croup mortality; he used both quantitative and anecdotal evidence and this claim did not resurface during the subsequent debate. In his turn, he referred to statistical evidence in favor of tracheotomy, the most weighty coming from a paper that had been read by Henri Roger and Germain Sée to the Société de Médecins des Hôpitaux and based on a comprehensive review of the 466 tracheotomies performed during the past nine years at the Hôpital des Enfants Malades. According to their figures, 27 percent of these operations (many by interns) were successful. In the 39 cases where doctors did not wait for total suffocation to begin but rather operated while it was still intermittent, the success rate was 64 percent.[85]

Malgaigne attacked these figures in various ways. He pointed to small inconsistencies in the reported figures and small differences between these figures and his own analysis of the hospital registers. He could also find no reasonable explanation for the fact that a nearly 100 percent mortality rate for tracheotomies before 1848 subsequently improved dramatically. But his main argument rested on plausibility. His reasoning ran as follows. Experience has shown that tracheotomies done in private practice had a very high mortality rate. Here he cited an informal poll of leading Parisian practitioners, including many academicians, carried out by Bouchut. This showed 312 deaths out of 346 operations, considerably higher than the mortality at Enfants Malades. Yet everyone knew that statistics for surgery in hospitals were always far worse than for those at home. The patients were almost always more affluent, better fed, and better cared for at home; and they did not face the unsanitary conditions and dangers of infection characteristic of hospitals, particularly Enfants Malades, one of the least salubrious hospitals in Paris. Malgaigne could come up with only one explanation. The statistics were so good because inexperienced interns were operating prematurely, long before parents would have allowed doctors to operate at home.

None of these objections stood up very well against the responses of Trousseau and numerous representatives of Enfants Malades. Using essentially anecdotal material, they disposed of Malgaigne's objections by arguing that major improvements in both surgical methods and patient care explained the recent successes of tracheotomy at the hospital. The staff of Enfants Malades also bombarded the academy with extensive denials that unnecessary or even premature surgery was being performed at the hospital. Trousseau was able to present new French and German statistics favorable to tracheotomy sent to him by other physicians. None of these arguments was overwhelming but their cumulative effect was to make Malgaigne back down so that by the end of the debate he was merely suggesting that Trousseau was putting too much stress on tracheotomy to the exclusion of other therapeutic modalities.[86]

As in the case of empyema, medical dictionaries pretty much replicated the results of the academy's discussions. In the twelfth edition of Littré's dictionary (1865),[87] the article on croup gave tracheotomy as the treatment of choice. It did not mention tubage, which was relegated to a separate negative and tiny (seven-line) entry.[88] But in this case debate in the academy does not seem to have been responsible for changing views, as it was in the empyema debate. It rather gave voice to an emerging consensus about the efficacy of tracheotomy and helped diffuse it through accounts of the debate published in medical journals. A comparison of the two debates also shows the continued pertinence of demonstrating the dangers of surgical procedures through animal experimentation.[89]

A major difference between the two debates was the virtual disappearance in the later one of appeals to the authority of major medical figures living or dead. But even more striking is the appeal to statistics, and the ease and assurance with which numbers were bandied about.[90] There was of course no real statistical sophistication. But if academicians were doing little more than simple counting, elite medical culture had nonetheless changed dramatically. How can we explain this development?

There have characteristically been two sorts of explanations for the early resistance and later acceptance of quantification in medicine. Both, incidentally, assume that Louis's numerism failed to gain acceptance in France before the twentieth century. Jacques Piquemal, for instance, sees the disappearance of Louis's school as an indicator of the rejection of numerical thinking at mid-century, a rejection that can at least in part be explained by inadequate numerical procedures.[91] Ian Hacking characterizes the success of numerism in France as brief and the use of statistics in French medicine as a tool of "rhetoric" rather than "science," due as much to lack of "techniques" as to opposition generated by medical theory.[92] I would, in contrast, suggest that counting was not merely occurring at mid-century but was providing convincing data in a limited number of cases. Quantification had become incorporated as one of several elements of clinical judgment.[93]

In a different vein, Terry Murphy has argued that the use of statistics in France began when therapies appeared whose effectiveness could be demonstrated by such methods.[94] This seems doubtful to me. Pleural drainage was neither more nor less effective, problematical, or dramatic than tracheotomy. What changed was the daily practice of many elite physicians. Physicians who had been too young to participate in the academic debates of the 1830s seem to have incorporated the recording of case information in quantifiable form into their practice, particularly their hospital practice. By the late 1850s the collection of statistics in hospitals was so widespread that the director of the Parisian hospital system created a statistical commission within his administration to coordinate and bring greater uniformity to the data being produced.[95] Such data were thus available to academicians in the 1850s.

But not all debates of the 1850s were cast in this form. The most important variable at work was the nature of what was being evaluated. Despite a sophisticated view of clinical counting emphasizing that it was valid only if it took clinical, pathological, and physiological data into account,[96] the procedure worked best to compel belief where such data were unnecessary. Surgical procedures like those just discussed were susceptible to counting because diagnosis, prognosis, and therapeutic result were relatively clear-cut. In fact such matters as disease entities and their cure were completely irrelevant. What was being counted was the incidence of death.

Nineteenth-century observers were fully aware that surgery was far more amenable to counting than was internal medicine.[97] The pioneering theoretician of probability, Lambert-Adolphe-Jacques Quetelet, had attributed this to the fact that surgical maladies were visible, whereas those of internal medicine remained hidden.[98] In actuality, it was not the visibility of disease that was critical but rather the possibility of perceiving immediate causal links between surgery and survival. This was by no means common.

The collection of surgical statistics in the middle decades of the century was widespread enough that these were frequently invoked in surgical debates of some considerable complexity. I refer specifically to discussions of surgical removal of cancerous tumors and of the puncturing of ovarian cysts.[99] But the numbers bandied about could not produce agreement in these cases because immediate death and survival were rarely at issue. Death if it occurred was months if not years removed from the surgical procedure. Furthermore, there was no way counting could take full account of all the different factors which participants themselves considered vital: types and sizes of growths, variations in survival time among both those operated on and those not, and cases of recurrence both in the short and long term. Nor were there recognized base lines that would permit comparison of these procedures with others or with nonintervention. Perhaps for that reason, by the 1870s one finds evidence of growing dissatisfaction with surgical statistics and calls for greater precision in categories commonly utilized.[100]

In the case of some of the internal therapies which were discussed during the 1850s and 1860s, such difficulties were multiplied. Nothing was stable—not the diagnostic category, certainly not the results, and sometimes not even the procedure itself. Consequently, academicians continued to treat them in the traditional way as complex and individualized entities. This meant that when they attempted therapeutic evaluations, they tended to rely on case descriptions. Frequently they avoided the issue of evaluation altogether to concentrate on whether a particular therapy "made sense." And in doing so they sometimes made use of scientific techniques that were far more sophisticated than counting.

Rheumatic Fever

In 1854 the hospital physician Martin-Solon read the academy a report evaluating a work submitted by Dr. Dechilly, a provincial hospital physician. In this work,

Dechilly advocated as a therapy for acute articular rheumatism—which came to be known as rheumatic fever[101]—the provoking of large blisters all along the affected joints. He argued on the basis of fourteen case observations that this procedure was more efficacious than some and less dangerous than other remedies currently in use. Martin-Solon reported that he had overcome his natural distaste for this treatment and had tried it on several patients. On the basis of only two of his own case observations, presented in considerable detail, Martin-Solon came to the conclusion that the method was not significantly more effective than other remedies and that, surprisingly, patients seemed able to tolerate so many large blisters. He concluded that it could be used as an alternative therapy in cases where the patient was too weak to tolerate bleeding or where diarrhea made internal medications inadvisable. He suggested that the academy vote to thank the author and to send his work to the publication committee.[102]

Many academicians found these conclusions to be excessively favorable. The hygienist Michel Lévy was particularly critical of the scanty and unrigorous case information which Dechilly (and Martin-Solon) had provided. He offered a far less positive conclusion—that the author be invited to pursue and "provide further details" of his research—which the academy voted in preference to those of the reporter.[103]

In reality, much of the debate surrounding this report had little to do with blistering, which almost everyone agreed was a common adjunct to existing therapies. Debate centered rather on the current use of intensive bleeding, a relic of Broussais's influence on Parisian medicine during the 1820s and 1830s. Both advocates and opponents of this therapy claimed the support of clinical experience for their respective views. Supporters of bleeding, most notably Bouillaud and Piorry, two eminent faculty professors of clinical medicine who were publicly disputing priority in the use and advocacy of massive bleedings, presented statistics in defense of this method. (Bouillaud cited 600 observations in which extensive and repeated bleedings were applied and Piorry 58.) But although their opponents had few statistics of their own to offer, no one, not even the other exponents of bleeding, took much notice of these figures. Those of Bouillaud in particular seem to have been quickly dismissed.[104]

Part of the difficulty in evaluating therapies in this case was that most patients recovered from the condition whether they were treated or not. Justification for therapy was provided by the cases that culminated in serious complications, chronicity, or cardiological tissue damage. By curing the condition more quickly, active therapies sought to minimize these dangers. Since the efficacy of therapies could thus not be directly tested, the debate hinged on the precise nature of acute articular rheumatism. Was it or was it not an inflammation? The response to this question could determine which therapy was the more rational response. If the condition was an inflammation or *phlegmasie*,[105] then bleeding was the traditional and obvious response. If it was not, something else was called for.

Everyone agreed that simple or traumatic arthritis was an inflammation. But acute articular rheumatism, which seemed closely related, was ambiguous. A number of academicians denied that it was an inflammation on various grounds: the uncharacteristic rapid movement of symptoms from one location to another; the apparent absence of lesions associated with inflammation; its sudden disappearance; the fact that pain could disappear while fever remained; the seeming absence of gangrene or suppuration in postmortem dissections. If the condition was not an inflammation, the obvious conclusion was that antiphlogistic therapies and particularly extensive bleedings were ineffective.

Just what should be used in their place was not so clear. Augustin Grisolle, professor of therapeutics at the Faculty of Medicine, advocated very light bleeding. He buttressed this conclusion with the examples of various historical figures, including Sydenham, Stoll, and Cullen, claiming they came to have serious doubts about the use of intensive bleedings.[106] The author of the original report, Martin-Solon, in contrast, insisted that acute articular rheumatism was a specific disease with a particular *cause rheumatismale* that accounted for its unique symptomatology. His therapeutic preference was for internal preparations, quinine sulfate and especially potassium nitrate, which he argued combated the rheumatismal cause.[107] This preference stemmed in part from his clinical experience; but it was also a logical consequence of his view of the disease. If the disease was caused by a "rheumatismal" element, it was not sufficient to merely diminish the quantity of blood through bleeding. The composition of the blood needed to be modified by a medication like potassium nitrate.[108] Malgaigne, who also questioned the inflammatory character of the condition, argued that discussion had become hopelessly confused since no one really understood the natural termination of the disease and because definitions of "cure" were highly imprecise.[109]

Proponents of the view that acute articular rheumatism was a mobile and generalized inflammation also provided evidence for their views. As Bouillaud pointed out, the tissues around the joints in articular rheumatism had the classical features of *phlegmasie* and inflammation, including redness, heat, and swelling. The general febrility was characteristic of angiotenic fevers. Most telling, chemical analysis of the blood found "a hard and consistent clot, covered by a thick membrane with a considerable augmentation of fibrine."[110] This was perfectly characteristic of blood during other inflammatory states. There was in addition analogy by cause. Like other *phlegmasies*, the disease seemed to result from "a chill when the body is sweaty." Piorry denied that the symptomatology of the condition was unique, arguing that the mobility of symptoms could also be found in other *phlegmasies* like pleurisy and pneumonia, which might also result in pericarditis. Bouillaud argued that inflammatory illnesses like pericarditis and endocarditis did not merely accompany acute rheumatism but resulted from the same basic cause. Piorry went even further by suggesting that the fibrine in suspension found in blood was the cause of inflammations as it moved through the body.[111]

The therapeutic conclusion was that heroic bleeding, the treatment of choice for inflammations, should be used in this case as well. Advocates of this procedure felt compelled to deny that Sydenham had abandoned bleeding nearly two hundred years before, indicating the continuing significance of historical medical authorities. But Bouillaud did not rely only on logical consistency or supporting opinions. He insisted that treatment had to be determined clinically and repeatedly cited statistics of various sorts, as did Piorry. These statistics, however, were not convincing to other academicians, so decisions were made on other grounds.

The advocates of extensive bleeding probably had the better of the argument. The evidence for the inflammatory character of the condition was powerful. The same therapy, massive bleeding, was advocated by everyone who viewed it as an inflammation. Their opponents could point to a number of unique features of the condition but they could not do much to explain the inflammatory characteristics. They were correct, we now know, in arguing for some specific cause (as were those who argued for a general inflammatory process) but they could offer no explanation of the cause. While there was considerable opposition to heroic bleedings, there was no agreement about alternatives. One academician believed in light bleeding, another in potassium nitrate, and yet others thought that nothing could be decided unless therapies were compared with expectant treatment. Little wonder that extensive bleedings continued to be presented as the treatment of choice for the condition in the 1865 version of Littré's *Dictionnaire*.[112]

The debate might appear at one level to have been "unscientific" in comparison with the surgical debates we have examined. But that seems to me to miss the main point. The discussion was messy to be sure because the subject was messy. However, sophisticated clinical reasoning and laboratory research were introduced in order to characterize acute articular rheumatism. Unable to bring much scientific expertise to bear directly on the issue of therapeutic efficacy, academicians brought their expertise to bear on matters of hematology and comparative symptomatology; on the basis of those results they used logic and experience to decide about therapeutics. This was not an isolated strategy, as we can see from the next case study.

Pulverization

During the 1850s, we saw earlier, the French system of spas underwent major expansion. As the number of patients increased, spa physicians began to experiment with new therapeutic procedures in an effort to increase the number of diseases they could treat. Given the ubiquitousness of respiratory maladies, it is not surprising that medical interest developed in the vapors emanating from mineral waters either naturally or by artificial means. Inhalation chambers were constructed at a number of spas and good results were reported. The Society for Medical Hydrology of Paris, recently established with the support of leading hydrologists in the Academy of Medicine, took a particular interest in these developments. A special commission to look into the matter was established under the presidency of the chemist Thénard. It prepared a questionnaire designed to stimulate research in this area and subsequently published it in the first volume of the society's new journal.[113] The society also offered a prize (never in fact awarded) for the best work submitted on the subject.

Soon after, the editor of a well-known medical journal, *La Revue médicale*, Jean Sales-Giron, published what was to be the first in a torrent of articles on the subject. He described a new inhalation chamber in the spa of Pierrefonds that was based not on vapors but on the "pulverization" of waters. Water at high pressure was directed at a pitted metal disk. It deflected off in the form of a cloud that was likened to a powder and that could be inhaled. Sales-Giron contended that while vaporization brought only volatile elements of a mineral water into contact with the respiratory system, pulverization permitted the water in its completeness to act therapeutically on the respiratory organs. It was thus to be preferred as a therapy for respiratory ailments. Because he pressed his claim for the superiority of pulverization over vaporization rather aggressively, Sales-Giron provoked considerable debate in the society. Working spa physicians were especially unhappy with Sales-Giron's criticisms of existing inhalation practices. A commission was appointed to resolve the issue experimentally.[114]

Meanwhile, Sales-Giron in 1856 sent a manuscript to the Academy of Medicine describing the new technique. Following normal institutional practice, the work was given to the leading academic hydrologists for evaluation. Ossian Henry, who did most of the academy's chemical analyses of new mineral waters, presented a report on behalf of himself and Philibert Patissier, a frequent author of annual reports for the mineral waters commission.[115] The report described Sales-Giron's method and claims and attempted to test what was considered their essence: that pulverized water, unlike vapor, did not lose any of its mineral properties in the process of pulverization. In order to do so, Henry placed paper impregnated with lead acetate around the pulverization chamber. The paper turned black or dark gray, indicating that the air was filled with enough sulfur to permit metallic sulfur to form. In a second stage the condensed liquid was analyzed chemically and was shown to contain all substances found in unpulverized waters. The conclusion was that "his method is founded on *rational principles*."[116] The therapeutic results of the method still needed to be established, Henry asserted. But since it was rational and since two German spas were already experimenting with the method, he hoped that other French establishments would set up pulverization facilities.

Henry's report was a classic academic response to a therapeutic innovation. Innovations were to be encouraged if they made sense and posed no dangers. Knowledge of efficacy would emerge from experience. Other writers, however, were calling both the rationality and safety of the procedure into question. Works on this subject were sufficiently numerous and contradictory to incite the chemist Antoine Poggiale, then serving as president of the academy's mineral waters commission, to undertake an evaluation of pulverization and the literature it had generated. He may also have been motivated by the desire to prevent the Society for Medical Hydrology from monopolizing evaluation of this new procedure. Poggiale's work was done parallel to that of the society and, indeed, there was cooperation in setting up certain experiments. But there may also have been a degree of institutional rivalry at work. It is difficult to attribute to coincidence Poggiale's presentation of his report to the academy just one day after a report on the same subject was presented to the Society for Medical Hydrology by Pierre-Oscar Reveil.

The two reports[117] are in many ways alike, though one represented the views of hydrologists in the academy and the other those of a more heterogeneous group including practicing spa physicians and urban hydrologists. Both reports evaluated the recent scientific literature on pulverization. Reveil's work followed the literature more closely in jumping from issue to issue. Poggiale's procedure was more systematic: he defined four central questions posed in the literature and then dealt successively with each. The results of the two reports were superficially similar but differed considerably in tone.

Poggiale's four fundamental questions were:

1. Do pulverized liquids penetrate the respiratory system?
2. Do they cool coming out of the apparatus?
3. Are sulfurous waters chemically modified by the process?
4. What are the therapeutic effects? [118]

Both reports did little to resolve the final question about therapeutic effects. Poggiale mentioned that of the writings sent to the academy four authors reported either no results or negative results while three others had positive results using the technique. Such great uncertainty, he said, underlined the need for further clinical research before any judgment could be reached. Reveil barely dealt with the issue at all, leaving it to the physicians attached to spas to resolve the matter. [119] The other three questions dealt with whether the procedure was rational and safe, criteria that would determine whether therapeutic research was worth pursuing. Unlike the question about clinical efficacy, these were tackled head-on.

Poggiale's second question dealt with a phenomenon that many writers had observed, the lowered temperature of pulverized waters. This challenged Sales-Giron's claims on two counts. It meant that the water being inhaled was not exactly like the water in its natural state. More important, however, was the possibility that such rapidly cooled waters might be the cause of respiratory problems. (Sudden cold was frequently blamed for a variety of maladies.) If this proved true, it might constitute a reason *not* to experiment with the therapy. Both reports reached substantially the same conclusions, not surprising since Poggiale had cooperated with the Reveil commission in setting up experiments to resolve the matter: there was a considerable decline in the temperature of water when pulverized but there was also a tendency toward equilibrium with the surrounding air. Consequently, Poggiale emphasized, the cooling effect could be controlled by saturating the surrounding air with vapor and maintaining it at a slightly warmer temperature than that of the mineral water before pulverization. The problem was clearly not seen to be significant enough to inhibit experimentation with the therapy. Nonetheless, designers of new pulverizers (and many were produced during the 1860s and 1870s) sought to deal with it by including devices to warm the pulverized water as it emerged from the apparatus.

Question number 3 about the loss of the more volatile sulfur compounds, particularly sodium sulfate, was handled in much the same way. Careful chemical analysis showed considerable loss of sulfurous elements through oxidation in certain waters though not in others. But while Reveil announced the results without comment, Poggiale suggested that the loss could be minimized if air-tight pipes were used to transport the water to the pulverizing apparatus.

This left question number 1 about the capacity of pulverized water to penetrate the respiratory system as the central and most contentious issue. For as Poggiale noted, therapy for respiratory ailments was possible only if the water actually came into contact with the affected organs. Here too the literature was contradictory. The two commissions thus made an effort to observe some of the experiments going on and to set up a number of their own.

Sales-Giron recognized that getting pulverized waters into the human respiratory system was not easy. The patient had to open his mouth wide, lean his head back, keep his tongue depressed, and inhale very deeply. Still he and his supporters could point to considerable experimental evidence suggesting it was possible. The most convincing was work by Demarquay and others showing that pulverized water was absorbed into the bronchi of rabbits. The standard procedure was to dissolve a chemical into water, force an animal to breath in the jet of pulverized water, and then, in a postmortem dissection, check the respiratory tract for traces of the chemical by means of a reactant. Although suggestive, this type of experiment was not definitive because small animals were used. Opponents of pulverization argued that the method of forcing animals to breath water was equivalent to drowning them and bore no relation to the way humans respired. Furthermore, one could not assume that what was true for rabbits applied to humans. Even less convincing were efforts to resolve the issue through the use of dummy models of the human respiratory system. Two efforts of this kind came in fact to opposite conclusions. But Poggiale dismissed all such experiments in principle. "We have operated on men and on animals; it is thus on men and on animals that one should have repeated our experiments, and not with tubes and flasks which have neither the suppleness nor elasticity of organic tissues."[120]

The animal experiments became more convincing in the light of an analogy and a single human experiment. Armand Trousseau, for instance, based his conviction that pulverized waters reached the lungs on an analogy with dust. Since we know that dust can enter the bronchi, the reasoning went, there is no reason to believe that water cannot.[121] Poggiale was able to confirm this, at least to his own satisfaction on one human subject. There came to his attention a nurse at the Beaujon Hospital who had undergone a tracheotomy and who was now breathing with the aid of a cannula. He had her inhale pulverized water containing a chemical and then introduced into the trachea by way of the cannula paper that had been treated with a reactant. This showed clearly that the pulverized water had indeed gotten that far. Poggiale assumed this proved that water could get into the bronchi. When confronted with the obvious objection that the experiment proved only that pulverized water could get as far as the trachea, Poggiale responded that given the evidence of animal experiments, it was up to opponents of pulverization to prove that water faced impenetrable obstacles in moving from the trachea to the bronchi.[122] The academy, in the end, voted its approval of Poggiale's report in spite of a lively debate in which opposition was spearheaded by the former spa physician Maxime Durand-Fardel.

The final report voted by the academy was a good deal more enthusiastic about pulverization than was the report of the Society for Medical Hydrology, though the actual conclusions were similar. The latter report, for instance, mentioned both the loss of sulfurous elements and the loss of heat without emphasizing that these phenomena could be minimized. It agreed that water could, under the proper conditions, penetrate the respiratory system but stressed only "in small quantities." And it pointedly asked: "but is this penetration sufficiently abundant to determine significant physiological phenomena and a useful therapeutic effect?"[123] It did not argue against the development of pulverization in spas but neither did it call for it.

The disagreement was not just about evidence. It pitted several academic hydrologists who were chemists (Poggiale and Henry) and who did not personally work with waters against working spa physicians or urban hydrologists (like Durand-Fardel) for whom therapeutic effects were paramount. (Trousseau was unique among

academic defenders of pulverization in having actually experimented with it therapeutically.) Both sides pretty much agreed that clinical evaluation needed to be done
in the course of spa treatments which required some prior investments in the technology. At issue was just how energetically it should be promoted given the
theoretical rationale for its use.

Both sides had institutional reasons for taking the positions they did. The academy, we have seen, tended to support the multiplication of therapeutic modalities so
long as these were not positively harmful. Responsible for regulating the entire
system of mineral waters, academicians also tended to support anything that could
bring new clients and greater affluence to the spas. Nor did they have much invested
in the existing vaporization chambers that had appeared over the last decade. For spa
physicians, however, what was at issue was the rejection of a technology many had
supported and worked with—vaporization—and its replacement by another whose
claims were largely theoretical. (Water in its complete state will have stronger therapeutic properties than the individual volatile elements in the water.) Even Armand
Trousseau, who was highly supportive of the therapy, was motivated by strong em-
piricist views to suggest that Sales-Giron was wrong to claim on theoretical grounds
that existing practices should be completely overturned.[124]

Furthermore, the two sides understood the theoretical rationale for pulverization
in different ways. Perhaps because the strong claim of opponents of pulverization
was that water could not get past the pharynx, Poggiale's allies believed that the mere
presence of pulverized water in the respiratory system made therapeutic effect possible and therefore worth testing. For the commission of the Society for Medical
Hydrology, in contrast, it was possible to concede the presence of water in the lungs
(and some members did not) without agreeing that the therapy was rational; it
was the *amount* of water which entered the lungs that was crucial. Since mineral
waters were considered a weak form of medication, large amounts were required to
produce any physiological effect. When the opponents visualized the process
of water therapy they did so in terms of bathing the body in a large volume of surrounding water or filling the organs of the digestive system with liquid. As
Durand-Fardel put it, water therapy "necessarily supposes large and easy access for
the medication, a veritable washing of the surfaces. . . . Without any doubt dusts
penetrate, but if they penetrate in the same quantities that pulverized waters must
penetrate, one would be immediately asphyxiated; and if pulverized waters only
penetrate as dusts do, what kind of effect could you expect?"[125]

In the end the academy voted in support of Poggiale's conclusions. But the victory was a partial one at best. Well-informed medical opinion did not slavishly repeat
the academy's conclusions. Littré's *Dictionnaire* of 1865, for instance, contained two
relevant entries. One titled *Pulvérisateur* referred to an apparatus very much like the
one popularized by Sales-Giron. It discussed the danger of cooling and the need to
keep room temperature high with vapor. But as far as absorbtion was concerned, it
stated that pulverized liquids "penetrate into the pharynx and larynx, as far as the top
part of the latter."[126] A second entry, titled *Pulvérisation*, was mainly about the pulverization of solids. But a short section on water mentioned the extensive loss of
sulfuric acid and added: "Mineral water inhalations are a major resource for the
treatment of maladies of the respiratory system. Pulverized water is very usefully

employed against anginas and chronic laryngitis, pulmonary hepatizations without the complication of tubercules, etc." [127] The strange claim that pulverized waters penetrated only as far as the larynx but that they were nevertheless useful for respiratory conditions, including several of the lungs, could be explained by the fact that we are dealing with two separate entries conceivably written by different authors. In future volumes of this work, however, the information was consolidated into a single entry without any attempt to reconcile the two views. Plainly opinion on the matter was divided.

In 1874 debate on the issue once again erupted, provoked by the annual report on mineral waters which spoke favorably about vaporization for respiratory ailments and suggested that pulverization should be employed only in "maladies of the isthmus of the throat, the pharynx, and the larynx." [128] It focused once again on penetration of the respiratory system, with speakers reiterating the opinions expressed twelve years before. Despite the invention of better machines, which broke up the liquid in smaller droplets, the only new elements in the argument were unsubstantiated claims by at least three speakers that clinical experience with the technique had not proven very successful.

In subsequent years the same lack of agreement seems to have prevailed but with the balance on the side of those who doubted that sufficient absorption took place. [129] Still pulverization seems to have spread to most of the large establishments primarily because it proved useful against throat ailments. What is striking about nearly everything written on the subject is the lack of concern with formal therapeutic evaluation and the focus on its condition of possibility, penetration. Even in 1948 a review of the new process of pulverization through aerosols by Justin-Besançon and Debray (both future members of the academy) emphasized this issue. [130] They cited experiments done in 1907 that demonstrated that penetration into the lungs in fact took place. [131] They discussed the new technique of producing aerosols and speculated that the lungs could not absorb enough water to be affected physiologically since waters were not very active pharmacodynamically. They too called for more physiological and clinical research. A popular work first published in 1963 also cited no clinical studies; it merely speculated that aerosols permitted deeper penetration of waters but that the quantity of water absorbed was if anything even smaller than that of other techniques of pulverization which did not propel water as deeply into the lungs. [132]

The focus on penetration instead of formal therapeutic evaluation in this case can largely be attributed to the difficulty of making precise therapeutic evaluations of thermal treatments. To the obstacles to producing such evaluations that were characteristic of internal medicine generally were added a variety of complications specific to mineral waters: the difficulty of evaluating symptomatic improvements in chronic illnesses, the loss of contact with patients after their treatment, and the general impossibility of controlling their behavior with respect to other simultaneous forms of treatment, to name but a few. This did not prevent spa physicians from making therapeutic judgments and it is probable that belief in the nonpenetration of pulverized waters reflected poor clinical results for respiratory illnesses. It is nonetheless striking that even such judgments were ordinarily framed in terms of penetration of the respiratory system rather than those of rigorous clinical evaluation. Overall, it seems evident that avoiding formal therapeutic evaluations that were fraught with difficulties was a common tactic not just in hydrology but in internal medicine generally.

These case studies suggest a number of fairly surprising conclusions to historians of medical science. The debates under review, for instance, show little of that famous therapeutic nihilism that was supposed to be characteristic of Parisian medicine during much of this period. The Parisian academic elite seemed on the contrary to take both existing and innovative therapeutics of all types with considerable seriousness. The elite was not merely not hostile to therapeutic innovation but was disposed positively toward it. This openness applies, to some degree at least, to methodological innovation as well. Animal experimentation at mid-century could be convincing where the issue was the danger of specific surgical procedures or the toxic qualities of certain substances. In most other cases, however, it ordinarily provided only indirect evidence that might be used in conjunction with deduction and analogy to make therapeutic judgments. Disagreements about the meaning of animal results in the pulverization debate illustrate clearly the limits of the animal analogy as a tool of scientific argument.

The claim that quantification was seriously set back by opposition to it during the 1830s (or by Claude Bernard's later critique) is difficult to credit on the basis of these discussions, which suggest its selective use as an instrument of clinical judgment. By the 1870s a medical dictionary could state categorically that the numerical method was a *cause gagnée*.[133] Its credibility, however, was determined primarily by the nature of the phenomenon being examined. Numbers remained far more difficult to use in matters of internal medicine than in surgery. It required a medication like the salicylates, which provided unusually striking symptomatic relief in cases of rheumatic fever, for numbers to be used in academic debates about internal medicine in the same unproblematic way they were used in surgery.[134]

In the case of both quantification and animal experimentation the problem for academicians was to decide under what specific conditions these procedures were capable of producing convincing results commanding general assent. The key seems to have been the production of results that were not ambiguous. That is why the most conclusive early debates using both numbers and animal experimentation revolved around life and death rather than symptoms. Once such results were produced, debate and negotiation about their *meaning* could take place. In the absence of such unambiguous results in the vast majority of medical situations, a variety of intellectual strategies were utilized, typically bypassing the thorny question of therapeutic effect and focusing on therapeutic rationale.

Ambiguity aside, it is hard to pinpoint the factors that allowed consensus to emerge in one case and not another. Quantification or animal experimentation might seem convincing in one case and not in another. The local context seems to have been determinant. Who presented the data (the quantification of Bouillaud, for instance, was usually greeted with incredulity), the nature of other corroborating or contradictory data, the extent to which the data called into question existing views of a disease—all could play a role, as could the fact that a specific procedure like tracheotomy was widely considered a "French" achievement.

Was the therapeutic consensus that the academy achieved in these cases, such as it was, socially constructed? Undoubtedly. Pretty much anything—ideology, professional interests, disciplinary concepts, intellectual values—could enter into the process, at one time or another. Certainly almost anything could be said; but not just anything could *compel agreement*. There was a concrete bottom line to all the bickering which had to do with the necessity of doing something for patients demanding relief without causing serious harm. What we have witnessed in these debates is the process by which an academic elite was seeking to resolve therapeutic issues while at the same time creating, on the fly, so to speak, more or less objective criteria for resolving such issues. All this was undoubtedly complicated by the proliferation of procedures and conceptual frameworks that were circulating at this strategic moment in medical history. But these processes are, I suspect, not qualitatively different from current efforts to cope with the messy immediacy of therapeutic judgments.

NOTES

1. The best discussions of nineteenth-century therapeutics are Charles Rosenberg, "The Therapeutic Revolution," *Perspectives in Biology and Medicine* 20 (1977), 485–506, and John Harley Warner, *The Therapeutic Perspective: Medical Practice, Knowledge and Identity in America, 1820–1885* (Cambridge, Mass., 1986). On debates about surgical therapeutics see Ulrich Tröhler, "'To Operate or Not to Operate?' Scientific and Extraneous Factors in Therapeutical Controversies within the Swiss Society of Surgery, 1913–1988," in *Essays in the History of Therapeutics*, ed. W. W. Bynum and V. Nutton (Amsterdam, 1991), pp. 89–113.

2. For the purposes of this chapter I define "major debates" as discussions that went on for at least four academic meetings. The changing mix of subjects is discussed in Chapter 3.

3. J. A. Rochoux, *BAM* 1 (1836), 533.

4. We do not, of course, have direct access to these debates but rely on written accounts. In this chapter I use the accounts published by the academy in *BAM*.

5. See, for instance, L. Guersant, "Thérapeutique," *Dictionnaire de médecine*, 2nd ed., vol. 29 (1844), pp. 606–20, esp. p. 617. For a more nuanced view see J.-B. Bouillaud, "Vitalisme," *Dictionnaire de médecine et de chirurgie pratique*, vol. 15 (1836), pp. 658–61.

6. It has been suggested to me by medical colleagues that this focus on appropriateness rather than direct efficacy continues to be characteristic of much therapeutic reasoning as a result of the need to come to practical conclusions, whether all the data are in or not.

7. N. Adelon, "Peut-on permettre l'établissement d'un dispensaire et d'un hôpital homéopathique?" *Annales d'hygiène publique et de médecine légale* 15 (1836), 435–49.

8. Many of the criticisms of Louis's numerism and Bernard's experimental medicine were not directed so much at the methods as at the spirit of exclusiveness motivating their spokesmen.

9. In conjunction with clinical observation, for instance, it allowed doctors to conclude that certain types of tumors might be helped by surgery while others would inexorably produce death. The structural features of ovarian cysts could, it was also believed, tell clinicians when it was advisable to drain these cysts and when they should be left alone.

10. G. Andral, "Observations sur le traitement de la fièvre typhoïde par les purgatifs, par M. de Larroque," *BAM* 1 (1836), 500.

11. The debate which broke out is in *BAM* 20 (1854–55). For a brief account of the major issues, see Ann La Berge, "Is the Microscope Useful for Pathology? A Mid-Nineteenth Cen-

tury Debate," paper presented at the annual meeting of the American Association for the History of Medicine, Cleveland, Ohio, May 3, 1991.

12. See the debate about the pulverization of mineral waters discussed below.

13. For examples relating to mineral waters see Chapter 6.

14. On some examples of this surgical tradition see Toby Gelfand, *Professionalizing Modern Medicine: Paris Surgeons and Medical Science and Institutions in the Eighteenth Century* (Westport, Conn., 1980), pp. 64–65.

15. The debate is scattered throughout *BAM* 3 (1838–39). It is discussed in John E. Lesch, "The Paris Academy of Medicine and Experimental Science, 1820–1848," in *The Investigative Enterprise: Experimental Physiology in Nineteenth-Century Medicine*, ed. William Coleman and Frederick L. Holmes (Berkeley, Calif., 1988), pp. 129–32.

16. *BAM* 3 (1838–39), 401–2, 414.

17. Ibid., 418.

18. Ibid., 872.

19. Ibid., 742.

20. Ibid., 414, 740.

21. Ibid., 414.

22. W. F. Bynum, "'*C'est un malade*': Animal Models and Concepts of Human Disease," *Journal of the History of Medicine and the Allied Sciences* 45 (1990), 401, 409.

23. Bynum argues that large-scale use of animals to develop disease models followed the widespread acceptance of the germ theory in the 1880s. Ibid.

24. In his rather hostile *éloge* of Magendie, Dubois d'Amiens suggests that in Magendie's case the cult of experimentation was carried to an extreme, "suppressing the doctor" and leading to therapeutic nihilism. F. Dubois d'Amiens, "Éloge de Magendie," *MEM* 22 (1858), xxvi–xxxi.

25. See the elaborate entry "Observation," in Émile Littré and Charles Robin, *Dictionnaire de médecine, de chirurgie, de pharmacie, des sciences accessoires et de l'art vétérinaire*, 12th ed. (1865), pp. 1023–24.

26. J. Raige-Delorme, "Observation," in *Dictionnaire de médecine*, 1st ed., vol. 15 (1826), p. 195. On Cabanis's defense of observational knowledge see Martin S. Staum, *Cabanis: Enlightenment and Medical Philosophy in France* (Princeton, N.J., 1980), pp. 103–9, and more generally, Erwin H. Ackerknecht, *Medicine at the Paris Hospital, 1794–1948* (Baltimore, Md., 1967), pp. 3–12.

27. See for instance, Ph. Pinel and I. Bricheteau, "Observation (histoire des maladies)," in *Dictionnaire des sciences médicales*, vol. 37 (1819), pp. 29–35; Raige-Delorme, "Observation," pp. 195–99.

28. Raige-Delorme, "Observation," p. 198.

29. Ulrich Tröhler, "Quantification in British Medicine and Surgery 1750–1830 with Special References to Its Introduction into Therapeutics," Ph.D. diss., University College London, 1978. Andrea A. Rusnock, "On the Quantification of Things Human: Medicine and Political Arithmetic in Enlightenment England and France," Ph.D. diss., Princeton University, 1990, came to my attention too late to be used in this discussion.

30. P.-S. Laplace, *Essai philosophique sur les probabilités* (1814). Mathematical probability in nonmedical statistics has its own history, which I will not go into here. Among recent works on this subject are Gerd Gigerenzer et al., *The Empire of Chance* (Cambridge, 1989) and Ian Hacking, *The Taming of Chance* (Cambridge, 1990).

31. P. C. A. Louis, *Recherches sur les effets de la saignée dans quelques maladies inflammatoires et sur l'action de l'émétique et des vésicatoires dans la pneumonie* (1835).

32. The same holds true for most public health statistics of the nineteenth century. See Bernard-Pierre Lécuyer, "Probability in Vital and Social Statistics: Quetelet, Farr, and the Ber-

tillons," in *The Probabilistic Revolution*, ed. Lorenz Kruger et al., 2 vols. (Cambridge, Mass., 1987), vol. 1, pp. 317–35.

33. Jules Gavarret, *Principes généraux de statistique médicale ou développement des règles qui doivent présider à son emploi* (1840).

34. F.-J. Double, "Recherches de statistique sur l'affection calculeuse, par M. le docteur Civiale," *CRAS* 1 (1835), 167–77.

35. This debate takes up a large chunk of *BAM* 1 (1836).

36. B. Risueño d'Amador, "Mémoire sur le calcul des probabilités appliqué à la médecine," *BAM* 1 (1836), 624. Also see Terry D. Murphy, "Medical Knowledge and Statistical Methods in Early Nineteenth-Century France," *Medical History* 25 (1981), 311.

37. A. F. Chomel in *BAM* 1 (1836), 724; J.-B. Bouillaud, ibid., 806.

38. See, for instance, the comments in J. Guérard, "Du Traitement de la fièvre puerpérale," *BAM* 23 (1857–58), 376.

39. F.-J. Double, *BAM* 1 (1836), 705.

40. J. A. Rochoux, *BAM* 1 (1836), 533. Variations of this statement recurred very frequently. See ibid., 550

41. Risueño d'Amador, ibid., 649; Double, 701.

42. Double, "Recherches de statistique," 173.

43. C. Navier, "Statistique applique à la médecine," *CRAS* 1 (1835), 247–51.

44. *BAM* 1 (1836), 541.

45. Chomel, *BAM* 1 (1836), 735; Rayer, ibid., 786–87.

46. Rayer, ibid., 780–81.

47. Ibid., 783–85.

48. Ibid., 784. Ann La Berge, "A Provincial Physician and the Tyranny of Numbers: An 1837 Debate," unpublished paper.

49. J. Raige-Delorme, "De la Discussion qui a lieu à l'Académie Royale de Médecine sur la statistique medicale," *AGM*, 2e sér. 14 (1837), 255–65.

50. John Rosser Matthews III, "Mathematics and the Quest for Medical Certainty: The Emergence of Clinical Trials, 1800–1950," Ph.D. diss., Duke University, 1992, chap. 2.

51. *BAM* 1 (1836), 764–68.

52. Ibid., 534. Bouillaud seems to have changed his position as the debate proceeded.

53. For instance, in early 1840 H. Husson, Baron, and Rayer presented a very lengthy and favorable report on a work based on statistics sent in by Jules Pelletan, a student of Bouillaud. *BAM* 4 (1839–40), 447–74. Pelletan's long essay was then published in its entirety by the academy. J. Pelletan, "Mémoire statistique sur la pleuropneumonie aiguë," *MEM* 8 (1840), 184–374.

54. *BAM* 1 (1836), 62–63. The report was cosigned by L. J. Sanson.

55. Unlike the British, who associated the term "empyema" with the collection of pus in the pleural cavity, the French used it to refer to all liquids. Furthermore, empyema for the French meant both the condition and the surgery to drain the liquid. I will use the word to refer to the condition and refer to the surgery as drainage.

56. This debate is analyzed in terms of its physiological content in Lesch, "The Paris Academy of Medicine," pp. 113–15.

57. *BAM* 1 (1836), 62–66.

58. Ibid., 122–23.

59. Ibid., 125.

60. Ibid., 142, 169.

61. J. Lisfranc, ibid., 189.

62. L. Castel, ibid., 143.

63. Ibid., 138; also D. Larrey, ibid., 159.

64. Notably J. Amussat, ibid., 145. That this was an issue for debate is somewhat surprising considering that the Oxford physiologists of the late seventeenth century knew quite well that puncturing the pleural membrane led to lung collapse. See Robert G. Frank, Jr., *Harvey and the Oxford Physiologists: A Study of Scientific Ideas* (Berkeley, Calif., 1980), p. 162. (I am grateful to Don Bates for bringing this point to my attention.)

65. P. J. Roux, *BAM*, 1 (1836), 166; A. Velpeau, ibid., 188; Lisfranc, ibid., 189.

66. Ibid., 140–42.

67. Ibid., 164–65, 184. Amussat also suggested on the basis of his experiments that blood injected into the lungs was usually absorbed; no one responded to this rather important distinction between blood and other liquids.

68. Ibid., 168.

69. P. A. Piorry, ibid., 180.

70. Ibid., 186

71. An important paper by G. Pelletan (ibid., 237) described experiments on dogs indicating that air penetrating the pleura indeed prevented breathing.

72. Ibid., 280–83.

73. As did the second edition of M. C. Sédillot's influential medical thesis, "De l'Opération de l'empyème" (2nd ed., 1841). Cited in Richard H. Meade, *A History of Thoracic Surgery* (Springfield, Ill., 1961), p. 235.

74. *Gazette médicale de Paris*, January 9, 16, and 23, 1841. Cited in Bricheteau's report on Trousseau, "Sur la paracentèse," *BAM* 11 (1845–46), 550.

75. See for instance the brief discussion following I. Bricheteau's positive review of Trousseau's work in *BAM* 11 (1845–46), 562–64.

76. Littré and Robin, *Dictionnaire de médicine*, p. 512.

77. Lew A. Hochberg, *Thoracic Surgery before the Twentieth Century* (New York, 1960), p. 251.

78. *BAM* 3 (1838–39), 908–17.

79. The *Dictionnaire de dictionnaires de médecine français et étrangers*, ed. Dr. Fabre (1850), vol 3, wrote in its entry on "croup": "The cures obtained in these desperate cases today place beyond doubt the usefulness, we almost said the necessity of this operation." In a review of the spread of these procedures internationally, Anne Hardy, "Tracheotomy versus Intubation: Surgical Intervention in Diphtheria in Europe and the United States," *Bulletin of the History of Medicine* 66 (1992), 536–59, overstates French opposition to the procedure by taking somewhat too literally some of Trousseau's own remarks.

80. Extracts from this paper were published in *BAM* 23 (1857–58), 1160–62.

81. *BAM* 24 (1858–59), 99–131.

82. Ibid., 420–21.

83. Ibid., 221.

84. Ibid., 149.

85. Ibid., 180.

86. Ibid., 343–44.

87. Littré and Robin, *Dictionnaire de médicine*, p. 389.

88. Ibid., p. 1563.

89. In both cases, as well, reports by veterinarians of artificially induced maladies in animals comparable to human maladies received no response from academicians.

90. Jules Simon in his article on croup in the *Nouveau Dictionnaire de médecine et de chirurgie pratique*, vol. 10 (1869), p. 368, indicates that statistics justifying tracheotomy continued to be produced at a rapid rate in the decade following the debate.

91. Jacques Piquemal, "Succès et décadence de la méthode numérique en France à l'époque de Pierre-Charles-Alexandre Louis," *France médicale* 250 (1974), 11–22, esp. 18–19.

92. Hacking, *Taming of Chance*, pp. 84–85.

93. The opposition of Claude Bernard to clinical quantification is frequently cited. One is hard-pressed to come up with the names of many other distinguished critics.

94. Murphy, "Medical Knowledge," 316.

95. *BAM* 27 (1861–62), 531–32. This committee introduced uniform and color-coded forms for each patient. H. Rey, "Statistique médicale," in *Nouveau Dictionnaire de médecine et de chirurgie pratique*, vol. 33 (1882). A debate on the salubrity of Parisian hospitals that agitated the academy in 1861 was almost entirely based on differential mortality statistics.

96. See the article "La Méthode numérique," in Littré and Robin, *Dictionnaire de médecine* p. 1018.

97. Rey, "Statistique médicale," p. 628.

98. Cited ibid., p. 627.

99. See, for instance, the debates on the curability of cancer in *BAM* 20 (1854–55) and on ovarian cysts and tumors in *BAM* 22 (1856–57).

100. A. Verneuil, "De Quelques réformes à introduire dans la statistique chirurgicale," *AGM* 6e sér. 22 (1873), 1–26, 275–309.

101. For an excellent review of the development of this disease concept, see Peter C. English, "Emergence of Rheumatic Fever in the Nineteenth Century," *Milbank Quarterly* 67 (1989), Suppl. 1, 33–49.

102. *BAM* 19 (1853–54), 665–83.

103. Ibid., 830–35.

104. A. Grisolle, ibid., 825, made reference to recent publications that had discredited Bouillaud's use of statistics.

105. *Phlegmasie* referred in the nineteenth century to an internal condition characterized by local overexcitation which drew excessive blood to the blood vessels of certain organs. The result was redness, swelling, heat, and pain in the affected area.

106. *BAM* 19 (1853–54), 716–17, 733–37.

107. Ibid., 682.

108. Ibid., 711, 737, 828.

109. Ibid., 774.

110. Ibid., 736.

111. Ibid., 707–8, 729–33, 738–40, 755.

112. Littré and Robin, *Dictionnaire de médecine* pp. 1313–14.

113. P.-O. Reveil, "Sur la Question de la pulvérisation des eaux minérales," *Annales de la Société d'hydrologie médicale de Paris* 8 (1861–61), 123–24.

114. Ibid., 126–27.

115. *BAM* 21 (1855–56), 1081–85.

116. Ibid., 1003. Italics added.

117. A. B. Poggiale, "Rapport sur diverses communications relatives à la question de la pulvérisation des eaux minérales et médicamenteuses," *BAM* 27 (1861–62), 267–97, was read on January 7, 1862. P.-O. Reveil, "Sur la Pulvérisation," 122–71, was read on January 6, 1862.

118. Poggiale, "Rapport sur diverses communications," 280.

119. Reveil, "Sur la Pulvérisation," 160.

120. *BAM* 27 (1861–62), 800.

121. Ibid., 781–82.

122. Ibid., 801.

123. Reveil, "Sur la Pulvérisation," 144.

124. *BAM* 27 (1861–62), 781–82. Poggiale interpreted the remarks as a criticism of chemistry and responded with his own attack on Trousseau's radical empiricism. Ibid., 809–11.

125. Ibid., 787.

126. Littré and Robin, *Dictionnaire de médecine* p. 1248.

127. Ibid., p. 1249.

128. I. Bourdon, "Rapport général sur le service médicale des eaux minérales de la France pendant l'année 1871," *MEM* 31 (1875), cxvii–clvi. (The quote is on cxxi.)

129. One medical dictionary concluded that there existed a strong likelihood that pulverized water did penetrate in sufficient quantities. (J.-M.-A. Beni-Barde, "Pulvérisation," *Nouveau Dictionnaire de médecine et de chirurgie pratiques*, vol. 30 [1881] pp. 147–56.) Another took no position in recounting the debate and added that many respected hydrologists preferred inhalation of vapors. ("Pulvérisation," *Dictionnaire encyclopédique des sciences médicales*, ed. A. Dechambre and L. Lereboullet, vol. 29 [1889], pp. 841–43.) A manual of thermalism did not include diseases of the lungs among the many indications for pulverization. E. Egasse and Dr. Guyenot, *Eaux minérales naturelles autorisées de France et de l'Algérie*, 2nd ed. [1892], p. 65.) The *Dictionnaire Littré* in the twentieth century continued to insist that pulverized waters penetrated to the upper part of the larynx but that they were useful for chronic inflammations of the lungs. E. Littré, *Dictionnaire de médecine*, 21st ed., ed. A. Gilbert (1905–8), pp. 1380–81.

130. L. Justin-Besançon and Charles Debray, "Les Aérosols en thérapeutiques hydrominérale en climatologie," *Presse thermale et climatique* 85 (1948), 1–9.

131. These were done in 1906–7 by Cany of La Bourboule, who left sheep in an inhalation chamber for two hours every day for twenty days. The animals were then killed and arsenic in the lungs was measured. (Arsenic was a major component of La Bourboule's waters.) These animals showed seven times the arsenic levels of controls.

132. Émile Duhot and Michel Fontan, *Que sais-je? le thermalisme*, 2nd ed. (1972), pp. 36–37.

133. Rey, "Statistique médicale," 629.

134. The discussion is in *BAM* 6 (1877).

8

The Posthumous Laënnec: Creating a Modern Medical Hero

The Academy of Medicine evaluated works of medical science in reports, prize competitions, and eulogies. It was not alone in this respect. Many other medical and scientific institutions performed similar functions. Wherever and however it took place, evaluation could occasionally merge into another characteristic scientific process: the elaboration of historical myth defining institutions, disciplines, or groups. In this chapter we shall examine this process in the evolution of a single medical reputation.

The subject of the chapter, Laënnec (1781–1826), inventor of mediate auscultation and the stethoscope, is generally recognized to be a charter member of the pantheon of medical greats.[1] I am not concerned here with Laënnec's life and works but rather with the evolution of his posthumous reputation, particularly in the century following his death. I will be seeking, more generally, to shed light on that process of collective judgment that leads to immortality for a select handful of doctors.[2] The protean capacity of such professional heroes to embody a variety of aspirations and concerns, I suggest, is crucial to this process.

The Academy of Medicine played a critical role in inventing the historical Laënnec. But my methodological strategy has been to situate the academy's contribution in the widest possible context. To chart Laënnec's reputation, I have thus searched out all books, articles, and speeches published between 1826 and 1876 and devoted specifically to his life and work. The bibliography that I have assembled is, I believe, practically exhaustive. I have, in addition, utilized passing references, and revealing silences as well, in the academy and in sundry books and articles. But since one can never be certain that such a collection of passing references is representative, let alone exhaustive, their primary purpose is to supplement and enrich our core sample of texts.

Studies specifically devoted to Laënnec appeared in three sequences in the half century following his death. A number of appreciations appeared just after his death

in some of the medical journals of the period. Surprisingly, there was little public reaction to his death in the Academy of Medicine or other elite medical institutions. A
second collection of appreciations, presented in the Academy of Medicine from 1837
to 1839, signaled the rise of his reputation and his growing status as an exemplar of
the discipline of pathological anatomy. A third series of hagiographic studies, largely
occasioned by institutional celebrations, appeared in the mid-1860s and consecrated
Laënnec's position as an authentic modern hero of French medicine.[3] By the time the
Academy of Medicine celebrated the centenary of Laënnec's death in 1927, the great
man's reputation had entered yet another incarnation. Laënnec now represented the
clinical and pathological traditions of a Parisian medical elite struggling to confront
the scientific revolution of the late nineteenth and early twentieth centuries.

The First Reactions

Laënnec's death in 1826 was noted in several important medical journals; but it received little attention in the two most significant medical institutions of the day, the
Academy of Medicine and the Paris Faculty of Medicine. Circumstances were partly
responsible. Laënnec's funeral took place in Brittany and was thus not attended by
the Parisian notables who at such occasions presented orations that were often subsequently published. As professor at the Paris Faculty of Medicine, Laënnec could
have expected a lengthy appreciation by one of his colleagues at the annual prize
giving ceremony of the faculty. The government, however, fearing student disorder,
had abolished these public ceremonies in 1823 and had replaced them with a small,
semiclandestine proceeding. At the ceremony of 1826 Jean Cruveilhier addressed the
assembled students and presented brief appreciations of five recently deceased professors, including Laënnec. This succinct tribute went virtually unnoticed in the
medical world.[4] Circumstances, however, cannot fully explain the silence of the
Academy of Medicine.

One of the major functions of the permanent secretary of the Academy of Medicine, we saw, was the presentation at the annual public assembly of the academy of
elaborate *éloges* devoted to the most illustrious of the recently deceased members.[5]
The permanent secretary of the academy, Etienne Pariset, inaugurated this task in
1824 with an *éloge* of Corvisart. In 1826, the year of Laënnec's death, he eulogized
the chemist Claude Berthollet, and a year later, when Laënnec might normally have
received an appreciation, he devoted his panegyric to Philippe Pinel, who had also
died in the previous year. This choice is understandable given Pinel's stature during
the first decades of the nineteenth century. But at that same meeting, Pariset also presented short eulogies of Edmé-Claude Bourru and Edmé-François-Chaudet
Beauchène. Neither was a household name in the Paris of the 1820s; the fact that
Pariset found them more worthy of tribute than Laënnec is curious.[6] Furthermore,
although *éloges* could be presented for several years after an individual's death,
Pariset did not make up for his omission at subsequent public meetings of the
academy.

Pariset was not an innovator in his choice of subjects for *éloges*. He usually
honored those who had already been honored by the medical and scientific establish-

ments. Laënnec was hardly the persecuted genius that some of his later biographers presented. But his credentials were somewhat incomplete and suspect. Of those whom Pariset eulogized, two characteristics stand out. First, every one of the men who received an *éloge* was one of the original members appointed to the Academy of Medicine during the winter of 1820–21. That is to say, all had a good deal of stature and seniority. Laënnec in 1820 was still a young man and had just published his *Traité de l'auscultation* the previous year; he was living temporarily in Brittany because of serious health problems. He was thus appointed not as a full member of the academy but as a corresponding associate. Full membership was not granted until 1823. The distinction is perhaps a subtle one, but the medical hierarchy was defined by such subtleties.

A second characteristic of some importance for Pariset was membership in the Academy of Sciences. During his tenure, members of the Academy of Sciences obtained 58 percent of the major *éloges* (over ten pages in length in their published form) at the Academy of Medicine and all ten of the *éloges* longer than twenty-five pages. The man who received the longest one was the biologist Georges Cuvier, not a physician and only marginally connected to the Parisian medical community. It would thus seem as if recognition of merit by Pariset depended largely on the prior recognition of merit by the elite of the scientific community. Laënnec's credentials in this respect were both incomplete and problematic. He had, for instance, failed on several occasions to be elected to the Academy of Sciences. There was nothing punitive about this. Many members of this academy had failed candidacies under their belts and Laënnec was still a young man competing against much more senior figures.[7] Nevertheless, Laënnec at his death lacked a crucial prerequisite for an *éloge*.

Laënnec did hold professorships at both the Collège de France and the Paris Faculty of Medicine, making him a visible member of the medical "establishment." But the honors in his case were tainted. He was appointed to the Collège de France in 1822 by the educational administration despite the fact that the faculty assembly had proposed François Chaussier for the chair while the Academy of Sciences, also consulted on the matter, had recommended François Magendie.[8] Worse, he obtained his chair at the Paris Faculty of Medicine as a result of the purge carried out by the government in 1822 which deprived eleven professors of their chairs. Laënnec had, in fact, been one of the chief architects of the subsequent reorganization.[9] This was an act which many found difficult to forgive.

If Laënnec's credentials were not of the sort to compel an *éloge,* neither was his stature in the medical community. The appreciations which appeared after his death reveal the ambivalence and controversy surrounding both his person and his scientific achievement. The two most positive eulogies were written by close associates in the enterprise of pathological anatomy: Antoine Laurent Jessé Bayle,[10] nephew of Laënnec's deceased collaborator Gaspard-Laurent Bayle, and the fellow Breton Jean-Alexandre Kergaradec,[11] who had done important work on fetal auscultation. Bayle, like Cruveilhier in his brief remarks to the faculty, insisted that auscultation was one of the most significant medical discoveries ever made and Laënnec one of the greatest physicians. Figures less closely associated with the inventor of the stethoscope were more reserved. A necrological notice in the British journal *The Lancet* was curiously noncommittal in recounting Laënnec's life.[12] In France, A. Boulland[13] and an anonymous author in the *Archives générales de médecine*[14] were more critical.

Despite their differing tones, all the necrologists were in substantial agreement about the nature of Laënnec's achievement. Everyone, for instance, recognized the brilliance of the *Traité de l'auscultation*. Even the very hostile notice in the *Archives générales de médecine* called the book "one of the finest productions of our epoch which assures Monsieur Laënnec a distinguished rank among the illustrious doctors of the nineteenth century."[15] For all who wrote about him, Laënnec had invented a diagnostic technique that brought rigorous clarity to diseases of the thoracic cavity.[16] But neither friend nor foe writing in 1827 saw auscultation as a radical departure in medicine or, in fact, as a major extension of pathological anatomy.

I am basing this statement in part on those eulogies of Laënnec which distinguish rigorously between his early work in pathological anatomy and auscultation as a diagnostic procedure. But I am also taking into account contemporary work in pathological anatomy where Laënnec was strangely absent. Gabriel Andral, for instance, who wrote the article on auscultation in the *Dictionnaire de médecine et de chirurgie pratique* (1829), published in the same year a major work on pathological anatomy.[17] The introduction emphasized his intention to link pathological anatomy and practical medicine without mentioning Laënnec as someone who had made a similar (and fairly successful) effort. In Jean Cruveilhier's article on pathological anatomy in another medical dictionary,[18] Laënnec is not mentioned in the text. His article of 1812 on pathological anatomy written with Bayle is listed in the bibliography but the *Traité de l'auscultation* is not. The lengthy review of the *Traité* in the *Edinburgh Medical and Surgical Journal*[19] recognized the pathological anatomy in the book but distinguished between Laënnec's clarification of morbid changes in the lungs and heart and his "method of distinguishing the several diseases of these organs." Laënnec's British translator actually separated out the sections on pathology from those on auscultation in the translation of the first edition.[20] Given the virtual consensus regarding the nature of Laënnec's achievement, how is one to explain the disagreements regarding his stature?

Some of the negative feelings about Laënnec plainly reflected political hostility. Notices critical of Laënnec all expressed displeasure with their subject's traditionalist monarchist and Catholic political views. *The Lancet* verbalized what many felt: "What appears most surprising, however, is that an individual with such powers of mind as Laënnec possessed, could, at the same time, have been a fanatic."[21] French writers were particularly disapproving of his role in the purge and reorganization of the Faculty of Medicine in 1822. Laënnec's supporters dealt with the charge by pointing out that Laënnec had not initiated events and had in fact protected certain professors from the wrath of the government. One of the most critical eulogists responded that having protected some professors "undoubtedly does great honor to Monsieur Laënnec; but it would have been more honorable still for him to have remained aloof from the secret maneuvers which resulted in the dismissals of men like Pinel and Chaussier as well as several other learned professors as esteemed for their virtues as for their talents."[22]

Personal factors also seem to have come into play. Laënnec was, by all accounts, a difficult man who did not endear himself to either opponents or colleagues. Ill health, moreover, prevented him from taking much part in the activities of the Academy of Medicine and forging ties of camaraderie with other members. Although many foreigners attended his clinic and lectures, his poor reputation as a teacher discouraged French students and doctors from attending in any numbers.[23] Consequently, unlike many of his competitors, he was without a loyal body of disciples to proclaim his greatness to the world.

Politically motivated hostility, personal animosities, and pedagogical failings were all real enough. But if Laënnec was largely unacknowledged at his death it was primarily due to *intellectual* reservations regarding his work. Despite its acknowledged brilliance, this work was perceived as limited in scope and distinctly old-fashioned. In the 1820s the new fashion in medicine was the physiological doctrines of François Broussais.[24] To most of the French medical world Laënnec seemed old-fashioned because he had vehemently and publicly opposed Broussais's doctrine. Broussais's popularity in 1827 was so great that even Laënnec's strongest defenders were forced to concede that he had perhaps rejected what was positive as well as what was negative about the physiological doctrine.[25] One did not have to be an unconditional supporter of Broussais (as Laënnec's anonymous eulogist in the *Archives générales de médecine* apparently was) to be perplexed by Laënnec's hostility. In his relatively more balanced necrology, Boulland said of his subject's rejection of Broussais's views: "How painful it is to see this sort of sentiment close all avenues toward the truth to the spirit of certain men!"[26]

Broussais's extraordinary popularity in the 1820s has been ably analyzed by Erwin Ackerknecht.[27] Whatever the failures of observation embedded in his system, Broussais's views were based on a powerful series of general principles: rejection of the traditional nosological categories, insistence that observation be anchored in theory, basing pathology on localism and physiology. His popularity was undoubtedly advanced by his liberal political views, widespread in the Parisian medical community of the 1820s. In contrast, Laënnec's medical views seemed those of a political and religious reactionary and seemed in some respects scientifically reactionary as well. Whereas Broussais prescribed relatively harmless leeching for most conditions, Laënnec was reproached for championing large doses of the dangerous emetic tartarus stibiatus (antimony potassium tartrate). While Broussais was perceived as a bold innovator breaking with tradition, Laënnec was viewed as a mere follower of the traditions established by Bichat, Pinel, and Corvisart.[28]

Above all, Laënnec seemed to lack something which Broussais clearly possessed: theoretical audacity. Over and over, contemporaries described Laënnec as a great observer who lacked the ability to generalize. Boulland referred to "the small reach of Laënnec's speculative views."[29] The *Dictionnaire biographique Panckoucke* of 1822 said of him: "If science does not count him among the doctors who have sought to generalize the views suggested by observation, it recognizes him as one of those who has contributed the most to enriching its domain."[30] In other words, Laënnec was one of those who described rather than explained. He discovered lesions and diagnostic signs with remarkable virtuosity but seemed to ignore the cause and nature of diseases. For all their acknowledged value, neither auscultation nor Laënnec's brand of pathology seemed capable of satisfying the widespread desire to better understand disease processes so that therapeutics could be improved.[31]

Rehabilitation

Laënnec remained unacknowledged by the major state medical institutions for another decade. In 1837 the section of pathological anatomy of the Academy of Medicine proposed to the entire academy that Laënnec be honored in the form of a statue or portrait to be placed in the main meeting hall. A special commission was named to examine the proposal and its report, presented in November 1837, was nothing less than a major appreciation of Laënnec's life and work.[32] Its recommendation for a bust or portrait was not in the end implemented. But by insisting that its report was not the *éloge* which the academy owed Laënnec, the report forced Pariset to belatedly honor Laënnec at the annual public meeting of the academy in December 1839.

A number of factors account for the timing of Laënnec's rehabilitation. In the decade following his death, auscultation, though not the stethoscope, had become widely accepted both in France and abroad. Time seems to have healed much of the bitterness surrounding Laënnec's role in the purge of the Faculty of Medicine in 1822. The reputation of Broussais had been in eclipse since 1831, leaving space for a new appreciation of Laënnec's achievement.[33] The great surgeon and pioneer of pathological anatomy Guillaume Dupuytren died in 1835. Since he had at one time been seen as a rival of Laënnec, his death focused attention on Laënnec as well. In 1837, Gabriel Andral published the revised fourth edition of the *Traité de l'auscultation*.

Most important, the discipline of pathological anatomy was in the process of achieving a new level of institutional acceptance. One must emphasize that it was the academy's section of pathological anatomy which initiated the effort to honor Laënnec. The commission report, like all appreciations of Laënnec during this period, stressed his role as a leading figure of the discipline, "one of the most zealous and most enlightened promoters of pathological anatomy."[34] It devoted almost as much space to his work in pathological anatomy as it did to auscultation. Seen in the 1820s uniquely as a diagnostic technique, auscultation was now interpreted as a major breakthrough in pathological anatomy.[35] In this context, the rehabilitation of Laënnec appears as part of the process of consecrating a new discipline by defining and honoring its pioneers and heroes.

Pathological anatomy had existed for some time as an integral part of clinical medicine.[36] But only in the 1830s did it begin to forge an autonomous institutional existence. One of the eleven new sections established in the Academy of Medicine as a result of the reorganization of 1829 was devoted to pathological anatomy.[37] In 1833 the academy created an annual prize, the Prix Portal, for the best work responding to a question in this subject. The first question to be posed was: Describe the influence of pathological anatomy on medicine from Morgagni to the present.[38] Plainly, the practitioners of the discipline were now prepared to evaluate, celebrate, and consecrate the history of pathological anatomy. A few years later readers of the *Mémoires* of the Academy of Medicine were treated to both the prize-winning and first runner-up essays dealing with this question. This celebration of pathological anatomy took up nearly one-half of the entire volume of 1837.[39] The winning essay by Risueño d'Amador, professor at the Faculty of Medicine at Montpellier, was a tour de force which argued that the recent work of Andral and Cruveilhier had enabled pathological anatomy to transcend narrow anatomical localism and to merge with older traditions of humoralism and vitalism. It was, in other words, now in the mainstream of medicine. Underlying such intellectual claims was a substantial institutional breakthrough. In 1836 the discipline had achieved mainstream status within medical education when Dupuytren's legacy to the Paris Faculty of Medicine led to the creation of a chair in pathological anatomy to which Jean Cruveilhier was appointed.

In seeking to upgrade Laënnec's reputation, practitioners of pathological anatomy were thus redefining the history of their field. They were associating it more closely with auscultation, which was by now widely accepted. In demanding posthumous honors for Laënnec they were, in effect, seeking official recognition for their discipline. Still, granted that practitioners of pathological anatomy were in search of precursors and heroes, it remains to be explained why Laënnec stood out from among the pioneers of the discipline. Although it makes Andral rather than Laënnec its main protagonist, the essay by Risueño d'Amador, suggests part of the answer. Laënnec had been among the few anatomists to make a significant contribution to one of the chief tasks of practical clinical medicine, diagnosis. He provided the missing link between the pathological laboratory and the clinic. This was how Risueño described Laënnec's accomplishment:

> Among the works of the school of pathological anatomy which we examine, there is not one which offers, as Laënnec's does, together with anatomical discoveries of the first order, a practical utility that is so immediate. For this admirable work is distinguished above all by its practical side. . . . Something that was apparently impossible has been done, and those least disposed to believe in the wonders of modern medicine have ended up yielding to the evidence and recognizing the immense superiority of a semiotic founded on pathological anatomy over the old semiotic.[40]

The glorification of Laënnec provided official recognition for the central role of pathological anatomy in clinical medicine and that of physical diagnosis in pathological anatomy. It thus sanctioned and gave form to a conceptual and methodological revolution that had been taking shape for several decades and which was coming to be seen as *the* distinguishing feature of the Paris school of medicine. Even as it was becoming a specialized discipline, pathological anatomy could remain firmly in the mainstream of clinical medicine.

Amid all the praise, the careful reader senses that a certain ambivalence to Laënnec persisted in some circles. There were still those, like Jean Bouillaud, who mixed hommage with sharp criticism.[41] The academy ignored its own vote to commission a statue or portrait of Laënnec. Pariset waited two years before delivering a somewhat lukewarm *éloge*.[42] Although he came to substantially the same conclusions about Laënnec's career as had the commission recommending a statue, his panegyric was comparatively short[43] and full of tangents; he contrived to end the section discussing Laënnec's work with comments on cardiology in which Laënnec was compared unfavorably to Andral.[44]

All of this suggests that Laënnec's reputation was in transition. The *Traité de l'auscultation* had already achieved the status of a classic. But Laënnec was still the contemporary of many of those writing about him, and personal animosities had not yet disappeared. Gabriel Andral, who had experienced the sting of Laënnec's barbed pen, could not restrain himself, in his introduction to the fourth edition of the *Traité de l'auscultation* from offering some criticism of Laënnec's temperament.[45] More significantly, perhaps, time had not yet made Laënnec's work so remote that he was seen only as a precursor of the modern. Leading pathological anatomists of the 1830s and 1840s were consciously reacting against what they perceived as the mistakes and inadequacies of an earlier generation, including Laënnec. Some viewed Laënnec as a narrow and descriptive organicist.[46] Andral, in contrast, saw him as a misguided vitalist who accepted that doctrine uncritically and who did not really understand pathological anatomy.[47] Organicist or vitalist, Laënnec was reproached for having neglected systemic physiology by a generation seeking to move pathological anatomy in that direction.[48] Yet pathological anatomists also claimed Laënnec and the practical success of auscultation for their discipline.

One sees this tension in a variety of contexts. Risueño d'Amador's prize-winning essay had many complimentary things to say about Laënnec, but the heroes of the piece were emphatically Cruveilhier and Andral. Laënnec was completely missing from the runner-up essay.[49] Similarly, Cruveilhier's very lengthy introduction to his *Traité d'anatomie pathologique générale*, published in 1849 and seeking to demonstrate the central importance of pathological anatomy to medicine, also did not mention Laënnec but insisted on two separate occasions that pathological anatomy had produced the clinical innovations of percussion and auscultation.[50]

One final example of this curious ambivalence is worth noting. In 1844 Frédéric Dubois d'Amiens, future permanent secretary of the Academy of Medicine, presented to that institution a survey of recent progress in French medicine. Laënnec was certainly one of the major stars of the piece. He was mentioned in several different contexts as the great genius of French medicine.[51] When it came to a specific discussion of pathological anatomy, Laënnec's name figured prominently for the "ingenious" and "profound" classification of organic lesions that he had proposed.[52] But in a footnote that is attached to Laënnec's name, Dubois presented a brief history of pathological anatomy which mentions everyone *except* Laënnec: Morgagni, Vicq d'Azyr, John Hunter, Bichat, Broussais, and, at particular length, Andral and Cruveilhier, who gave "pathological anatomy a decided preeminence in the school of Paris." Placing the history of the discipline in a footnote and reserving the text for Laënnec's work on classification is indicative of both the desire to identify Laënnec with the discipline of pathological anatomy and the difficulty writers were having integrating his work in any account of the historical development of the discipline.[53]

Glory

During the 1840s and 1850s little was published about Laënnec. A medical thesis prepared in Montpellier, another appreciation by the loyal Kergaradec, and an article in an American medical journal represent the sum total of work devoted to the inventor of auscultation.[54] He was, of course, discussed in textbooks and figured prominently in Dubois d'Amiens's *éloge* of Broussais before the Academy of Medicine in 1848.[55] But if Laënnec was not exactly ignored during these two decades, neither was he especially celebrated. Two biographical dictionaries of the 1850s were generally complementary and praised auscultation for introducing a new era in medicine; but there is a notable absence of exaggerated claims for Laënnec's stature. One of these dictionaries, Michaud's *Biographie universelle*, even included a long criticism of auscultation for fostering an excessively narrow organicism and an obsession with scientific methods which neglected the individual and the vital principle.[56]

Several decorative details give some indication of Laënnec's status during this period. By 1856, we saw earlier, the Academy of Medicine contained many artistic and decorative objects, including eighteen statues of deceased academicians. Laënnec's was not among them.[57] When the artist Charles Müller was commissioned in 1848 to paint several murals to decorate the academy, Laënnec discovering auscultation was one of the subjects considered for representation. Due to budgetary constraints, however, only two murals were completed: Pinel causing the chains of the insane to be removed at the Bicêtre and Larrey operating on the battlefield. In other words, Laënnec's achievement was considered worthy of representation but did not have first priority.[58] He had not yet become *the* symbol of the Parisian clinical school.

This situation changed during the mid-1860s. Two events occurred which firmly established Laënnec's stature as an emblematic hero of medical science. In 1865 the Paris Faculty of Medicine sponsored a program of eleven popular lectures in the history of medicine.[59] Paul-Emile Chauffard, then an *agrégé* but soon to be appointed professor of general pathology (1870), presented a major evaluation of Laënnec in the only lecture devoted to a nineteenth-century figure. At roughly the same time, the major national association representing the medical profession, the Association Générale des Médecins de France (AGMF), was engaged in a public campaign to raise funds in order to commission a statue of Laënnec. The statue was unveiled in Paris as part of the 1867 World Exposition and a year later a well-publicized ceremony celebrated the statue's unveiling in Laënnec's hometown of Quimper. Many of the speeches and appreciations presented on that occasion were subsequently published, as were a number of other works occasioned by the festivities.[60]

These two events were certainly connected in that they both expressed and generated new interest in Laënnec. But each occurred in the context of rather different institutional developments. The lecture series on the history of medicine was meant to inspire Parisian students of medicine. As one faculty spokesman explained, the goal was to instill an appreciation of theoretical and scientific achievements in medicine.[61] It must be seen in the context of the wider movement taking shape to reform medical education through science.[62] The course of lectures also reflected a growing interest in the history of medicine. In 1863 the Paris Faculty of Medicine had appealed to the administration for a course in the history of medicine.[63] The appeal was rejected; but a year later Charles Daremberg was appointed to teach the subject at the Collège de France, and the year after that the faculty launched its program of popular lectures. In 1871 Daremberg was finally named to a new chair of medical history at the Faculty of Medicine.[64]

That the history of medicine was identified with a more scientific orientation in medicine may seem surprising. But for many physicians of the mid-nineteenth century, both history and scientific research were alternatives to a narrow focus on medical *practice*. History centered the attention of students on great moments in the production of medical knowledge and provided a reasoned view of the past which made possible a more informed *theoretical* understanding of medicine. Medical history could also focus attention on the achievements of French medicine, which appeared to many during this decade to have been left behind by developments in Germany. It could thus stimulate greater French effort while at the same time defending the reputation of France in the scientific competition among nations. This was one of the roles of the Laënnec myth in the 1860s and during the Third Republic.

Discussions of Laënnec during this period inevitably emphasized that the inventor of auscultation was a representative of *French* medicine, his nation's candidate for medical immortality. In his lecture of 1865 Chauffard insisted that Laënnec was France's main claim to scientific glory. The great medical discoveries of an earlier period had occurred in other nations. "Auscultation emerging perfect from the hands of Laënnec provided us with a dazzling revenge." It had made "the medicine of the world our tributary."[65]

Chauffard had more on his mind than France's scientific glory. His lecture amounted to a major revision of Laënnec's reputation and was the first step in the retrospective constitution of a nineteenth-century tradition for his own brand of vitalism. Chauffard challenged the lingering belief that Laënnec's genius had been exclusively one of empirical observation rather than theoretical innovativeness. He repeatedly emphasized the theoretical elements in Laënnec's work.[66] It was a doctrine, one is not surprised to learn, not unlike Chauffard's own. It was based on a respect for medical tradition combined with openness to scientific innovation. It systematized existing knowledge in pathological anatomy and was concerned with etiology and nosology as well as local diagnosis. Chauffard also challenged the by now widespread view that Laënnec had been a localist blind to the insights of vitalism by emphasizing the provisional and heuristic nature of Laënnec's localism and his openness to systemic and vitalist explanations.[67] Laënnec, in other words, was the major modern precursor of that tradition of medicine of which his own brand of vitalism was the most recent manifestation. He would develop this argument a decade later in his classic study of Gabriel Andral,[68] which established a line of scientific filiation between himself and Laënnec through the person of Andral.

In this case Chauffard's attempt at revision does not seem to have been particularly successful. An article on Laënnec written in 1879 repeated the old saw that Laënnec lacked the genius of induction and generalization.[69] And the connection between Laënnec and vitalism never appears to have become widely accepted. It required the rediscovery of the manuscripts of Laënnec's lectures at the Collège de France to prove that Chauffard had in fact been correct.[70]

Planning for the Quimper ceremonies got under way in 1864 and may well have influenced the choice of Laënnec a year later as the subject of Chauffard's historical lecture. These ceremonies represented considerably more than a local initiative; they were part of a wider effort to organize the French medical profession nationally. In 1858 longstanding attempts to establish a national medical association finally came to fruition when the AGMF was established. Its professional role would prove to be fairly limited in the decades to come, and some of its most important activities had to do with fostering a national medical identity.[71] The executive of the AGMF enthusiastically took up the suggestion to sponsor a subscription to raise funds for a statue of Laënnec. Its president, Pierre Rayer, who was also First Physician to Napoleon III, took it upon himself to obtain the emperor's authorization for the festivities. Within a few years a sum of 20,000 francs was collected from private donors and the sculptor Lequesnu was commissioned to begin work. Although there was a local program committee in Quimper, the financing and the planning of the celebrations were predominantly coordinated by the AGMF.[72] The Academy of Medicine was also involved through the activities of one of its members, H. L. Roger, a leading organizer of the event. The academy sent four representatives to the festivities and associated itself "with this dazzling hommage rendered to one of the greatest *gloires* of our institution and of French medicine."[73] Of the eight speeches presented, four were by members of the academy; Roger's own oration was made in the name of the academy and was subsequently published in its *Bulletin*.[74]

The AGMF's involvement so early in its history in this project seems to have been an effort to define the history of French medicine and to win for it appropriate public recognition. The academy's role in this initiative reflected its support of these larger professional aspirations but also early efforts to emphasize its own scientific status; these would peak during the following decade with Chauffard's plan to restructure the institution.[75] Laënnec was not the only possible centerpiece for such a celebration. At the same time the AGMF was raising funds for Laënnec's statue, the departmental council of the Haute Vienne was seeking to raise funds for a statue of Dupuytren in the latter's hometown of Pièrrebuffière.[76] In 1867 a drive was also launched for funds to commission a statue of Trousseau at the Paris Faculty of Medicine.[77] Despite such competition, Laënnec remained the most obvious symbol of medicine's claim for greater public recognition. He had contributed something practical and concrete to medicine and to humanity, something increasingly visible on a daily basis to both doctors and their patients.[78] His achievement demonstrated that the interests of medicine were identical with those of society, as well as affirming "what this great art can do for the welfare of mankind when it is inspired, when it is honored by the teachings of a master like Laënnec."[79] In his reports on the planning of the Quimper festivities, Roger characterized the forthcoming events as an opportunity for France to demonstrate that she attached as much importance to celebrating the achievements of medicine and science as she did to glorifying military prowess. The number of public statues of healers indicated in quite precise fashion the degree to which medicine was recognized by society.[80]

The significance of the ceremonies had to do with their national and profession-wide character. Laënnec was transformed from a hero of pathological anatomy to the major figure of French medicine. In line with this, the language of celebration escalated. Auscultation was now described as "the finest discovery which science has placed in the service of humanity."[81] Laënnec himself had now become the greatest doctor of modern times, the French Hippocrates and a benefactor of humanity. He had given doctors the power to "read . . . the alterations hidden in the depths of the body."[82] But more important, he had invented a method that had made medicine scientific, "which continues to exist and thanks to which medicine has become positive and moves ever closer to the exact sciences."[83] He had also become the real father of pathological anatomy and the Paris clinical school more generally. All those who had preceded him were reduced to the role of precursors. There were in fact two versions of this interpretation. The one that was dominant in the 1860s was that Laënnec together with Broussais had founded the Paris clinical school. This brings us to the issue of Broussais's posthumous reputation, only slightly less fascinating than that of Laënnec himself.

In the aftermath of his death, Broussais posed a problem for instant historians of medicine. There remained fervent supporters of the great reformer, though fewer than before. There were also far more writers willing to criticize his physiological doctrine. Many others just could not make up their minds. Representatives of official institutions had particular difficulty responding to the death of this controversial figure. The Paris Faculty of Medicine, for instance, sent two representatives to speak at Broussais's funeral. The dean, Mateo Orfila, gave a brief speech made up of conventional regrets and platitudes. He left a more substantial appraisal to Broussais's erstwhile disciple, Jean-Baptiste Bouillaud.[84] The representatives of the Academy of Medicine at Broussais's funeral and at a statue-unveiling ceremony at Val-de-Grâce hospital in 1841 simply refused to be pinned down.[85] In the second case, especially, Etienne Pariset, who spoke in the name of the academy, said a few nice things about his subject's extraordinary qualities, launched into an elaborate disquisition on the nature of God and the universe, and insisted that a full evaluation of Broussais required the passage of time and distance from the controversies he had generated. He never did present the full academic *éloge* that Broussais's stature seemed to demand. The evidence suggests that his neglect was deliberate and that the academy's administrative council commissioned someone else to do the job.[86]

One can appreciate the difficulties of evaluating Broussais by examining an *éloge* which was presented in 1839 by the professor of physiology Pierre Bérard at the annual prize-giving ceremony of the Faculty of Medicine.[87] Bérard tried to have it both ways. The physiological doctrine was wrong but Broussais was nevertheless a great figure. Bérard supported this judgment by distinguishing between the doctrine and the physician with major clinical insights, by suggesting that even mistaken theories advance science through the research and controversy which they generate, and by pointing out that whatever its limitations Broussais's doctrine supported localism. Reading this convoluted and lengthy piece one cannot help but sympathize with eulogizers who refused to take a clear stand.

A decade later the issue had been resolved. Pariset's successor as permanent secretary of the Academy of Medicine, Dubois d'Amiens, had no doubts about Broussais's stature or the nature of his achievement.[88] One of the first *éloges* which he presented after his appointment was devoted to the "the great reformer." It was no longer possible to take the doctrines themselves seriously, but Broussais was nonetheless presented as one of the two founders of pathological anatomy, the other being Laënnec. Broussais's contribution was essentially negative. Almost singlehandedly he had destroyed the edifice of eighteenth-century medicine. He had also championed and popularized many of the principles on which scientific medicine would be based. But he did not himself develop the full implications of these principles. It was left to Laënnec to fulfill this task and to create a truly scientific medicine.

Chauffard challenged this by now dominant interpretation of the origin of pathological anatomy. According to him, Broussais and Laënnec were definitely not complementary figures pursuing a common enterprise. Rather, they were as they had appeared to their contemporaries: antagonists who represented contradictory principles, the one retrograde and reactionary, the other progressive and scientific. In Chauffard's narrative, Laënnec pulled medicine into the modern world despite the reactionary influence exercised on French medicine by Broussais.[89]

The opinion that Broussais and Laënnec were two giants who complemented each other did not disappear overnight. It was a convenient literary technique for describing the struggle between the two men that was both aesthetically and psychologically pleasing. It resolved their conflict in a higher synthesis, an attractive literary gambit, and explained how so many of the brightest minds of a generation had been seduced by the physiological doctrine. A report on the recent progress of French medicine published in 1867 repeated this view.[90] A year later Bouillaud's lengthy appreciation of Laënnec presented in Quimper reiterated it with considerable force and erudition. Nevertheless, it was Chauffard's perspective which came to prevail. By the early twentieth century Laënnec was usually presented in France as *the* originator of the French school of pathological anatomy and of scientific medicine in general.[91] Broussais, in contrast, was relegated to the ranks of a minor and slightly ridiculous curiosity.[92] This was the situation in 1953 when Erwin Ackerknecht published his classic article on Broussais, which reminded professional historians at least of Broussais's seminal influence on the development of the Parisian clinical school.

Laënnec in the Early Twentieth Century

In 1879, on the sixtieth anniversary of the publication of the *Traité de l'auscultation*, the Paris Faculty of Medicine sponsored a new edition of that work while the Parisian hospital administration named a new hospital after its author. From then on, the number of new works about Laënnec increased exponentially. It is virtually impossible to examine all the publications dealing with Laënnec that appeared after 1880. The reputation of the inventor of the stethoscope was no longer dependent on official activities, though these continued to take place. What is more, foreigners were almost as likely as the French to express their interest and homage. Laënnec was now in the public domain, available to anyone searching for a subject or a precursor.

If a full examination of Laënnec's reputation in the twentieth century is thus not feasible, it is nevertheless possible to view it within the more narrow confines of the Academy of Medicine. The centenary of Laënnec's death in 1927 provided the occasion for yet another institutional tribute to the inventor of auscultation. The academy's own centenary celebration in 1920 seems to have awakened a taste for festivities commemorating its most famous members. The first one in 1922 was devoted to Louis Pasteur, born a century before. The next two honored British figures who predated the academy, Edward Jenner (1923) and Thomas Sydenham (1924), followed in 1925 by a commemoration of Jean-Martin Charcot's birth. The celebration of Laënnec's death two years later thus represented the third tribute since 1920 to illustrious members of the academy.

At a public meeting presided over by Minister of Public Instruction Edouard Herriot, with a large number of foreign visitors present,[93] five speakers rehearsed various aspects of the great man's career. They were immeasurably aided by the recent publication of Rouxeau's biography, from which they borrowed liberally.[94] Hyperbolic claims for Laënnec's genius still abounded. One speaker called him "perhaps the greatest medical genius of all humanity."[95] Another attributed to him "the prodigious progress accomplished by medicine during the past century."[96] The "Frenchness" of Laënnec's achievement was emphatically asserted, as part of the effort to demonstrate that France took a back seat to no nation when it came to medical science.[97] A professor of medical history later explained that his inaugural lecture in that subject at the Paris Faculty of Medicine in 1919 had commemorated the centenary of the *Traité de l'auscultation* because

> I wanted to show in this way how the role of the professor of the history of medicine was to magnify, by making known their works, our national medical heroes [*gloires*]. "That is," I said, "the primary obligation of our teaching and I would willingly add in imitation of our venerable Joachim du Bellay: the chair of history of medicine of the Faculty of Paris should have as its motto: *the defense and illustration of French medicine.*[98]

The centenary celebrations continued in this mode. Edouard Herriot referred to Laënnec as a "purely French genius"[99] while Charles Achard could reduce the medical history of the nineteenth century to the work of three Frenchmen—Laënnec, Claude Bernard, and Louis Pasteur.[100]

If all this was only an intensified version of claims made during the Laënnec tributes of the 1860s there was one profound difference. The intellectual context for celebrations of Laënnec's achievement had changed dramatically since the nineteenth century. During the 1860s Laënnec could be taken as a model for the most advanced medical science of his time. By 1927 he was a historical figure whose achievements had been overshadowed by those of Claude Bernard and Louis Pasteur. Bernard had been drawn into the medical pantheon soon after his death. For the medical reformers who achieved institutional power during the 1870s and 1880s and who sought to introduce experimental science to medical education and practice, Bernard was an emblematic figure. At his death, he was the subject of a lengthy funeral oration in the name of the Academy of Medicine.[101] Seven years later, Jules Béclard devoted a substantial academic *éloge* to Bernard, whose views were presented as the inspiration for the revolutionary changes transforming European medicine.[102] Pasteur's trajectory, however, was more complex.

Unlike Bernard, who had little to do with the Academy of Medicine, Pasteur directly challenged the academy from the moment of his election as an *associé libre* in 1873. He questioned its institutional practices and scientific orthodoxies. By the time of his death in 1895, there were few academicians who doubted the basic premises of the germ theory, although they might disagree about particular applications or general consequences for therapy. It is thus surprising to note that there was no necrological notice in the academy in response to his death. Even more astonishing, there was no academic *éloge* devoted to Pasteur until 1914, nearly twenty years after his death. Though retrospective *éloges* had become common, they were seldom delayed this long in the case of someone so illustrious.

The silence of E. J. Bergeron, permanent secretary at Pasteur's death, is perhaps understandable. He was rather elderly when Pasteur died (he had been born in 1817) and was nearing the end of his tenure as permanent secretary. He was also by all accounts not much of a scientist or scholar[103] and an informed discussion of Pasteur's work may have been beyond his capabilities. But his successor, Sigismond Jaccoud, was in a different league altogether. Erudite and well-informed, he was quite capable of reviewing Pasteur's scientific corpus. If he did not do so, it was because he chose not to.

There were, I would suggest, two major reasons for not honoring Pasteur with an *éloge*. First, the great man was neither a doctor nor a full member of the academy but a chemist and an *associé libre*. There was little pressure to eulogize Pasteur because other scientific institutions in which he was a full member assumed the task. Second, Pasteur's genius was widely recognized. It seemed more urgent at the turn of the century to acknowledge the French medical men whose contributions to bacteriology were being ignored. It is thus no accident that the first bacteriologist honored with an *éloge* was J. A. Villemin, an army doctor who had presented his findings on the transmissibility of tuberculosis to the Academy of Medicine. Jaccoud's treatment sought to demonstrate the magnitude of Villemin's achievement and emphasized that his contribution was far more important for disease prophylaxis than Koch's discovery of the actual microorganism.[104] But if the *éloge* was explicitly a defense of French as opposed to German scientific achievement,[105] it can also be read as a claim for the contributions of French medicine to the development of bacteriology and public health. Jaccoud strengthened his case two years later with an *éloge* of the veterinarian-bacteriologist Edmond Nocard.[106]

On the one occasion when Jaccoud did deal with Pasteur, it became clear that he, like many clinicians of his generation, had reservations about the germ theory of disease, at least as it was sometimes expounded. He did not doubt that microbes caused many specific diseases or that bacteriology was an important resource for medicine. But he was disturbed by what he saw as the tendency to reduce all disease to microbes and all medicine to bacteriology. Furthermore, Jaccoud was a believer in the vitalism propounded by his mentor Malgaigne, which emphasized the importance of the individual as the terrain of disease and healing. By accentuating the role of an outside agent in causing illness, bacteriology could be seen as an attack on this traditional but still vibrant view. This was certainly Jaccoud's perspective and in the review of nineteenth-century medical developments which he presented soon after taking office, he devoted a generous amount of space to Pasteur. But his Pasteur was a quasi-vitalist who, unlike the nameless devotees of "bacteriology," admitted that the organism could sometimes spontaneously produce bacterial disease and emphasized the importance of "vital resistance" in determining receptivity to disease. "We find," he concluded, "in Pasteur the vitalism of Malgaigne."[107]

Jaccoud's reservations about bacteriology and unorthodox views of Pasteur were not shared by his successors, Georges Debove and Charles Achard. In 1914 Debove devoted his first *éloge* after becoming permanent secretary to Pasteur; there is nothing in his treatment to suggest that bacteriology was in any way problematic for medicine.[108] At the academy's centenary celebration in 1920, Pasteur appeared in talk after talk as the dominant influence in recent medicine, surgery, and public health, while his work was represented as "the most beautiful page in the history of the academy in the nineteenth century; it will remain for our company its greatest claim to honor."[109] Two years later the centenary celebrations of Pasteur's birth completed the appropriation of Pasteur by the Academy of Medicine and French medicine generally.

It is in this context that the celebration honoring Laënnec took on a bittersweet flavor. For the pertinence of Laënnec's achievements to the new medicine taking shape was not at all clear. Was his achievement, in the words of one speaker, no more than a historical date, irrelevant to a medicine revolutionized by the germ theory and physiological discoveries pertaining to the functions of the glands?[110] What was at stake was nothing less than a century-long tradition of clinical medical research and practice in France. In one form or another various speakers tried to confront this question. Paul Bar addressed it most explicitly by making Laënnec—not for the first time—the symbol of clinical observation. If Pasteur was the personification of "induction," Laënnec represented "observation," which "will always remain the supreme law":

> It is thanks to it that the doctors living in the medical atmosphere of their times can indicate to the men of the laboratory, to researchers, the inadequacies of their insights or can consecrate the progress of which they [researchers] are the promoters. It is thanks to it, finally, that medicine approaches most surely its goal, the most noble of all those which man's activity is required to attain: to alleviate human suffering.[111]

Emile Sargent was even more specific. The anatomoclinical method, he argued, remained, despite all the acquisitions of science, the "most certain and most solid foundation for the interpretation of morbid signs" and was perfectly compatible with newer physiological methods. In fact, the essence of Laënnec's method was not to replace one technique with another but to bring together and consider the results of all possible techniques:[112]

> Do not tamper with the great principles of the anatomoclinical method. Let us remain loyal to the teachings of the Master who founded the great French clinical school and who established the rules and the principles according to which we must search for the demonstration and the value of our findings.[113]

In the potted history of medicine which the academy's secretary, Charles Achard, presented, three Frenchmen were responsible for the three great revolutions that had transformed modern medicine: the first was Laënnec, who had created hospital medicine on the anatomopatholological model; the two other were Claude Bernard, who had introduced experimental physiology into medicine, and Louis Pasteur, who had inaugurated the stage of etiology which in turn opened the way for therapeutics.[114] On one level this vision of history can be seen as a reflection of the scientific nationalism that was so characteristic of French medicine during this period. But read carefully, it can also be seen as part of the effort to associate French clinical medicine with the laboratory discoveries that had revolutionized medicine. In Achard's account, the latter two innovations did not replace the anatomoclinical model but rather built on it. In fact, Achard went on, these three stages were also the stages of clinical investigation. The clinician begins by observing symptoms using far more precise techniques than had been available to predecessors. He then goes on to try to explain the symptoms by grouping them into syndromes, using anatomy to determine organ lesions and physiology for those of functions. His next step is to determine the cause of the disorder, often using experimental methods, and to conceptualize the entire morbid process. He is then in a position to attack actively the cause of the disease.[115]

In this vision, traditional clinical methods are not abandoned but added to by accretion.[116] Even more important, experimental laboratory science is integrated into clinical medicine but on the latter's terms. It is the logic of the clinic that prevails and that determines how physiology and bacteriology are utilized. Achard made this point even more explicitly a year later at the centenary celebration of the birth of the neurologist Alfred Vulpian. The subject of the celebration, it was said, had combined the skills of a clinician, anatomopathologist, and experimental physiologist in a harmonious way, applying with particular success the latter disciplines to clinical interpretation.[117] These three types of competence, Achard argued, "have become the necessary attributes of the great doctor."[118]

This of course was not the only possible view. The elderly Georges Hayem (b. 1841), whose own research career had been notably shaped by laboratory methods, spoke about Vulpian's clinical work at the same ceremony. He admitted that medicine was now entering an exciting new "humoral" phase based on chemistry.[119] He nonetheless affirmed that traditional anatomoclinical methods continued to be fruitful and especially appropriate for hospital doctors in a position to do postmortems. Even more vigorously he praised Vulpian the clinician. "A great clinician is a man who is completely exceptional, before whom one must bow as deeply as before the most illustrious savants."[120] If Hayem was more sympathetic than the younger Achard to the intellectual traditions of the academic elite (which were those of his youth), he too was responding in his way to the need to situate these traditions within the context of medicine's recent scientific revolution.

I have suggested in this chapter that the foundations for Laënnec's near legendary status were laid between the late 1830s and mid-1860s. This leaves us with an obvious question. Why did this process occur, and why was Laënnec rather than someone else chosen for professional canonization?

The quality of Laënnec's discovery provides part of the answer. By "quality" I allude to far more than its unquestionable brilliance and fruitfulness. I refer as well to its simplicity, to its ability to be captured in such formulas as "auscultation," the "stethoscope," and more elaborately "the application of sound to diagnosis." One did not have to understand the roots of Laënnec's activity in pathological anatomy. Like the germ theory, auscultation could be grasped in a simple form. It could also be grasped physically by every doctor on an increasingly routine basis. It would in fact be difficult to find a medical discovery that intruded so regularly and ubiquitously on the doctor–patient relationship. That it was aimed against diseases of the chest cavity, and especially tuberculosis, the great scourge of the nineteenth century, undoubtedly contributed as well to Laënnec's stature. The fact that auscultation was unquestionably a French invention made its inventor a particularly suitable candidate for canonization.[121] Finally, his early death ensured that the kind of myth-building which depends on the demise of the hero for its full expression began without delay. The contrasting case of Andral, who outlived his scientific achievements by nearly forty years, is highly instructive.

As a result of all these factors, Laënnec evolved during the half century following his death from the inventor of auscultation, to the man who had linked pathological anatomy to clinical medicine, and then to one of two founding fathers of the Paris school and the greatest French physician of the nineteenth century. This reputation was forged at a series of public ceremonial occasions at which various groups sought to identify themselves with the practical benefits of auscultation. Laënnec was in a sense their candidate for greatness and his success was theirs as well.

By the twentieth century, Laënnec's reputation took on different, rather more complex burdens. The inventor of the stethoscope had become the single founding father of the Paris school. He had also become the standardbearer for the clinically centered, eclectic research traditions of the Parisian medical elite. These traditions by now appeared somewhat old-fashioned and their adherents were struggling to redefine them in the wake of the recent successes of the experimental laboratory. The celebration of Laënnec's reputation affirmed the continuities between research traditions old and new.

The basis of Laënnec's complex and many-layered reputation was a medical discovery that was, by any standards, extraordinary. But it evolved in the way it did because various groups at different times found it necessary to create histories for themselves, histories graced with heroes. Laënnec's great achievement meant essentially that he was available for such appropriation.

NOTES

1. René-Théophile-Hyacinthe Laënnec was born in Brittany in 1781 and moved to Paris in 1799 to pursue medical studies. He received his MD in 1804 and practiced and taught privately in Paris. In 1816 he was appointed physician at the Necker Hospital, where he began serious research on auscultation. In 1819 he published his classic *Traité de l'auscultation médiate*, 2nd rev. ed. (1826). He was appointed professor at the Collège de France in 1822 and the Paris Faculty of Medicine in 1823.

2. There have been few detailed studies of medical reputations. Some exceptions are Richard H. Shryock, "The Medical Reputation of Benjamin Rush," *Bulletin of the History of Medicine* 45 (1971), 507–52; L. S. Jacyna, "Images of John Hunter in the Nineteenth Century," *History of Science* 21 (1983), 85–108; Robert G. Frank, Jr., "The Image of Harvey in Commonwealth and Restoration England," in *William Harvey and His Age: The Professional and Social Context of the Discovery of Circulation*, ed. Jerome J. Bylebyl (Baltimore, Md., 1979), pp. 103–43. On the reputations of leading French scientists, see Dorinda Outram, "Scientific Biography and the Case of Georges Cuvier: With a Critical Biography," *History of Science* 16 (1978), 153–78, and Bernadette Bensaude-Vincent, "A Founder Myth in the History of Sciences? The Lavoisier Case," in *Functions and Uses of Disciplinary History*, ed. Loren Graham, Wolf Lepenies, and Peter Weingart (Dordrecht, 1983), pp. 53–78.

3. I will be primarily concerned with Laënnec's reputation in France. Few studies devoted to Laënnec were published outside France before about 1880.

4. An exception was *Nouvelle Bibliothèque médicale* 4 (1826), which published Cruveilhier's speech (442–50).

5. On academic *éloges* see Chapter 5; on the thematic content of Pariset's *éloges* see Chapter 9.

6. All of these were published in *MEM* 1 (1828). They are reprinted in Etienne Pariset, *Histoire des membres de l'Académie Royale de Médecine*, 2 vols. (1850).

7. The most serious biography of Laënnec presents his dealings with this academy as a consistent series of snubs. (Alfred Rouxeau, *Laënnec après 1806* [1920], pp. 198, 260, 275, 284.) But this view seems unjustified. On the occasion of both of his candidacies for membership to the Academy of Sciences, Laënnec was defeated by much more senior men, in 1822 by Chaussier, aged seventy-six, and in 1825 by Boyer, aged sixty-five.

8. Laënnec, in fact, had been the first choice of the Academy of Sciences's medical section for this chair. But when the entire academy voted, it elected François Magendie. Maurice Crosland, *Science under Control: The French Academy of Sciences, 1795–1914* (Cambridge, 1992), p. 233.

9. Rouxeau, *Laënnec après 1806*, p. 285. More generally on these events, see Charles Odic, "Les Événements du 18 novembre 1822," Thèse en médecine, Université de Paris, 1921. Political connections were also behind Laënnec's appointment to a hospital position in 1816. See André Finot, "Louis Becquey, découvreur de Laënnec," *Histoire des sciences médicales* 3–4 (1970), 167–73.

10. A.L.J. Bayle, *Notice historique sur Laënnec* (1826). Bayle was best known for work on the organic causes of mental derangement.

11. J.-A. Lejumeau de Kergaradec, *Notice sur le Professeur Laënnec* (1826).

12. "Biographical notice of the late Professor Laënnec," *Lancet* 11 (1826), 44–45.

13. A. Boulland, "Notice sur le professeur Laënnec," *Journal des sciences médicales* 1 (1827), 284–94.

14. "Notice sur M. René-Théophile Laënnec," *AGM* 13 (1827), 620–25.

15. Ibid., 623.

16. In addition to the works already cited, which all make this point, see the review of the second edition of the *Traité de l'auscultation* in the *Edinburgh Medical and Surgical Journal* 26 (1826), 406–43.

17. Gabriel Andral, *Précis d'anatomie pathologique* (1829).

18. *Dictionnaire de médecine et de chirurgie pratique*, vol. 2 (1829), pp. 346–72.

19. *Edinburgh Medical and Surgical Journal* 26 (1826), 406–43.

20. Audrey B. Davis, *Medicine and Its Technology: An Introduction to the History of Medical Instrumentation* (Westport, Conn., 1981), p. 89. British understanding of Laënnec is analyzed in greater detail in Russell C. Maulitz, *Morbid Appearances: The Anatomy of Pathology in the Early Nineteenth Century* (Cambridge, 1987).

21. *Lancet* 11 (1826), 45.

22. *AGM* 13 (1827), 621.

23. See, for example, the evaluation of Laënnec's teaching in Félix Ratier, *Coup d'oeil sur les cliniques médicales de la Faculté de médecine et des hôpitaux civils de Paris* (1827), p. 330. On Laënnec's popularity among foreign doctors see M. D. Grmek and Pierre Huard, "Les Élèves étrangers de Laënnec," *Revue d'histoire des sciences* 26 (1973), 315–37. On his British students, see Russell C. Maulitz, "Channel Crossing: The Lure of French Pathology for English Medical Students, 1816–36," *Bulletin of the History of Medicine* 55 (1981), 475–96, esp. 485.

24. François Broussais (1772–1838) was probably the last of the great medical systematizers. His physiological doctrine was based on the notion that all illnesses were due to

irritation of organs and especially of the gastrointestinal tract, from which they spread to other parts of the body through "sympathies."

25. Kergaradec, *Notice*, p. 15, and Bayle, *Notice historique*, p. xxxi.

26. Boulland, "Notice," 290.

27. Erwin H. Ackerknecht, "Broussais, or a Forgotten Medical Revolution," *Bulletin of the History of Medicine* 27 (1953), 320–43. More recent studies of Broussais are Jean-François Braunstein, *Broussais et le matérialisme: médecine et philosophie au XIXe siècle* (1986) and Michel Valentin, *François Broussais, empereur de la médecine* (Dinard, 1988).

28. This is especially stressed in the notice in *AGM* (n. 14) and Erwin H. Ackerknecht, *Medicine at the Paris Hospital, 1794–1848* (Baltimore, Md., 1967), p. 98. Also see Jacalyn Duffin, "Laënnec: entre la pathologie et la clinique," Thèse 3è cycle, Université de Paris I, 1985.

29. Boulland, "Notice," 289.

30. *Dictionnaire des sciences médicales: biographie médicale*, 7 vols. (1820–25), vol. 5, p. 471. The entry is signed by F.-G. Boisseau.

31. In his article "Anatomie pathologique" in the *Dictionnaire de médecine*, 2nd ed. 30 vols. (1832–46), vol. 2, p. 556, J. Dezeimeris divides the discipline into two schools: one, stemming from Hunter, Bichat, and Broussais, had tried to link anatomical lesions to physiology, while the other, led by Laënnec, had been purely descriptive. The former had made serious errors but was by far the more fruitful, according to the author. This analysis was repeated more than thirty years later in J.-M. Guardia, *La Médecine à travers les siècles* (1865), pp. 35–37.

32. H. Husson, "Rapport sur la convenance de placer le buste de Laënnec dans la salle des séances de l'Académie," *MEM* 7 (1838), 30–44.

33. Jacques Piquemal, "Le Choléra de 1832 en France et la pensée médicale," *Thalès* 10 (1959), 69.

34. Husson, "Rapport," 30.

35. Ibid., 44.

36. The best study of the early history of this discipline in France and Britain is Maulitz, *Morbid Appearances*.

37. The influence of pathological anatomy in the academy extended beyond this section, since many practitioners of the discipline were in the sections of medical and surgical pathology.

38. *MEM* 3 (1833), 44.

39. *MEM* 6 (1837).

40. B. Risueño d'Amador, "Influence de l'anatomie pathologique sur la médecine depuis Morgagni jusqu'à nos jours," *MEM* 6 (1837), 444–45.

41. J.-B. Bouillaud, *Essai sur la philosophie médicale et les généralités de la clinique médicale* (1836).

42. In *MEM* 8 (1840), 19–40. Reprinted in Pariset, *Membres de l'ARM*, vol. 2, pp. 240–74.

43. It ran to twenty-two pages in the version published in *MEM*. Fourteen individuals had received or were to receive considerably longer *éloges* from Pariset.

44. Pariset, *Membres de l'ARM*, vol. 2, pp. 271–72.

45. Andral, preface to *Traité de l'auscultation*, 4th ed. (1837), pp. viii–ix.

46. Risueño d'Amador, "Influence," 460–61.

47. Andral, preface to *Traité*, 4th ed., pp. viii–ix. Despite Andral's comments, the notion that Laënnec had taken a stand behind localism in opposition to vitalism was extremely prevalent.

48. Laënnec took physiological theory very seriously in his Collège de France lectures, of course. But since the lectures had not been published, it is doubtful whether their content was known to most Parisian physicians of the late 1830s.

49. C. Saucerotte, "Mémoire à la réponse à cette question: Quelle a été l'influence de l'anatomie pathologique sur la médecine depuis Morgagni jusqu'à nos jours?" *MEM* 6 (1837), 494–604.

50. *Traité d'anatomie pathologique générale* (1849), pp. 28, 36.

51. F. Dubois (d'Amiens), "Des Progrès récents de la médecine en France comparés à ceux de la chirurgie," *MEM* 11 (1845), esp. ciii.

52. Ibid., xcvi.

53. This treatment makes more sense if we remember Dezeimeris's distinction, mentioned in note 31, between a physiological school of pathological anatomy and a purely descriptive one. The nineteenth-century members of the descriptive school are excluded from the historical résumé.

54. These were J.-B. Soudres, *Études médicales sur Laënnec*, medical thesis, Montpellier, 1851; J.-A. Lejumeau de Kergaradec, *Notice sur Laënnec* (Rennes, 1852); A. Flint (no title) in the *New Orleans Medical News and Hospital Gazette* 6 (1859–60), 736–56.

55. *MEM* 14 (1849), i–xxviii.

56. "Laënnec," *Biographie universelle ancienne et moderne*, ed. J.-F. Michaud, 2nd ed., 45 vols. (1843–65), vol. 22, pp. 435–39. This entry is signed by Didier. Also see the entry on Laënnec in *Nouvelle Biographie générale*, ed. J.-C. Hoefer, 46 vols. (1855–66), vol. 28, pp. 657–61, by C. Saucerotte.

57. Louis Peisse, *La Médecine et les médecins; philosophie, doctrines, institutions, critiques, moeurs et biographies médicales* (1857), vol. 2, pp. 307–38.

58. See Chapter 5 for a discussion of this episode.

59. One of the lectures about Jean de Wier by Alex. Axenfeld provoked so much political controversy that Minister of Public Instruction Victor Duruy canceled the series.

60. Among the most important were J.-B. Bouillaud, *Éloge de Laënnec* (1869); A. Lecadre, *Étude comparative; Broussais et Laënnec* (Le Havre, 1868); D. de Thizan, *Le Docteur Laënnec* (Quimper, 1868). The shorter speeches made at the Quimper ceremony were published in *Union médicale*, 3e sér. 6 (1868).

61. *Union médicale*, 2e sér. 25 (1865), 546.

62. On this movement see George Weisz, "Reform and Conflict in French Medical Education, 1870–1914," in *The Organization of Science and Technology in France, 1808–1914*, ed. Robert Fox and George Weisz (Cambridge, 1980), pp. 61–94.

63. The request was discussed by the commission of educational inspectors, meeting of October 29, 1863, AN F17 13071. Also see C. Daremberg, *Histoire des sciences médicales comprenant l'anatomie, la physiologie, la médecine, la chirurgie et les doctrines de pathologie générale* (1870), pp. 6–7. Denise Wrotnowska, "Documents inédits à propos de la création de la chaire de l'histoire de la médecine à la Faculté de Paris," *Histoire de la médecine* 11 (1956), 75–79.

64. After Daremberg's death the government financed the academy's purchase of his private library. See Chapter 2.

65. P.-E. Chauffard, *Laënnec: conférences historiques de la Faculté de Médecine* (1865), p. 27. Also see E. J. Bergeron, "Éloge de H. Roger," *MEM* 39 (1900), 8.

66. Chauffard, *Laënnec*, pp. 4, 40, 47.

67. Ibid., pp. 16, 30.

68. P.-E. Chauffard, *Andral: la médecine française de 1820 à 1830* (1877).

69. A. Chereau, "Laënnec," *AGM*, 7e sér. 4 (1879), 51–65.

70. See Jacalyn Duffin, "Vitalism and Organicism in the Philosophy of R.-T.-H. Laënnec," *Bulletin of the History of Medicine* 62 (1988), 525–45, and her "Laënnec."

71. On the AGMF, see Jacques Léonard, *Les Médecins de l'ouest au XIXe siècle*, 3 vols. (Lyon, 1978), vol. 2, 1004–53.

72. Reports on the preparations were regularly made at AGMF annual meetings and published in *Union médicale*.

73. Letter from Roger in *BAM* 33 (1868), 348.

74. *BAM* 33 (1868), 754–60.

75. This is discussed in Chapter 2.

76. There seems in fact to have been some competition between the two fundraising efforts. See Roger's report to the assembly of the AGMF in *Union médicale*, 2e sér. 29 (1866), 133.

77. *Union médicale*, 3e sér. 4 (1867).

78. According to Stanley Joel Reiser, *Medicine and the Reign of Technology* (Cambridge, 1979), p. 38, the stethoscope achieved widespread acceptance in Great Britain and the United States by the 1850s. In fact, we know little about the extent of its use. As late as 1885 the eleventh edition of J.-B. Barth and H. L. Roger's *Traité pratique d'auscultation* (1885) treated use of the stethoscope as opposed to the ear as a matter of personal preference or circumstances. The *Index to the Surgeon General's Catalogue*, ser. 1 (Washington, 1880–95), contains ten pages of listings on auscultation (vol. 1) but devotes less than one page to the stethoscope (vol. 13). Forty years later M. Laignel-Lavastine wrote that French doctors used immediate auscultation more frequently than mediate auscultation. "Sur le Centenaire de la mort de Laënnec," *Bull. Soc. Fr. hist. méd.* 21 (1927), 99–108.

79. Speech by A. Tardieu, president of the AGMF, at Quimper, August 15, 1868, published in *Union médicale*, 3e sér. 6 (1868), 250.

80. Roger to the AGMF in *Union médicale*, 2e sér. 29 (1866), 133.

81. Tardieu in *Union médicale*, 3e sér. 6 (1868), 250.

82. Roger in *BAM* 33 (1868), 757.

83. Ibid., 759. Also see *Union médicale*, 3e sér. 6 (1868), 300.

84. M. Orfila, *Discours prononcé au nom de la Faculté de Médecine de Paris sur la tombe de M. Broussais* (1838); J.-B. Bouillaud, *Discours prononcé au nom de la Faculté de Médecine de Paris sur la tombe de M. Broussais* (1838). Both speeches can be most easily located in AN AJ16 6511.

85. These were J.-B. Nacquart, whose oration was published in *BAM* 3 (1838), 266–69, and Pariset, whose oration is in *BAM* 6 (1840–41), 1038–44.

86. Meeting of the administrative council, January 11, 1848, in AM Liasse 13. The incident is discussed in greater detail in Chapter 5.

87. P. Bérard, *Discours prononcé dans la séance publique de la Faculté de Médecine de Paris du 4 novembre 1839* (1839).

88. F. Dubois, "Éloge de Broussais," *MEM* 14 (1849), i–xxviii.

89. Chauffard, *Laënnec*, pp. 44–45.

90. J. Béclard and A. Axenfeld, *Rapport sur le progrès de la médecine en France* (1867), pp. 2–3. Lecadre's study of the two men is cast in the same mold. Thirteen years later, Béclard in his *éloge* of Andral maintained this interpretation despite the fact that he relied heavily for detail on Chauffard's book about Andral. Jules Béclard, *Éloge d'Andral* (1880), p. 6.

91. See, for example, C. Achard, "Le Rôle de Laënnec dans l'évolution de la médecine," *BAM* 96 (1927), 455–67; Lion Meunier, *Histoire de la médecine depuis ses origines jusqu'à nos jours* (1911), p. 415.

92. See, for example, H. Folet, "Broussais et le broussaisme," *Bull. Soc. fr. hist. méd.* 5 (1905), 239–305. The Academy of Medicine failed to celebrate the centenary of Broussais's death in 1938.

93. The list of foreign delegates took up pages 467 to 470 of *BAM* 95 (1926).

94. Alfred Rouxeau, *Laënnec avant 1806: l'enfance et la jeunesse d'un grand homme* (1912); and *Laënnec après 1806*.

95. C. Mirallié, "Les Origines médicales de Laënnec," *BAM* 96 (1926), 424.

96. M. Letulle, "Laënnec anatomo-pathologiste," *BAM* 96 (1926), 425.

97. This theme in further discussed in my discussion of Achard's *éloges* in Chapter 5.

98. Pierre Ménétrier, "L'Enseignement de l'histoire de la médecine à l'École de Santé et à la Faculté de Médecine de Paris," *Bull. Soc. fr. hist. méd.* 24 (1930), 384.

99. *BAM* 96 (1926), 462.

100. Achard, "Le Rôle de Laënnec," 458–60.

101. A. Moreau in *BAM* 7 (1878), 128–32.

102. J. Béclard, "Éloge de Claude Bernard," *MEM* 35 (1887), 1–24, esp. 19.

103. Achard described him as a "clinician of the first order . . . but a little remote from the scientific movement that was transforming medicine. . . ." C. Achard, "Jaccoud à l'Académie," *BAM* 104 (1930), 614.

104. S. Jaccoud, "Éloge de Villemin," *MEM* 40 (1906), 1–18. He first developed this theme more briefly in "Un adieu à la rue des Saints-Pères," *MEM* 40 (1906), 11–12.

105. Jaccoud said of Koch that he discovered the agent of transmission "announced" by Villemin and established the pathogenic specificity of his baccillus "en suivant fidèlement le programme de Pasteur . . ." in "Éloge de Villemin," 15.

106. "Éloge de Nocard," *MEM* 41 (1910), 1–23.

107. Jaccoud, "Un adieu," 20–21.

108. G. Debove, "Éloge de Pasteur," *BAM* 72 (1914), 375–90. For Achard's judgment of Jaccoud's views see C. Achard, "Jaccoud à l'Académie," *BAM* 104 (1930), 645–46. A more detailed and nuanced discussion of Jaccoud's views can be found in P. Ménétrier, "François-Sigismond Jaccoud," *BAM* 104 (1930), 607–08.

109. A. Chauffard, "Un siècle de médecine à l'Académie," *Centenaire de l'Académie de Médecine, 1820–1920* (1921), p. 161.

110. P. Bar, presidential address, *BAM* 96 (1926), 410.

111. Ibid., 411.

112. Sargeant, "Laënnec clinicien," *BAM* 96 (1926), 444–49.

113. Ibid., 449.

114. Achard, "Le Rôle de Laënnec," 458–60.

115. Ibid., 461–62.

116. In a different manner, A. Chauffard made a similar point in his talk at the tricentenary celebration in honor of Sydenham's birth. The great clinicians like Sydenham and Trousseau should not be forgotten, he said, because "it is to them that we owe our methods of clinical examination which are the necessary prologue and obligatory accompaniment of laboratory medicine." *BAM* 91 (1924), 647.

117. C. Achard, "La Médecine de Pinel à Vulpian," *BAM* 97 (1927), 753.

118. Ibid., 754.

119. His own research career had been notable for his contributions to hematology.

120. G. Hayem, "Vulpian médecin," *BAM* 97 (1927), 730–31.

121. Frank, "Image of Harvey," pp. 134–36, suggests that Harvey's reputation derived in part from similar nationalistic sentiments in England. Frank also emphasizes the conceptual accessibility of Harvey's achievement as a component of the latter's developing reputation.

9

The Self-Made Mandarin:
The Eulogies of Pariset

In this chapter I will examine the *éloges* and funeral orations of Etienne Pariset,[1] the first permanent secretary of the Academy of Medicine, serving from 1823 until his death in 1847. My intent is to ascertain through these writings the values and self-images of the medical elite during the first half of the nineteenth century. I do not claim that Pariset's depictions of medicine and its practitioners are necessarily "true" in any literal sense. I merely suggest that they constitute one representation among many of the medical elite of this era. This representation, however, was uniquely in-fluential because of its thematic coherence and because it was reiterated regularly by the authorized representative of the most prestigious medical institution in France. Pariset's eulogies undoubtedly distort reality; but the very distortions are richly evo-cative of the collective beliefs and values of the newly emergent medical elite.

Technical medical and scientific discussions comprise the bulk of academic *éloges*, though not of funeral orations.[2] However, I will concentrate here on the way in which medical *careers* are depicted in Pariset's corpus. To understand what was conventional and what was innovative in Pariset's thematic treatment of this subject, I shall compare his eulogies with those of two of his prerevolutionary predecessors: Antoine Louis, who prepared panegyrics for the Académie Royale de Chirurgie from 1740 to the mid-1780s,[3] and Félix Vicq d'Azyr,[4] who performed the same service for the Société Royale de Médecine from 1776 to 1790. We shall also occasionally con-sult the *éloges* written by Georges Cuvier for the Academy of Sciences between 1800 and 1830.[5]

Because eulogies were highly formalized literary productions, themes and vocabulary did not change radically from one eulogist to the next. Whether in the eighteenth or twentieth century, intelligence and hard work led to professional achievement. Altruism characterized the lives of subjects and stoic lucidity the hour of their death. Yet small but significant alterations did in fact creep in. I will argue that these alterations added up, in Pariset's corpus, to a social vision significantly different from that of the eighteenth-century medical eulogists.

Pariset added to the standard biographical motifs of the eighteenth century a relatively new topos: the myth of the self-made man, bringing together two elements, virtue and fortune, traditionally considered to be antithetical.[6] A variant of fortune, political power, was uniquely problematic. Unlike riches, it could not even be directly acknowledged. But Pariset did introduce politics indirectly through another new motif, courage in defying the mob. He developed as well a complex vocabulary of medical virtue in order to describe his subjects and express professional ideals. The result was a literary corpus singularly permeated with thematic tensions.

Medical *Éloges* of the Eighteenth Century

Both Louis and Vicq d'Azyr ordinarily began their *éloges* with the birth of the subject. Between the name of the subject and details of birth, Vicq d'Azyr frequently placed a predicate clause listing the titles and honors accumulated by the subject during his life, thus immediately establishing the subject's claim to a panegyric. The juxtaposition of professional titles and birth information is without any sense of contrast; it expresses a vision of social reality in which the social distance traveled between birth and death was in fact minimal.

In the eighteenth-century medical academies, personal merit was considered more significant than social origins. In his *éloge* of Gerard Van Swieten, Louis emphasized that his subject's merit made it unnecessary to discuss his distinguished background, "from which he did not derive any advantages. The man who is capable of being appreciated for himself, whose virtues and talents have rendered him estimable, does not require the vain display of a genealogical table."[7] Louis's own eulogist would express similar views about the elevated social background of his subject.[8]

What both men found most compelling about family backgrounds were instances of talent, learning, and eminence, particularly, though not exclusively, in medicine. Subjects were perceived to have inherited not wealth or position but models of behavior that led to professional success. Nevertheless, the extent of family wealth is of some significance to both eulogists; each in his own way expressed the view that too much or too little wealth served as a barrier to medical greatness. Vicq d'Azyr expressed the disadvantages of the two extreme states with wonderful clarity:

> One must above all count among these obstacles [to becoming a savant] the excessive favors of fortune, and its excessive mediocrity. The first accelerate the progress of passions, hamper that of ideas; they teach to feel rather than to think; they offer the senses the prestige of pleasure, and the soul, seduced, no longer dares to deliver itself either to reflection or to work. The second stops the march of the spirit; it withers the bud, depriving it of the sap without which it cannot either grow or fortify itself; it stifles those fortunate dispositions which men receive more often than they profit from.[9]

In this vein, Vicq d'Azyr affected surprise that Albrecht Haller achieved greatness despite his high social rank.[10] Likewise, Louis insisted that the disadvantages of Van Swieten's Catholicism mitigated his noble birth.[11] For those born to excessively low rank, a life of scholarship was possible only if a relative or patron intervened to provide the resources necessary for study.[12] This placed the subject in a passive role at the mercy of fortune. Individuals did not themselves overcome their social conditions. To be sure, adversity built character. In several *éloges*, Vicq d'Azyr presented early reversals of family fortune as a stimulus to industriousness.[13] These stories, however, differ fundamentally from the classic rise from modest origins.

Throughout their lives, the subjects of Louis and Vicq d'Azyr worked hard, as their educations trained them to do. The *éloges* are filled with such words as *laborieux, assiduité, zèle, ardeur*. But for both authors work took place in the context of a classically well-ordered life. An individual was productive because of "the moderation and exactitude of his regimen"[14] or "the exact observance of the laws of temperance."[15] Work habits reflected both classical ideals of moderation and Hippocratic ideals of health.

For Louis, excessive labor had several negative connotations. In one *éloge*, it was associated with a busy surgical practice and a consequent lack of scientific achievement.[16] Elsewhere he associated excessive fervor with unseemly ambition that led to attempts at self-promotion. He wrote, for instance, of a deceased personal enemy who had led "the most active and most laborious life," that the same sentiment that led his subject "to sacrifice his time, his rest, his fortune, his very health, to the progress of science, made him search for his reward in the publicizing of his works."[17] For Vicq d'Azyr, immoderate exertion destroyed the individual's health and consequently his capacity to contribute to science. Since his subjects were somewhat less inclined to be governed by the rules of moderation, he regularly warned of the self-defeating effects of excessive labor.[18] He centered his *éloge* of Jean-Baptiste Bucquet on the early demise of his subject, "exhausted by his immoderate work . . . devoured by his own ardor." The piece is set as a morality tale whose conclusion is:

> His death will always be a lesson for the small number of savants who give themselves up to study with too much ardor: it will teach them that one frequently misses one's goal in hurrying too much to attain it; that great works and great reputations are the fruit of long years; and that finally, in dedicating oneself through excessive fatigue to a certain and premature death, one risks losing all rights to immortality.[19]

There is, however, a profound ambiguity in Vicq d'Azyr's *éloges*. The subjects' death in the line of duty is presented as a normal occurrence. One such case led Vicq d'Azyr to celebrate at length the self-sacrifices of the medical profession.[20] Figures like Haller are portrayed without comment as excessively devoted to work.[21] Elsewhere Vicq d'Azyr tells another tale of ardor resulting in premature death. But his conclusion is ambiguous:

> With less love for study and for the celebrity which is its reward, Monsieur [Charles] le Roy would possibly have had a longer and more peaceful life; but does happiness depend so much on that tranquillity which some turn into a lifeless idol? . . . Monsieur le Roy had the pleasure of being useful in this double manner, and he enjoyed the true happiness of which weak humanity is capable. We should thus not find fault with or pity him but make efforts to imitate him.[22]

In this as in other respects, Vicq d'Azyr seems to have been a transitional figure oscillating between traditional images of medicine in the eighteenth century and emerging stereotypes that would be characteristic of the nineteenth. It may well be, however, that even in the eighteenth-century context, medical *éloges* were atypical of the genre because of their professional concern to promote good health. The *éloges* of the Académie des Inscriptions et Belles Lettres, for instance, describe men martyred by their single-minded devotion to literature.[23]

Work led to achievement for the subjects of *éloges* but the extent of worldly success varied enormously. In the vast majority of cases, it was modest. A minority of individuals, however, achieved fame, wealth, and prestigious office—what Louis liked to call *gloire*. Louis took in his stride the fact that a small number of his subjects (usually foreigners) attained great position. What was troublesome was the manner in which advancement to any level was pursued. Excessive interest in worldly advancement was manifestly a bad thing in his estimation. He did not shrink from criticizing some of his subjects for their relentless pursuit of worldly success.[24] The figures Louis admired made worldly or financial sacrifices for medicine and science. Honors came automatically to them despite their natural modesty and lack of avarice.

Vicq d'Azyr, in contrast, never admitted that any of his subjects selfishly sought material gain or advancement. But he was ambivalent about great wealth and position, perhaps because it was a realistic prospect for many physicians of the Société Royale. For Vicq d'Azyr, the attainment of too much wealth and position was rather unseemly; it was even worse to live in luxury, which set an individual apart from his colleagues and patients. He gently chided one of his subjects (Bucquet) for acquiring a taste for luxury; such behavior made the practice of medicine impossible since patients inevitably considered the physician too elevated to concern himself with their illnesses.[25]

Vicq d'Azyr's views expressed the sense of stable social position that was so much a part of corporate behavior in the eighteenth century. Great wealth and position lifted the physician out of his natural state and out of the natural *confrérie* of medicine. It might even lift him into the worlds of court and nobility, viewed with a mixture of horror and fascination. Wealth of this magnitude was acceptable only if individuals behaved *as if* they did not, in fact, possess it. Vicq d'Azyr justified Haller's great wealth, for instance, by insisting that his subject continued to live frugally in spite of it.[26] Similarly, the wealth of Joseph Lieutaud increased "without augmenting his expenditures."[27] In the latter case, in fact, Lieutaud faced the ultimate risk of uprootedness from the medical *confrérie* when he was appointed to a medical position at the royal court, a place in which "simple and straightforward men are always alien." However, Lieutaud resisted the tempest; "[he] was one of those rare men found in small numbers at courts; he remained always the same, and was never anything but a doctor and an anatomist."[28] In the same vein, Louis says of François Quesnay that he lived at court as a cenobite, "without any passion other than work of the mind."[29]

Vicq d'Azyr developed an imagery of polar contrasts to express his ambivalence toward worldly success. He repeatedly contrasted the peace, happiness, and productivity that resulted from the disinterested search for knowledge with the difficulty, unhappiness, and discomfort produced by the pursuit of glory. The former condition was frequently identified with life in the provinces, represented in terms of pastoral simplicity; the latter was symbolized by Paris, where ambition, rivalry, jealousy, and bitterness were men's common lot. This polarity was mobilized, for instance, to describe the refusal of some of Vicq d'Azyr's subjects to be sucked into the maelstrom of Parisian ambition. Because Pierre Navier resisted the lure of Paris, "he saw pass peacefully the days which a jealous rivalry would have filled with bitterness, if ambition had distanced him far from the home of his fathers."[30] Others, like Le Roy, succumbed finally to the attractions of the capital:

> What a change! an immense city to cross each day; a large number of rivals to balance; everyone needing to be satisfied at once; responding to the crowd of the curious whose love of novelty determines confidence and fashion; resisting the torrent of nuisances; confounding criticisms; braving envy; that is the painful task which a doctor imposes on himself when, called to the capital, his talents carry him immediately to the pinnacle of celebrity. . . .[31]

Mention of such rivalries actually occupied a double role in Vicq d'Azyr's universe. On one level, it provided a clear warning against the ambition for glory. On another, the very unpleasantness of the quest justified whatever glory was achieved; it was the heavy price which the subject had payed for his success. The eighteenth-century cult of great men, we know, demanded suffering from its heroes.[32]

In a variety of ways, therefore, the *éloges* of the eighteenth century exhibited considerable tension with regard to the theme of fortune. Fortune itself, for Vicq d'Azyr, and the pursuit of it, for Louis, were fundamentally incompatible with love of truth and duty to patients. But the stresses generated within these *éloges* were never very intense because "fortune" was not very visible. The theme was not avoided but neither did it occupy center stage. In Pariset's eulogies, however, "fortune" came into its own.

Pariset: The Rise from Humble Origins

Pariset devoted considerably more attention to his subjects' family background than did his predecessors. In many *éloges*, he followed the conventional practice of locating among family members and ancestors models of talent and virtue. He established connections between the subject and other eminent figures through common regional origins or year of birth. However, the most striking motif in Pariset's treatment of early backgrounds is that of modest social origins; ten or so individuals (out of thirty-three eulogized subjects) are cited as exemplars of a new kind of medical hero who overcomes humble origins to achieve greatness and fortune.

Pariset was not breaking new ground. This form of bourgeois romance began to take shape in several *éloges* presented by Cuvier to the Academy of Sciences after 1810. The latter's treatment of François Fourcroy (1811), for instance, centered primarily on the tension between science and political life; but a secondary theme was the rise from humble origins.[33] This theme takes center stage in Cuvier's treatment of the surgeon and hospital reformer Jacques Tenon (1817), whose entire life was that of a man

> at grips with fortune and nature, and succeeding, by force of perseverance, in winning over one and the other durable victories. . . . Born in poverty, practically in indigence, he did better than enrich himself; he became for our country one of the principal benefactors of the poor, by ameliorating the refuges of misfortune.[34]

In both cases wealth was permissible because of extenuating circumstance. In the case of Fourcroy, it did not lead to happiness; in the second, it served to benefit the unfortunate.

In Pariset's *éloges*, this theme was ubiquitous, shorn of reservations, and turned into a codified literary formula. Here is what Pariset had to say about the early poverty of Baron Dubois:

> Strange but honorable conformity with the foremost men of his time, Portal, Corvisart, Pinel, Fourcroy, Chaussier, who, born poor but laborious, tireless, and full of genius, in the end opened for themselves the road to riches and celebrity![35]

He said of Double:

> It is from such modest beginnings that rises one of the most brilliant careers ever traversed by a man of our profession. The same as Linnaeus, in Sweden, and P. Franck in Germany; the same as Dupuytren, Chaussier, Fourcroy, Vauquelin, among us, Double was in a profound indigence; he only got out of it by his work. It is from his work, and work of the most obstinate sort, that he obtained everything. He owed nothing to chance; he owed nothing to either intrigue or favor.[36]

This element of bourgeois romance in these *éloges* undoubtedly owed something to the fact that Pariset, unlike Louis and Vicq d'Azyr, who came from privileged backgrounds, was himself of modest origins. He was, it can be argued, especially susceptible to a plot structure which recounted and glorified his own social itinerary. However, one finds the same plot in eulogies written by other academicians during this period. It is a commonplace of the literature of these decades as evidenced by the work of Stendahl and Balzac, who explored its darker side.[37] Even political debates assumed the existence of considerable social mobility in French society.[38]

Pariset's rhetoric did not so much reflect differences in social origin as it did transformed circumstances. The fathers of most of Pariset's subjects practiced many of the same occupations as did those of Louis and Vicq d'Azyr; they were country doctors, pharmacists, skilled artisans, and magistrates. But whereas these states were viewed as *honnête*, or unremarkable, in the eighteenth century, they were now identified with poverty, at least in comparison with the success that would be achieved. Underlying the bourgeois romance is not so much increased social mobility in the nineteenth century but rather changing contexts and perceptions. That is to say that the bourgeoisie of the eighteenth century felt itself to be blocked from the highest rungs of the social ladder. Individuals could raise their economic and social status through merit but only up to a point. There was always a level beyond which one had to renounce bourgeois class identity.[39] In the early nineteenth century, whatever the actual reality, mobility *seemed* to be without limits. In addition to wealth, which had always been somewhat attainable, political influence, administrative responsibilities, and even noble status now seemed within reach of talented and hardworking individuals.

The medical elite was one of the most spectacular instances of this change of context and perception. During the eighteenth century, positions at the royal court could bring brilliant worldly success; but few such positions existed and these tended to be the preserve of men from affluent families. Even those closest to the ruling classes were essentially personal servitors of the great rather than recognized servants of the state. After the French Revolution, however, the medical elite was consolidated around state institutions like the Paris Faculty of Medicine, the hospitals, and the Academy of Medicine. With state posts and a recognized public health role to fill, members of the medical elite became something like *hauts fonctionnaires*, who perceived themselves to be the equals of other elite groups in French society. Under the Empire and Bourbon Restoration, many could even expect to be ennobled. Having reached such heights, their social origins inevitably appeared modest.

The theme of humble origins served two rhetorical purposes. It introduced a contrast that heightened the individual's achievement while at the same justifying that success. Such cases demonstrated that neither wealth nor family connections were behind professional success. Only talent and hard work could explain a change in fortune of this magnitude. Pariset's eulogies celebrated individual instances of social mobility in order to convey a message: success was possible if one obeyed certain rules. Here is what Pariset wrote about Gilbert Breschet's early career:

> I insist, gentlemen, on these beginnings, as I did for Pinel, for Vauquelin, for Dupuytren, for Chaussier, for Esquirol, because it is at the beginning of these laborious careers that the value and character of men reveals itself most vividly, and because it is always *a propos* to show by these examples how poverty nobly emancipates itself from its dependence through work; in other words, how the poor man raises and honors himself by rendering himself, not merely useful, but even necessary to his fellows.[40]

The unstated message was equally evident: those who had failed to reach the professional summit lacked either the ability or necessary vigor. Pariset had taken an emerging literary cliché and had made it central to the professional self-image of the new medical elite.

Literary appropriation, however, did not just move in one direction. The myth of the self-made man in France was from the beginning closely associated with medicine. It is not accidental that famous Parisian physicians are portrayed by Balzac as having risen from humble origins.[41] Nor is it fortuitous that the two examples of this motif in Cuvier's *éloges*, Fourcroy and Tenon, were both medical men. The theme of social mobility was particularly congruent with elite medicine. Aside from the truly humble origins of certain academicians, careers based on lifelong advancement through public competitions and elections fostered a self-image emphasizing social ascent through merit and hard work. Careers in the state administration, organized along very different lines, do not seem to have fostered similar self-images.[42] Not all academicians, of course, had been born poor. But this was inconsequential since poverty became generalized during medical studies and early years of practice.

For most of Pariset's subjects, as for those of his predecessors, the choice of a medical calling did not require any special struggle or conversion experience.[43] But it did require sacrifice. Once embarked upon medical studies, Pariset's subjects went beyond the conventional industriousness of the eighteenth century to engage in an exhausting frenzy of activity exercised in conditions of extreme poverty. Such poverty was not just the fate of those from modest backgrounds. It was a natural condition through which all aspiring members of the medical elite had to pass. The long years of study on meager family allowances, the poorly paid faculty and hospital posts, provided even those born to affluence an opportunity to overcome hardship. These hardships formed an integral part of the struggle for knowledge, described with zest and not a little nostalgia. Dupuytren, for instance, survived as a laboratory assistant in Paris, according to Pariset, by sharing with a friend

> a small room, three chairs, a table, some bread, water; and to the side several volumes of classical authors which the two friends reread with delight, a sort of bed on which they forgot for an instant the exhausting activities of the day. In the summer, these exhausting activities sometimes began at four in the morning, an example which, with many others, can teach youth at what price successes are purchased. . . .[44]

By defying his father's wish that he study law, Corvisart had to break with his family and make his own way. He came to Paris "alone and without support, without either recommendations or resources." As a young teacher he endured grinding poverty:

> His annual salary did not exceed 100 écus; and more than once he was reduced to the painful necessity of borrowing. . . . All the same, a single thought occupied him during his distress, that was to live for knowledge and to improve his knowledge by experience.[45]

Increasingly in Pariset's panegyrics this early period was treated as a romanticized initiation. In his 1844 *éloge* of Esquirol, the son of a wealthy businessman, Pariset describes his subject's arrival in Paris:

> He was on his arrival almost as poor as were on theirs Portal and Vauquelin, and Pinel, and Dupuytren, and so many others for whom work was the road to glory and opulence. . . . Each day, for two years, Esquirol came from Vaugirard to the Salpêtrière clinic, to the classes of the Jardin des Plantes, to the lessons of the Faculty of Medicine; rugged trails during the winters; but during the other seasons, a little bread and some fruit made them charming. . . . [H]appy time of poverty, work and hope, the memories of which still charmed the last years of Esquirol's life.[46]

This myth of initiation brought together the special dedication that seemed necessary for an elite medical career with a temporary bohemian poverty becoming fashionable in literary and artistic circles. Balzac's Cénacle circle was the literary prototype of this myth of poverty and dedication which served both as a means to and indication of future greatness. In Pariset's *éloges* this myth justified later worldly success by emphasizing the obstacles that had been so valiantly overcome. But like all initiations, it also served as a principle of common identity, founded on shared experience and nostalgia.

Pariset: Advancing Careers

In many regards Pariset discussed the careers of his subjects in conventional ways. Yet with only slight changes in vocabulary he managed to distance himself considerably from the eighteenth-century vision of medical achievement, particularly with respect to two subjects: hard work and worldly success. There is no ambiguity surrounding excessive devotion to work in the eulogies of Pariset and other medical writers of the period. Subjects are confirmed workaholics who run themselves into the ground in paroxysms of self-sacrifice. The scientist's laboratory, viewed in the eighteenth century as a bucolic and pastoral refuge from worldly struggles, becomes yet another one of the many locations in which individuals exhaust themselves. Medical heroes pursue glory in a blaze of exalted self-abnegation.

In a funeral oration, Nicholas Adelon honored his friend P. Rullier: "[You sacrificed] to the study of your art, to the service of your patients, I would say not only the interests of your fortune, and that of [worldly] pleasures, but care for your health."[47] This motif of constant labor and self-sacrifice is one of the most enduring topoi in the medical eulogies of the nineteenth and twentieth centuries. It is as if the high status of the medical elite could be justified only by constant labor. But the theme also seems to have expressed very real professional ideals. An unpublished proposal to reform medical education prepared in the early 1820s by the surgeon-academician Philippe Pelletan suggested that the summer vacation shortening the school year should be eliminated because "the exercise of medicine does not permit any vacation, and young men must become accustomed early to devoting themselves entirely and without reserve to an art whose exercise is a continual process of study and uninterrupted practice."[48]

Visiting patients by day, writing at night, the subjects of *éloges* had ample opportunity to indulge their passion to help others. The words "abnegation" and "sacrifice" recur constantly in these *éloges*. Military surgeons had particularly good opportunities to display these virtues on a heroic scale. Percy's military life was one of "fatigue, privations, suffering and perils." What devotion, Pariset declared, "what constant forgetting of oneself! or rather, what abnegation."[49] Civilians were given the opportunity to exhibit martial virtues of self-sacrifice during epidemics.[50]

Such labors led inevitably to successful careers. In a few cases success was modest. Most often, however, individuals attained the professional summit. In Pariset's *éloges*, the accumulation of honors and wealth was neither an exceptional condition nor the somewhat suspect reward for a life spent in pursuit of glory. It was rather the *natural* condition of hard work and merit. Individuals had no need to seek it because its arrival was inevitable. This theme is not without its tensions. Pariset retained the classical ambivalence toward ambition, as well the suspicion that professional success was not always merited. Like his predecessors, he regularly insisted that posts and honors that had been obtained by subjects owed nothing to unmerited patronage and intrigue. In his telling, worldly rewards and honors were never actively pursued; they simply came to hard-working individuals who, if truth be told, would have preferred to avoid them.[51]

When Vauquelin obtained a faculty chair in 1809, he "triumphed without combating and the chair came to him rather than he to it."[52] When Bourru was appointed to the Academy of Medicine "this honor which he did not expect was conferred as a result of his reputation, as had been those which he had previously received and which came to him without his having to seek them."[53] Certain individuals were constitutionally incapable of building careers but happily found patrons who recognized their worth.[54] Academicians were no more interested in money than in position. Some, like Charles Marc and Claude Berthollet, refused to profit personally from their discoveries. Nor did they utilize their posts to gain wealth; like Nilamon Lerminier, their hearts were open to humanity and their hands closed to gold. They had only one objective—"to forget themselves in order to help the unfortunate."[55] No one was more unfortunate than the poor. As in the eighteenth century, serving as a physician to the poor was considered morally superior to serving the rich. A model practitioner like Marc always gave preference to his poor patients.[56]

On one occasion, Pariset met head-on persistent rumors that Baron Portal, founder and first president of the academy, had early in his career utilized methods bordering on charlatanism in order to attract clients. His only fault, Pariset explained, was "during his first years, to be mistrustful of the future, to not believe in the natural effect of his talents, to have wanted to attach wings to his fortune, in order to precipitate its flight."[57] It was not Portal's actions or motives that constituted his error. Rather, he did not *believe* in "the natural effect of his talents" and tried to *precipitate* his natural rise. This is precisely what the majority of Pariset's subjects, in his telling at least, managed to avoid doing. Success, rather, was the natural consequence of merit and hard work.

The frequency with which Pariset repeated this theme reflected, I suspect, the social tensions provoked by the emergence of a postrevolutionary medical elite possessing enormous prestige and not a little power. How could one control the inevitable rivalries and conflicts which resulted from fierce competition for "glory" on this new scale? Pariset's bourgeois romances did not merely portray members of the medical elite as having overcome every conceivable obstacle while remaining indifferent to worldly rewards. As explicit efforts to present models of professional behavior to the living, they also sought to check and sublimate the naked ambitions that were always threatening to tear apart the medical community. They carried a message: unbridled competition for glory did not merely make individuals unhappy, as Vicq d'Azyr had counseled; it was positively counterproductive. Against all the available evidence, this message insisted that glory awaited not those who clawed their way to the top but rather those who devoted their Herculean labors (for nothing less would do) to science and to their patients.

The inevitability of success, the necessary link between virtue and fortune, is so all-pervasive in these eulogies that one is struck by the existence of a single eulogy during Pariset's tenure as secretary that follows a radically different narrative logic. Significantly, it is one of two long *éloges* which Pariset delegated to others.

Nicholas Chervin died in 1845; his *éloge* was presented by Pariset's future successor as permanent secretary, Frédéric Dubois d'Amiens.[58] The reason that Pariset avoided this particular *éloge* is apparent: Chervin was his great opponent in the contagionist controversies of the 1820s and 1830s. One also suspects, however, that Pariset would have been incapable of creating an *éloge* out of such material. In his universe, individuals suffered only temporary reversals of fortune. If worldly success was not distributed equally, if it faced the occasional unjust setback, it was nonetheless roughly commensurate with talent and hard work. Chervin's life broke all these rules.

Dubois's *éloge* of Chervin contained many of the same thematic elements found in those of Pariset, especially the portrayal of relentless hard work in pursuit of disinterested truth. But in contrast to Pariset's heroes, Chervin carried disinterested love of truth in the form of his anticontagionist crusade to such extremes that he forfeited the honors and fortunes (though not the fame) that were his due. Having exhausted his inheritance and far too preoccupied to earn a decent livelihood, Chervin had lived and died in abject poverty. Dubois related his experience as part of a delegation sent by the Academy of Medicine to pay its respects to Chervin, then convalescing from a first attack of apoplexy:

> It was then and for the first time that was revealed to us this noble distress. We climbed to the fifth floor into a modest furnished room where he had lived for more than fifteen years; a bed, a commode and several chairs constituted all his furniture; several books, the tools of his trade, filled a small shelf above his commode.[59]

One finds similar descriptions in Pariset's discussions of student life or early years of practice. But there is no room in his universe for such poverty at the end of an illustrious man's career.

This myth of the solitary prophet is no less a form of romance than Pariset's bourgeois variant. The struggle for truth is paid for not merely by endless labor and a brief period of youthful poverty but by lifelong poverty and social marginality. It is in many ways far more effective as myth because it does not have to reconcile idealistic self-abnegation with the struggle for worldly success. Nevertheless, it was rarely utilized in the eulogies of the Academy of Medicine. The model of immoderate adherence to doctrinaire beliefs was not one that Pariset found congenial. Nor did it apply easily to the visibly successful and even celebrated men who, by definition, made up the membership of the academy.

Domesticating Conflict

One consequence of the need to master the violent energies which threatened constantly to tear apart the medical elite is the virtual absence of a theme that was fairly ubiquitous in the *éloges* of Louis and Vicq d'Azyr: professional rivalries and public polemics. In the *éloges* of the eighteenth century, Parisian medicine was portrayed as a world of violent public conflicts. The acknowledgment of public controversies in which subjects had become embroiled provided an occasion to show that such controversies caused enormous pain to participants and damage to the profession.[60]

Such public conflicts virtually disappear from Pariset's universe. The prodigious public combats between, say, Laënnec and Broussais are not mentioned. It is as if the openness of the eighteenth century about such matters could not survive the new conditions of the nineteenth. Such occurrences had become literally unspeakable. They could be mentioned only if they had occurred in the distant past or if the subject of the *éloge* could be portrayed as an innocent victim. If mention of specific individuals could be avoided, Pariset might state matters more clearly. The demise of a medical society, for instance, was used to illustrate the destructive behavior that should be avoided by academicians.[61] Most often, the subjects of *éloges* were innocent of such behavior. The intense rivalry between the schools of Pinel and Corvisart, according to Pariset, owed nothing to the great chiefs of the schools. "Pinel did not tolerate if anyone dared to murmur before him a word against Corvisart. Corvisart suppressed with the full extent of his severity any shadow of an insinuation against Pinel. . . ."[62]

Pariset hinted at the tensions wracking the medical community when he discussed his subjects' traits of character. In a brief character sketch of the deceased which he, like many eulogists, tried to draw, he was able to indirectly address rules of professional conduct. Since such sketches were intended as inspirational models of behavior, the character of the deceased had to be described in essentially positive terms. At the same time, they had to be recognizable to listeners who had been colleagues of the deceased. Eulogists resolved the dilemma by treating minor flaws in such a way as to draw moral lessons from the subject's life.

The descriptive terms favored by Pariset to portray his subjects were not dramatically different from those of his predecessors. Both he and they were drawing on venerable models of virtue; many of the terms they used go back to the chivalric literature of the medieval period.[63] But Pariset's usage is particularly systematic and codified. Brief character portraits usually appear at the end of discussions of careers as a technique of conclusion and summary. They utilize a limited number of formulaic terms in different combinations. To introduce Pariset's vocabulary of character and virtue I should like to begin with his *éloge* of the alienist Esquirol, in which the moral evaluation is both uncharacteristically glowing and especially elaborate. It appears at the very beginning of the *éloge* and provides the piece with much of its thematic unity.

To know Esquirol is to love him—this is Pariset's less-than-inspired opening. The panegyrist then elaborates a long list of virtues culminating in a final summary passage which demarcates those traits of character that are particularly worthy of emulation. Esquirol was

> an excellent man, whose actions and published works honored France, and who, in order to render our sense of his loss, can I say more sweet? should I say more bitter? left us within his memory something like a perpetual lesson *de droiture, de modération, de désintéressement et de bonté.*[64]

Esquirol's life thus provides a lesson in four virtues which I deliberately leave untranslated. At the two ends of this list are *droiture* and *bonté*; sandwiched between are *modération* and *désintéressement.*

Droiture is defined by the *Dictionnaire Robert* as a quality which compels an individual to conduct himself in conformity to "moral laws" and duty.[65] Among many equivalents are *rectitude, franchise, probité* and *justice.* It is thus a commitment to abstract principle—law, duty, truth, reason—and has hard masculine connotations, especially when it is associated by Pariset with words like *sévérité* and *fermeté.* Sometimes associated with this complex of virtues is *courage,* the willingness to brave danger in pursuit of duty or truth. In one form or another, all these terms represent transcendence of normal human passions and self-interest in the pursuit of higher values.

Bonté is defined by *Robert* as that moral quality which leads one to do good on behalf of others. It is a response not just to abstract imperatives but to human need. *Altruisme, philanthropie,* and *humanité* are synonyms with which it is associated, as are terms like *pitié, charité, bienfaisance, compassion, tendresse, douceur,* identified with a tradition of Christian charity. Some of these words, notably *bienfaisance,* have especially close association with women's charitable activities, and indeed many of the terms in this complex of terms have nurturing and feminine connotations. Some of the words also convey a strong emotional response to suffering and need.

Modération, the most classic of the traditional virtues, is defined as the absence of excess in conduct or emotion. It connotes remoteness from extreme passions, violent language, and excessive ambition. But Pariset used the term primarily in the context of social relations, particularly those involving professional peers. *Modération*, for the eulogist, is a requirement of human sociability reducing the possibilities of friction and conflict. It is one of many related social virtues in Pariset's moral vocabulary; these include *simplicité, modestie* and *bienveillance*. In specific contexts, terms associated with the first two categories of virtue, *franchise, bonté, douceur*, for instance, can have connotations of affability and sociability with respect to colleagues.

The final term, *désintéressement*, is the sacrifice of self-interest. This is probably the most fundamental medical virtue. Self-sacrifice, in Pariset's moral world, underpins the attachment to duty, the desire to attenuate suffering, and even the smooth workings of the social group. Words like *sacrifice, abnégation*, and *oubli de soi* convey a similar meaning within his moral vocabulary.

These four complexes of related terms (with some terms overlapping several complexes) underlie most of Pariset's character descriptions. The description of Pinel's character, for instance, touches on all four:

> And do not think that these peaceful virtues of Pinel, his *bonté*, his *candeur*, his *modestie*, this *désintéressement* that is so perfect, this intense *compassion* for misfortune of which he gave so much proof, do not think that this sage practice of never attacking and respecting the rights of the other in order to have his own respected was incompatible with *courage*.[66]

The terms used break down as follows according to the four categories we have been discussing:

Principles	Humanity	Sociability	Altruism
courage	*bonté*	*candeur*	*désintéressement*
	compassion	*modestie*	
		n'attaquer	
		respecter	

Once again, attachment to principles and to humanity forms the outer limits of the description, with terms of sociability and altruism in between.

In his introduction to the funeral oration honoring Lerminier, Pariset begins with a list of the professional virtues which the subject possessed: *"le savoir, le courage, le désintéressement, l'humanité la plus tendre, la loyauté la plus délicate."*[67] Aside from knowledge, which is usually taken for granted, the virtues closely follow the pattern found in the *éloge* of Pinel.

Principles	Humanity	Sociability	Altruism
courage	*humanité*	*loyauté*	*désinteréssement*

The first two categories—attachment to principles and attachment to humanity—are variations of the old distinction between justice and mercy. They can be viewed as elemental professional virtues which coexist in fundamental tension and govern the relationship of the healer to his patient: firmness and principle, on one hand, and humanitarian compassion, on the other; suppressing emotion in order to function effectively and responding with feeling to human suffering. This dualism of imperatives is most evident in Pariset's treatment of military surgeons, who frequently performed in extreme situations. Here is his opening to the eulogy of Baron Larrey:

> [A]nd think for a moment about the noble qualities which form the military surgeon, *patience* and *courage*, *douceur* and *fermeté*, the most tender *pitié* and the most inflexible *sévérité*; an inexhaustible *vigilance*, an entire *oubli de soi-même*, an absolute *dévouement* to the unfortunate. . . .[68]

Here the two categories of qualities are explicitly juxtaposed: passivity and courage, firmness and feeling, gentleness and severity—in short, justice and mercy. The tableau concludes with the altruistic qualities on which the first two rest.

These three qualities are so fundamental to our notions of medical devotion, it seems astonishing that qualities of sociability, apparently so much more superficial, are given equal emphasis and in fact predominate in many eulogies, as the examples from Pariset's eulogies of Pinel and Esquirol suggest. Elite medicine was perceived as a collective enterprise in which individuals worked together in a variety of institutions. This collective activity was threatened constantly by the forces of individual ambition. The ubiquity of his message of sociability was his invariable response to them.

Nevertheless, the category of sociability was not really as fundamental as the other three. For the panegyrist was able, within limits, to talk about its opposite— unsociability—among certain subjects. No eulogist could refer to the opposite of probity, courage, or altruism in his subjects without provoking scandal, but the opposite of sociability could be discussed tactfully. It was less serious and it seems to have been widespread, making it difficult to ignore if a recognizable portrait was to be presented.

We can better understand unsociability by examining its opposite, "sociability," more closely. Probably no one embodied sociability more fully than did the dermatologist Alibert:

> Gentle [*doux*] with his own, inoffensive and obliging with everyone, never a word of hatred, never an act of vengeance, even when most justified, ever escaped from him. To pardon, forget wrongs, is the height of *modération*; and this *modération* he had, even without thinking about it. What *tendresse* he showed his patients! And to what point did he carry *bienfaisance*! His house was the refuge of the unfortunate.[69]

Here, the hard, severe, and manly virtues are conspicuously absent. Social virtues, with moderation identified as the capacity to pardon and forget insults and wrongs, slide effortlessly into humanitarian virtues like tenderness for patients and good works. The link between social and humanitarian virtues is not fortuitous; both reflect similar benign feelings for colleagues and patients. Specific words like *doux* and *bienveillant* can be used in both senses, depending on the context.

There seems, however, to be real tension between the hard virtues of principle and those of sociability, as if those attached to principle are unlikely to be much concerned with social niceties. In the description of Pinel quoted above, we saw social and humane virtues appearing in alternating order with, at the very end, Pariset's insistence that Pinel's notable "peaceful virtues" did not reflect lack of courage; this becomes the pretext for describing some of Pinel's activities during the Revolution. The rhetorical point depends on the apparent incompatibility between manly virtues of principle and softer qualities of humaneness and sociability. It is true that terms like *franche* can express both a passion for truth and an ideal of masculine camaraderie. But in Pariset's moral world, attachment to abstractions is frequently inimical to tolerance of colleagues.

This relationship between manly virtues and sociability had of course to be expressed delicately in the context of eulogies. Here is Pariset's treatment of the pharmacist Pierre Robiquet, whose duties as treasurer of the Paris School of Pharmacy left ample scope for the virtues of justice and order:

> [T]his *vigilance*, this *fermeté*, this spirit of *justice* and *ordre* which, putting everything in its place, made negligence and confusion disappear; this happy mixture of *bienveillance* and of *sévérité*, that made him at one and the same time loved and respected by the professors, feared and cherished by the students. . . . He was a man passionate about his art and about the honor of the profession; an upright (*intègre*) administrator bringing to his accounts all the *droiture* of his soul; sensitive to excess to evidence of affection, taking umbrage at the slightest sign of malevolence, but easy to get on with, debonair, and as quick to forget wrongs as he was to feel them.[70]

Virtually all the qualities described are hard and masculine (vigilance, firmness, justice, order). The closest Pariset comes to a humanitarian virtue or sociability is *bienveillance*, in this case referring to benevolence shown colleagues and students and somewhat weakened by its explicit association with severity. But passion for abstractions of many different sorts turns quite naturally in this account into an excessive sensitivity and tendency to easily take offense. This honesty is almost too much and the eulogist retreats quickly to catalogue more sociable qualities (easy to get on with, quick to forget wrongs), which almost balance the quick anger.

The link between the attachment to principle and unsociability is developed more explicitly in Pariset's treatment of the veterinarian Jean Huzard:

> Never has a man carried *désintéressement* further, and shown a more severe *probité*. This *probité ombrageuse*, too quick, perhaps, to suspect that of others, sometimes gave his speech a harshness [*rudesse*] which was belied by the kindness of his heart.[71]

In the first sentence, disinterestedness is coupled with "the most severe probity." In the second, probity has been turned from a virtue to a weakness by the addition of the adjective *ombrageuse* (quick to take offense) and the phrase "quick to suspect" the probity of others. The result is a harshness of speech masking kindness of the heart. The distinction between language and heart characterizes unpleasant behavior as a superficial phenomenon which need not be taken too seriously. It is a form of the spatial metaphor of surface/content which Pariset frequently used to make palatable weaknesses of character. So long as they were just surface features which hid the fundamentally humane and sociable traits underneath, weaknesses of character could be discussed by the eulogist without undermining the self-image of the medical elite. They served in fact as negative lessons in professional sociability.

Politics and Courage

Pariset's eulogies, like those of Louis and Vicq d'Azyr, have little to say about the political and administrative activity of subjects. However, the relative silence of the eighteenth-century eulogists results primarily from the exclusion of medical men from political and administrative power. These might, in rare instances, hold high *medical* posts at court and be in a position to benefit medical institutions. Thus Louis lauded Van Swieten's measures to end charlatanism while Vicq d'Azyr expressed regret that Lieutaud never used his position as the King's First Physician to unify and reform French medicine.[72] But subjects were not, by and large, seen as significant political actors. Consequently, the characteristic tension of Vicq d'Azyr's *éloges* pits medical research and practice (pastoral happiness) against thirst for medical notoriety and high medical position (urban ambition). Political and administrative power is never an explicit alternative.

The French Revolution brought large numbers of scientists and doctors into positions of political and administrative prominence. The world of power became a realistic alternative for men of knowledge; politics in turn impinged directly on professional life. Political power was a central element in Cuvier's *éloges* which were a sustained meditation on the relationship between science and political power.[73]

In Pariset's *éloges*, silence surrounds the world of politics. There are, to be sure, abundant indications of the author's own belief in enlightened authoritarian rule. Pariset portrayed the French Revolution as a time of calamity characterized by mob rule. Kings and emperors, in contrast—especially those who supported scientists and savants—came off well. In accordance with the cult of Napoleon already developing during the Restoration, Napoleon was usually portrayed as a heroic and sympathetic personality. Among his greatest virtues was his willingness to honor merit in medicine as in other spheres.

But if Pariset's own views are transparent enough, silence surrounds his subjects' political beliefs and activities, including those relating to medical institutions. The work of Cuvier and Portal in creating new medical institutions is largely passed over, as are the admittedly brief political careers of Vauquelin and Percy. In two other cases political activity and beliefs are mentioned only to be condemned.[74] The silence regarding politics becomes especially evident if we compare Pariset's treatment of Cuvier with Cuvier's own discussion of Fourcroy. The latter is clearly comfortable with a life devoted to political and administrative activity, whereas the former is not. One could as easily compare each man's *éloge* of Corvisart. It is practically inconceivable that Pariset would ask even rhetorically, as Cuvier did, whether Corvisart might not have been able to use his influence on Napoleon to moderate the emperor's excessive ambitions.[75]

Some of Pariset's reticence may have reflected the fact that the medical men who were his subjects were considerably less likely than were Cuvier's scientific subjects to be active in politics. However, I would also suggest that Pariset was at least in part responding to inherent tensions in the role of the medical elite as representatives and often appointees of the state at a time when regimes were changing so rapidly. Silence about politics helped project an image of political neutrality, which supported the claim that changes in regime had no bearing on the status of the medical elite. In an extremely revealing statement, Pariset justified Dominique Larrey's willingness to serve under each successive regime in terms that emphasized the political neutrality of the physician:

> A doctor worthy of the title, a surgeon sees in men only the beings whom he must relieve [of pain, illness]. He can carry affections in his heart but he does not have preferences. . . . Do not be astonished then to see Larrey not refuse his services to any of the governments which succeeded one another. His art made him a citizen of the world and servant of all men.[76]

It was not that doctors could not hold political beliefs. But these were irrelevant to the practice of medicine. Consequently, another panegyrist could commend his subject, Adrien de Lens, for remaining "loyal to his principles and to his political attachments" after being purged from his post by the July Monarchy.[77] Political beliefs were admirable so long as they did not affect the doctor's obligation to humanity. Men in power, unfortunately, did not always understand the neutrality of medicine, and many of Pariset's subjects were in fact victims of political vendettas and purges. Pariset's descriptions of these cases are brief and completely lacking in detail. They suggest the flimsiness of and lack of rational foundation for the case against purged individuals.[78]

Political events intruded on subjects' lives in yet another way by forcing them to exercise qualities of personal courage and heroism. Physical courage, we saw, was a major part of the medical self-mage of the early nineteenth century. This was almost certainly due to close relations between medical institutions and the military under the Revolution and Empire. It may also have been an expression of the embrace by the middle classes of aristocratic notions of honor and martial prowess that led during this period to the spread of dueling.[79] Whether on the battlefield or in the fever ward of a civilian hospital, doctors were expected to risk their lives regularly for the benefit of patients. But the doctors' courage could also be more directly political. Although exercised in the name of humanity rather than a political creed, such courage enabled the individual to defy unjust powers.

Pariset, like Cuvier and most men of science, viewed the revolutionary terror as a time of "political calamities" characterized by unjust tribunals "who breathed only blood." A few of Pariset's subjects took solace in scientific and medical work. Many others defied an unjust regime. Acts of defiance ranged from Nicholas Deyeux's refusal to hide from the authorities on the grounds that he would in so doing betray a recently executed brother[80] to the more significant act of hiding and helping to escape those facing certain death. Jean-Baptiste Louyer-Villermay, Pinel, Pierre-Francois Percy, and Vauquelin were among those who are said to have sheltered or in some way aided political prisoners, emigrés, or foreign troops.[81] Such actions were not represented as political but rather as extensions to the political domain of medical ideals. The very words used by Pariset to describe Vauquelin's motives, "acute sentiment of *humanité*" and "*pitié*," are standard elements in his vocabulary of medical devotion. In another context Pariset directly linked such actions with medical care for the poor and unfortunate, saying of one of his subjects (Bourru): "always the same eagerness to provide care for the poor, to aid the unfortunate, to defend the oppressed."[82]

The preceding quotation referred to Bourru's successful efforts to restore the property of an order of nuns recently dispossessed by revolutionary authorities. Pariset's subjects did not just labor in secret to save lives; they openly confronted unjust authorities in order to restore justice. At the height of revolutionary violence, Pinel managed to secure a pension for the disgraced and doomed Condorcet. Berthollet was asked by revolutionary authorities to chemically analyze a particular *eaux de vie* believed to be poisoned. Knowing that his interlocutors were seeking a guilty verdict in order to confiscate the proprietor's fortune, Berthollet nonetheless insisted that he could find no irregularities. "The irritated tyrants forced him to come to them and, in a ferocious tone," asked him to reconsider. Berthollet, of course, refused. "Is it not natural that the man inspired by such courage would also have the courage which one brings into battle?"[83]

The resistance to injustice was never directed at the established authority of kings. The authorities defied are portrayed as enraged, ferocious mobs which have lost the capacity for reason. Resistance is thus more than courage, it is a form of inner strength and power which overwhelms the force of the mob. When his uncle was arrested by revolutionary authorities, Charles-Louis Cadet de Gassicourt "flew to the Commune, then absolute sovereign; he pressed, he beseeched, and his executioners, softened, handed over their prey to him."[84]

Pariset elaborated on this theme in his funeral oration for Esquirol, who, while with the army in Narbonne, took it upon himself to come to the aid of the persecuted. "He dared present himself before one of those ferocious tribunals of those unhappy times and, without being an advocate, spoke on behalf of a detainee who was being badly defended by his advocate."[85] Completely successful, he refused a reward and soon after defended a worker accused of setting fire to a state workshop. The eulogist reflects: "In times of Furor, what would become of peoples if God did not provide them here and there with some courageous virtues?" In his later *éloge* of Esquirol at the academy, Pariset tellingly referred to the same incident as "the triumph of Orpheus, who tamed the tigers."[86] The courage of the medical hero is the courage to face down the irrational beast within the people. Just as he cures their illnesses he can, by virtue of moral superiority, soothe their savage rage and move them to pity. He possesses, in other words, a special kind of power.

In the perspective of the emerging middle class, the mob constituted an ever-present threat demanding heroic resistance. Here is Breschet during the Revolution of 1830:

> During the sacking of the archbishop's palace, he dared immerse himself in the fury of the people in order to calm it, to pull it out of its frenzy, in order to open its eyes to the harm it was doing to itself. . . . [T]he people, moved, yielded.[87]

During the same Revolution of 1830, Larrey faced down a mob ready to break into his hospital. "This firmness stopped them, they retreated."[88] In his *éloge* of Lerminier,

Pariset juxtaposed two anecdotes. First he told how, during the revolt of Madrid, Lerminier faced down a mob of rebels: "he owed his safety only to his energetic firmness against the rebels who surrounded him." Pariset immediately went on to describe how, with Moscow in flames, "Lerminier alone rushed headlong through the furors of the fire, reached the Kremlin and saved his compatriots."[89] In both instances the medical hero has faced down and brought order to violent natural energy gone out of control.

Apart from his occasional political pronouncements, therefore, Pariset's *éloges* make a number of significant political statements. The world of politics is ideally excluded from medicine, which retains its own sphere of autonomy. Individuals hold political beliefs and may even participate actively in politics. But rather than being a source of dramatic tension, as it was for Cuvier, this fact is simply irrelevant. To be sure, politics intrudes on men's lives. It can unfairly take away legitimately earned honors and fortunes. It has frequently presented the medical hero with the need to combat injustice and face down the animal passions of the enraged mob. In so doing, he demonstrates his own power, moral superiority, and right to elite status. He is a true bourgeois hero who has overcome all obstacles in order to attain honor and wealth and whose courage and strength help preserve the social order from anarchy.

Pariset's eulogies are richly evocative of the competing values, impulses, and metaphors from which the self-image of the French medical elite was cobbled together in the early nineteenth century. Images of military and political courage, economic mobility, chivalric and Christian concepts of medical virtue—all coexisted within the somewhat artificial framework that held them. The myth of the self-made mandarin in particular married two elements tugging in opposing directions. There was, first, the traditional theme of disinterested devotion to truth or to curing, devotion which did not admit of worldly ambition. To this inherited theme Pariset added the relatively new plot of social and professional mobility. This plot did not merely justify elite status. It was psychologically satisfying because it was congruent with lived experiences of ascent through the ranks of the professional hierarchy. But the marriage of elements was a tense one because worldly success cannot easily be divorced from worldly ambition. The disparate elements in Pariset's *éloges* seem occasionally to be held together by an effort of will. But they reflect the rich and complex nature of elite medical identity in the first half of the nineteenth century.

NOTES

1. On Pariset's life and career see George D. Sussman, "Etienne Pariset: A Medical Career in Government under the Restoration," *Journal of the History of Medicine* 26 (1971), 52–74; Paul Busquet, "Pariset," *Biographies médicales* 1 (1927–28), 229–45; F. Dubois d'Amiens, "Éloge de Pariset," in Etienne Pariset, *Histoire des membres de l'Académie Royale de Médecine*, 2 vols. (1850), vol. 1, pp. ix–20.

2. The distinction between *éloges* and funeral orations is discussed in Chapter 5.

3. Antoine Louis, *Éloges lus dans les séances publiques de l'Académie de Chirurgie, 1750–1792*, ed. F. Dubois d'Amiens (1859). I am grateful to Toby Gelfand for making avail-

able to me his microfilm copy of this book. On Louis's life and work see P. Sue, "Éloge de Louis," in *Eloges de Louis*, pp. 416–49.

4. F. Vicq d'Azyr, *Oeuvres de Vicq d'Azyr, recueillis et publiés avec des notes et un discours sur sa vie et ses ouvrages*, ed. J. L. Moreau de la Sarthe, 6 vols. (1805). For his biography see J. L. Moreau de la Sarthe, "De la Vie et des ouvrages de Vicq d'Azyr," in *Oeuvres de Vicq d'Azyr*, vol. 1, pp. 1–88.

5. Georges Cuvier, *Recueil des éloges historiques lus dans les séances publiques de l'Institut Royale de France*, 3 vols. (Strasbourg, 1819–27). On his *éloges* see Dorinda Outram, "The Language of Natural Power: The *Éloges* of Georges Cuvier and the Public Language of Nineteenth Century Science," *History of Science* 16 (1978), 153–78, and on his career, Dorinda Outram, *Georges Cuvier: Vocation, Science and Authority in Post-Revolutionary France* (Manchester, 1984).

6. See James D. Garrison, *Dryden and the Tradition of the Panegyric* (Berkeley, Calif., 1975) esp. chap. 2; and O. B. Hardison, Jr., *The Enduring Monument: A Study of the Idea of Praise in Renaissance Literary Theory and Practice* (Chapel Hill, N.C., 1962).

7. *Éloges de Louis*, p. 233.

8. Sue, ibid., pp. 416–17.

9. *Oeuvres de Vicq d'Azyr*, vol. 3, pp. 140–41 (Navier). Also see *Éloges de Louis*, p. 63.

10. *Oeuvres de Vicq d'Azyr*, vol. 2, p. 305.

11. *Éloges de Louis*, p. 233.

12. *Oeuvres de Vicq d'Azyr*, vol. 3, p. 141 (Navier) and p. 381 (Buttet).

13. Ibid., p. 368 (Planchon), and vol. 2, p. 306 (Haller).

14. Ibid., p. 32 (Lieutaud). Vicq d'Azyr used almost the exact same language to describe de Nobleville. Vol. 2, p. 180.

15. *Éloges de Louis*, p. 41 (Malaval). Also see p. 70 (Roeder), p. 214 (Morand).

16. Ibid., p. 33 (Bassuel).

17. Ibid., p. 140 (Lecat).

18. *Oeuvres de Vicq d'Azyr*, vol. 3, p. 65 (Buttet).

19. Ibid., vol. 1, p. 276.

20. Ibid., vol. 3, p. 136.

21. Ibid., vol. 2, p. 348.

22. Ibid., vol. 3, p. 446 (le Roy).

23. See H. Duranton, "L'Académicien au miroir," *L'Histoire au dix-huitième siècle* (Aix-en-Provence, 1975), pp. 449–78.

24. For instance, in the *éloges* of Petit, Lecat, David.

25. *Oeuvres de Vicq d'Azyr*, vol. 1, pp. 270–71.

26. Ibid., vol. 2, p. 346, note 1.

27. Ibid., vol. 3, p. 30.

28. Ibid., p. 20.

29. *Éloges de Louis*, p. 263.

30. *Oeuvres de Vicq d'Azyr*, vol. 3, p. 168.

31. Ibid., vol. 2, p. 444. Also see his remarks on Lieutaud. Vol. 3, p. 15.

32. Jean-Claude Bonnet, "Naissance du Panthéon," *Poétique* 33 (1978), 51–52; Modal Osso, "Le Panthéon: l'École normale des morts," in *Les Lieux de mémoire: I, La République*, ed. Pierre Nora (1984), p. 142.

33. Cuvier, *Recueil des éloges* vol. 2, p. 5.

34. Ibid., pp. 269–70.

35. Pariset, *Membres de l'ARM*, vol. 2, p. 572.

36. Ibid., p. 590.

37. *Le Rouge et le noir* and *Illusions perdues* are well-known. Less enduring are novels like Balzac's *Jean Louis* (1822) and Michel Masson's *Le Grain de sable* (1832), which also prominently feature this motif.

38. For an example see George Weisz, "The Politics of Medical Professionalization in France, 1845–1848," *Journal of Social History* 12 (1978), 3–30. On the importance of mobility in bourgeois thought see Adeline Daumard, "Caractères de la société bourgeoises," in *Histoire économique et sociale de la France*, ed. F. Braudel and C. E. Labrousse, vol. 3 (1976), pp. 840–41.

39. This point is made in many studies of eighteenth-century French society. See, for instance, R. Lion, "Les Nouvelles élites," in *Histoire économique et sociale de la France*, ed. F. Braudel and C. E. Labrousse, vol. 2 (1970), pp. 634–40.

40. Pariset, *Membres de l'ARM*, vol. 2, p. 603. Among Pariset's other *éloges* with this theme are those of Chaussier, vol. 2, p. 47, and Vauquelin, vol. 1, p. 319. Also see François Mérat's oration honoring Huzard, *BAM* 3 (1839), 302.

41. José Bozzi, *Balzac et les médecins dans La Comédie Humaine* (1932).

42. In an impressionistic survey of the eulogies in the *Annales des Mines* during Pariset's tenure, I did not find a single instance of this theme applied to the state corps of mining engineers. Aside from the fact that members of this corps undoubtedly came from more affluent backgrounds than did doctors, advancement does not appear to have been perceived as a change of professional status, as it was for doctors. The essential status, of these engineers was secured when they graduated from the École des Mines. Subsequent promotions followed naturally.

43. The *éloges* of the Academy of Sciences in the eighteenth century tended in contrast to emphasize the need to defy paternal opposition in order to undertake a career in science. Charles B. Paul, *Science and Immortality: The Éloges of the Paris Academy of Sciences (1699–1791)* (Berkeley, Calif., 1980), p. 59. A similar motif in Cuvier's *éloges* is discussed in Dorinda Outram, "Before Objectivity: Women, Wives and Cultural Reproduction in Nineteenth-Century French Science," in *Uneasy Careers and Intimate Lives: Women in Science, 1789–1968*, ed., P. Abir-Am and D. Outram (New Brunswick, N.J., 1987). Similarly, the *éloges* of the Académie des Inscriptions et des Belles Lettres emphasize that vocations for literature had to overcome a variety of obstacles before they became careers. Duranton, "L'Académicien au miroir."

44. Pariset, *Membres de l'ARM*, vol. 2, p. 106.

45. Ibid., vol. 1, p. 100.

46. Ibid., vol. 2, p. 428–29.

47. *BAM* 1 (1837), 775. Also see Jolly in *BAM* 11 (1845–46), 507 (de Lens).

48. In *Enquêtes et documents relatifs à l'enseignement supérieur*, vol. 37, ed. A. de Beauchamp, (1890), p. 210. The emphasis on industriousness is characteristic of bourgeois society more generally during this period. William H. Sewell, *Work and Revolution in France: The Language of Labor from the Old Regime to 1848* (Cambridge, 1980). But there is probably something special about the role of this motif in medicine that makes doctors exemplars of the work ethic for Barrington Moore, "Historical Notes on the Doctor's Work Ethic," *Journal of Social History* 17 (1984), 547–71.

49. Pariset, *Membres de l'ARM*, vol. 1, p. 291.

50. Funeral oration for Double, *BAM* 7 (1841–42), 883.

51. See, for instance, the funeral orations for Robiquet, *BAM* 5 (1839–40), 196; Petit, 157; Double, *BAM* 7 (1841–42), 883.

52. Pariset, *Membres de l'ARM*, vol. 1, p. 330.

53. Ibid., p. 277.

54. Pariset, *Membres de l'ARM*, vol. 1, pp. 167, 199 (Berthollet); *BAM* 2 (1838), 646–47 (Laurent).

55. Pariset, *Membres de l'ARM*, vol. 2, p. 568.

56. Ibid., p. 367.

57. Ibid., p. 35.

58. F. Dubois d'Amiens, "Notice historique sur M. Chervin," *MEM* 12 (1846), xxxvii–lix.

59. Ibid., liv.

60. For examples, see Louis's *éloges* of Petit, Lecat, Haller, and Fleurant, and Vicq d'Azyr's *éloges* of Maret, Haller, Navier, and Dubourg. For examples in the *éloges* of the Academy of Sciences see Paul, *Science and Immortality*, p. 95.

61. Pariset, *Membres de l'ARM*, vol. 1, p. 276.

62. Ibid., pp. 246–47.

63. Maurice Keen, *Chivalry* (New Haven, Conn., 1984), pp. 2–3, 10–11.

64. *Membres de l'ARM*, vol. 2, p. 425.

65. I have used a number of major dictionaries in determining the meanings of these words. These include *Grand Larousse de la langue française*, 7 vols. (1971–78): *Le Grand Robert de la langue française*, 2nd ed., 8 vols. (1985); *Trésor de la langue française*, 15 vols. (1971–92); and Émile Littré, *Dictionnaire de la langue française* (1956–58).

66. Pariset, *Membres de l'ARM*, vol. 2, p. 255.

67. Ibid., p. 567.

68. Ibid., p. 483.

69. Ibid., p. 582.

70. Ibid., p. 587.

71. Ibid., p. 357.

72. *Éloges de Louis*, p. 242; *Oeuvres de Vicq d'Azyr*, vol. 3, p. 26.

73. See, for instance, Cuvier, *Recueil des éloges*, vol. 3, p. 3, and Outram, "The Language of Natural Power."

74. *Membres de l'ARM*, vol. 1, p. 159, where Cadet de Gassicourt is criticized for radical political views, and vol. 2, p. 200, which condemns Desgenettes's youthful involvement in a secret student society.

75. Cuvier, *Recueil des éloges*, vol. 3, p. 376.

76. Pariset, *Membres de l'ARM*, vol. 2, p. 517.

77. *BAM* 11 (1845–46), 509.

78. For instance, *BAM* 1 (1837), 548 (Dubois), 386 (Desgenettes); Pariset, *Membres de l'ARM*, vol. 1, p. 331 (Vauquelin); and, by other eulogists, in *BAM* 11 (1845–46), 509 (de Lens).

79. Robert A. Nye, *Masculinity and Male Codes of Honor in Modern France* (Oxford, 1993), chap. 7.

80. *BAM* 1 (1837), 858.

81. *BAM* 2 (1838), 323 (Louyer-Villermay); Pariset, *Membres de l'ARM*, vol. 1, p. 255 (Pinel); p. 308 (Percy), p. 328 (Vauquelin).

82. Ibid., p. 278.

83. Ibid., pp. 202–203.

84. Ibid., p. 137.

85. *BAM* 6 (1840–41), 329–30.

86. Pariset, *Membres de l'ARM*, vol. 2, p. 427.

87. *BAM* 10 (1844–45), 684.

88. Pariset, *Membres de l'ARM*, vol. 2, p. 519.

89. Ibid., p. 568.

10

Elite Medical Careers in the Nineteenth and Twentieth Centuries

Members of the Academy of Medicine may not have been the best doctors in France but they have certainly been among the most successful. A close look at the academy's membership thus provides an illuminating perspective from which to view the professional and social conditions of success in French medicine. Since many different types of professional powers have traditionally been concentrated in the hands of these academicians, or doctors very much like them, an examination of this sort may also prove relevant to understanding both the strengths and weaknesses of French medicine during the nineteenth and twentieth centuries.

This chapter, like the one that follows, is based on the results of a prosopographical study of the members of the Academy of Medicine at four moments in time: 1821, 1861, 1901, and 1935. I have limited myself to titular members, who clearly represented the summit of the Parisian medical hierarchy.[1] The total population is approximately four hundred individuals, all male. The methodology was to collect biographical information about all members during these years by searching through a wide variety of published biographical sources and administrative archives of many different sorts. All the collected data were brought together and then analyzed by computer.

This chapter uses the collected data to describe the career structures of elite medicine in Paris. It will be argued that the careers of academicians became increasingly rigid, uniform, and competitive during the course of the nineteenth century. In Chapter 11 I will extend my focus to the changing social characteristics of academy members and to the place of the Parisian medical elite in French society.

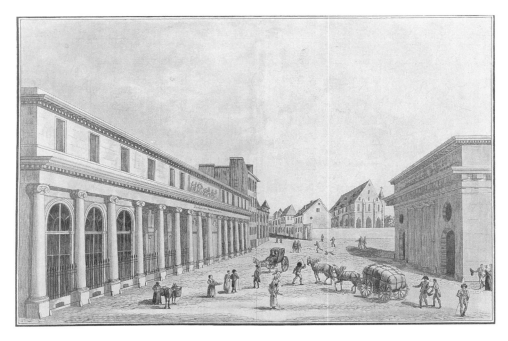

FIGURE 10.1. The Paris Faculty of Medicine in the early nineteenth century. (Musée Carnavalet)

Career Paths

Academicians in the early nineteenth century, we saw in Chapter 2, represented a wide range of medical careers. As time went on, however, they were increasingly likely to be professors in public institutions of medical or scientific education and research, with the majority at the Paris Faculty of Medicine. If they were not professors, academicians were usually holders of senior posts in the public hospitals of Paris or junior appointments at the Faculty of Medicine. For all but a few marginal categories of academicians, the growing dominance of professors in the academy was part of a broader tendency toward increased career uniformity at all levels of the system.

Increasing uniformity began with medical training. Academicians in 1821 had a relatively wide variety of educational backgrounds. A little less than one-third of the men in this cohort received their first medical degree before the reconstitution of postrevolutionary medical education in 1794. Many of those with postrevolutionary degrees were trained in the military. On their return to civilian life they took the examinations of a faculty for the MD diploma, which was a legal prerequisite for civilian medical practice. Most academicians obtained the MD from a faculty of medicine. One-fifth had surgical diplomas from the prerevolutionary Collège de Chirurgie and another fifth had degrees in either pharmacy or veterinary medicine.

About 20 percent of the academicians of 1821 received their medical degrees outside Paris, the majority at the Faculty of Montpellier; another 25 percent or so came to the Paris Faculty of Medicine after having begun their studies at a provincial institution or in the military. In the three later populations, over 90 percent of the members obtained their degrees in Paris in spite of the fact that the number of medical faculties increased from three to seven during the last decades of the nineteenth century. The proportion beginning medical studies elsewhere before coming to the capital also decreased substantially.[2]

Future academicians needed to study in Paris because career success was becoming progressively more dependent on student clerkships in the Parisian hospitals. Throughout the nineteenth century small numbers of medical students were appointed each year on the basis of their performance in a special competition (*concours*) to four-year hospital internships (*internat*).[3] They were chosen from a

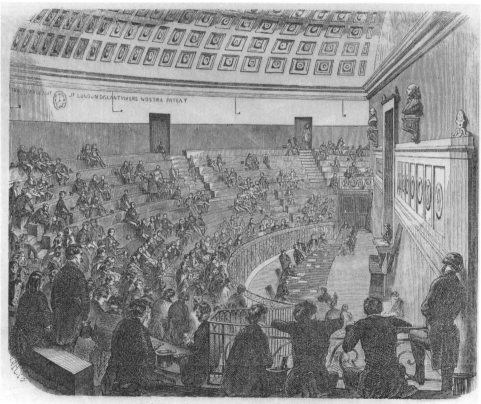

École de médecine de Paris. — Le grand amphithéatre.

FIGURE 10.2. The main amphitheater of the Faculty of Medicine in the mid-nineteenth century. From E.-A. Texier, *Tableau de Paris* (Paris, 1852). (Bibliothèque Nationale)

larger pool of students who had spent one or more years (usually two) in a junior nonresidency clerkship, the *externat*, also obtained through a *concours*. These interns received room and board in the hospital and a small stipend which raised them out of the poverty characteristic of student life in the Latin Quarter. More important, they underwent a remarkably intense clinical apprenticeship under the direction of the leading physicians and surgeons of the day. Increasingly, it was the *internat* which governed entry to elite medical careers.

Founded in 1802 (though it had precursors among ancien régime surgeons), the *internat* came to play a very similar role in medicine to the one played by the *grandes écoles* in science and engineering; it assured a high-quality education for an elite, making the caliber of training for the mass of students a less than pressing issue. Like the *grandes écoles*, it produced a powerful esprit de corps among those who went through it. The *internat* experience was clearly intense, as evidenced by the great warmth and fondness with which it is discussed in memoirs and autobiographies.[4] Within medical culture as a whole, the *internat*, symbolized by the *salle de garde* (common room), achieved something like mythic status:

> One says *salles de garde* as one says the artists' studios of Montmartre, as one says the literary groups of Bohemian Paris, and this word evokes the image of a laborious and extravagant youth, seedbed of the illustrious and the failed, but always of the unusual [*des fantaissistes*].[5]

As this quotation suggests, exceptionally rich clinical experience was only one attraction of the *internat*. The young men who filled these posts had, somewhat

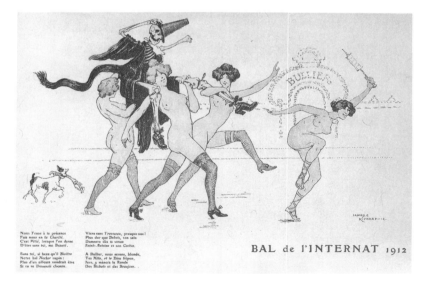

FIGURE 10.3. Poster advertising the annual interns' ball. The poem at left plays on the names of the major Parisian hospitals. (Musée de l'Assistance Publique)

unusually for trainees, a great deal of responsibility and even authority within the hospital since their medical superiors were absent for most of the day. They were, moreover, on the road to career success.[6] Their liminal status as part elite physicians and part students gave them freedom from social constraints that would disappear once they entered fully into the middle-class world of the medical elite. Some *salles de gardes* attracted small coteries of writers, artists, and *demimondaine* ladies who were socially several cuts above the street prostitutes of the Latin Quarter.[7] The annual intern's ball became, by the end of the nineteenth century, a lively and ribald Latin Quarter institution featuring scantily clad young women. Perhaps the best indication of how positively the *internat* was viewed is the fact that in their fourth and final year, interns competed intensely among themselves for a gold medal which allowed the winner to continue serving as an intern for an extra year.

The *internat* was too new an institution to have had much impact on the academicians of 1821 but it was well established among those of 1861, when half of all doctors and pharmacists passed through it.[8] In the sample of 1935 about three-quarters of all MDs in the academy (and virtually all of the surgeons) and two-thirds of the pharmacy graduates were former interns.

Much more, however, became expected of the future elite. Nearly 20 percent of the academicians of 1901 had during their student years held a junior laboratory or clinical post at the medical faculty or School of Pharmacy; among those of 1935 the

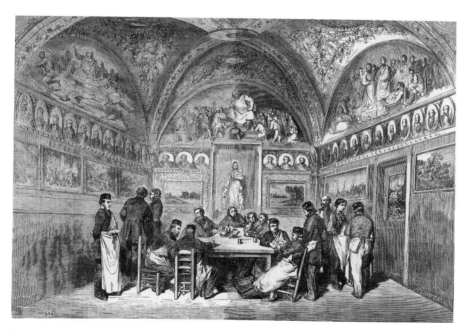

FIGURE 10.4. *The Interns' Room at the Charité Hospital*, by Gustave Doré, 1867. (Collection Roger-Viollet)

figure was 34 percent. As well, one-third of all MDs in the academy in 1901 and 1935 had won at least one of the very competitive student prizes granted by the faculty or the hospital administration. Over half the pharmacists in the academy in 1935 had obtained an equivalent prize. Those interns interested in the laboratory sciences had to find time and a laboratory where they could begin research. Last but not least, it became a tradition for interns to offer private classes to students preparing to compete in the *internat* competition. Teaching was both a way to review and synthesize material for the more advanced competitions coming up and an opportunity to hone the pedagogical skills that were so prized in clinical instruction.

Life became even more hectic after graduation. Characteristically, private practices were established soon after the diploma was obtained. A well-placed patron within the faculty or hospital system might refer wealthy patients, find one a job with a medical journal or as secretary to a senior medical figure, and facilitate publication and election to prestigious but restrictive societies like the Société de Biologie that brought one in contact with the leaders of medical science. A patron could also aid those with elite aspirations to keep a toehold within official institutions. In the early nineteenth century, many future academicians made a reputation by teaching private courses. Their successors were appointed to formal positions in teaching institutions. (Increasingly, *concours* replaced discretionary professorial appointments.) About 20 percent of the academicians in 1901 had at the postdoctoral level held junior posts in the laboratories and clinical wards of the Faculty of Medicine. Among the academicians of 1935 the figure was over 40 percent; if one includes those academicians who had held equivalent posts at the School of Pharmacy or in the laboratories of scientific institutions, the figure for the later sample is about 50 percent of all academicians.

Only a small minority of academicians took more than one higher degree (see Table 10.1). The number of MDs with other medical degrees was never large, but from the middle of the nineteenth century higher degrees in science assumed some importance for elite medical careers; about 10 percent of MD academicians acquired doctorates of science. Surprisingly, the proportion changed little from the population of 1861 on, despite the expanding role of science in medicine and the growing proportion of academicians working in institutions of science and research.

For pharmacists in the academy,[9] however, the doctorate of science gradually became a crucial second degree (see Table 10.1). In our two twentieth-century

TABLE 10.1 Multiple Degrees				
Degree	*1821*	*1861*	*1901*	*1935*
MD				
% with pharmacy	4	3	4	1
% with veterinary medicine			2	
% with DocSc	1	8	11	10
Pharmacy				
% with MD	20	15	27	9
% with DocSc	27	31	82	73
% with MD and DocSc	7	8	27	9

TABLE 10.2   Later Positions Held by Academicians, by percent of Academicians

Position	1821	1861	1901	1935
MD, hospital	48	51	59	65
MD, *agrégation*	9	42	56	51
MD, hospital and *agrégation*	7	34	46	40
Pharmacy, hospital		8	1	45
Pharmacy, *agrégation*		30	45	64
Pharmacy, hospital and *agrégation*		8	18	27

populations, about three-quarters of the pharmacists had science doctorates. Among the cohort of 1901 medical diplomas remained pertinent, with over one-quarter of the pharmacists accumulating both medical *and* science doctorates, but the former seem to have lost their value for the pharmacists of 1935. This pattern provides some indication of the symbiotic relationship—based on the fundamental role of chemistry—that developed between elite pharmacy and the world of institutional science in the late nineteenth century.[10]

Most academicians, however, did not go on to other degrees but rather prepared for the various *concours* which governed appointment to the next rungs of the medical ladder, posts in the Parisian hospital system and the *agrégation* of the Faculty of Medicine and School of Pharmacy (see Table 10.2). If one excludes the extremely diverse cohort of 1821, future academicians were characteristically appointed to one or both of these positions while in their early or mid thirties, frequently after several unsuccessful *concours*. Although it was occasionally possible to be elected to the academy with only one of the titles, the two usually went together. Over 70 percent of the hospital physicians had the *agrégation* and over 80 percent of the *agrégés* held hospital posts. A similar pattern developed among academician-pharmacists. A hospital post did not often lead to the academy in the absence of a teaching or research appointment.[11] By the same token, the only large group of academicians with only the *agrégation* were professors of basic science.

Unlike hospital appointments, which were permanent, appointment to the *agrégation* introduced in 1823, was for a limited nine-year term. This made the small number of positions at the Faculty of Medicine at any one time (twenty-four in 1826, forty in 1896) more accessible if fleeting. *Agregés* were not assigned definite functions until the 1860s when they began to serve as junior teaching staff. The *agrégation* was valued primarily because it was prestigious enough to attract affluent clients to a physician's private practice and because it provided access to professorships. It became increasingly rare for appointments to faculty chairs to be made without prior acquisition of the *agrégation*.[12] Most *agrégés* in our samples made it into the academy because they had gone on to become professors at the Faculty of Medicine. Only about 20 percent of them in 1861 and 1901 had not gone on to a teaching chair, with the figure declining to 9 percent among academicians in 1935. Even combined with a hospital post, the title was no longer sufficient for membership in the academy.

Exceptionally, during the July Monarchy appointment to faculty chairs had also been effected through *concours*. But this was abandoned under the Second Empire for a system of ministerial appointment based on faculty recommendations. Subsequently, once an individual became an *agrégé* and obtained a hospital post, the period of formal *concours* was at an end. Here is how a long-time dean of the Faculty of Medicine, Henri Roger, described his successful attainment of these titles: "It was in the year of grace 1892 when I was delivered from the horrible nightmare which had, since the beginning of my medical studies, troubled my existence, halted my initiatives, paralyzed my efforts."[13]

Roger's bitterness suggests some of the hostility which the system of career advancement provoked. First, it was based on memory and rhetorical ability. Characteristically, candidates had to prepare and memorize answers to a large number of quasi-canonical questions and then deliver the response orally to fill a specific time allotment, which grew longer as one advanced through the hierarchy. In addition to memory, fluent speech was vital. At the instigation of his mentor Georges Debove, Charles Achard took lessons in diction from an actor at the Odeon Theater.[14] For many of those who aspired to German-style research careers, the time devoted to preparation was a major impediment to scientific productivity. It was also a barrier to early specialization since these *concours* were encyclopedic. Many and perhaps the majority of academicians did not share Roger's hostility to the system, but a succession of reformers did try to mitigate its worst features by making research productivity an element of competition.[15]

A second criticism that was frequently raised was that the various competitions were not fair because "patrons" on the examination juries systematically favored their own students and disciples. The importance of patronage in facilitating the long and grueling process was widely acknowledged. Charles Achard mentions matter-of-factly that he failed on five occasions to become a hospital physician. He was typed, he reported, as one of those good candidates waiting for his jury. Sure enough, on his sixth try, with two of his patrons on the jury, he was successful.[16] Discussion of the advantages and disadvantages of such patronage was widespread, with defenders suggesting that long-term personal knowledge of individuals was a far more accurate indicator of merit than a brief *concours*.[17]

Once past the stage of *concours*, individuals had considerably more freedom to pursue their personal interests. Nevertheless, future academicians continued to compete for the next rung of the career ladder: professorial chairs of higher education. This meant that in addition to their hospital services, to which it was traditional to devote a good part of the morning, and private practices, to which most academicians devoted their afternoons, a variety of other activities occupied elite practitioners. Some taught in junior positions in the medical schools and, less frequently, institutions of science. More often, *agrégés* and hospital physicians taught private courses at the *école pratique* of the Faculty of Medicine or in the Parisian hospitals. As medical faculties became influenced by the German model of higher education, candidates for chairs had to emulate their colleagues in scientific institutions by demonstrating a capacity for research. This meant in practice that they had increasingly to compile a fairly lengthy record of publications.[18] When a chair at the faculty did become available, candidates had to be prepared to "visit" leading professors in order to try to win their vote while patrons worked feverishly in the background.[19]

Even at this stage, formal competition was not at an end. Future academicians (starting with the population of 1861) frequently competed for the prizes awarded by the Academy of Medicine and the Academy of Science. The latter were particularly sought-after and they were plentiful.[20] The number of academicians who won at least one cash award or, in a few cases, a medal, rose from 41 percent in the sample of 1861 to 62 percent in that of 1935. The prizes awarded by the Academy of Medicine were obtained less frequently because they were not very numerous until the last decades of the nineteenth century and because individuals ceased to be eligible for such awards once they were elected to the academy. Still nearly 40 percent of the academicians of 1935 had obtained a cash award from the academy. Only 30 percent of the members in that year did not win at least one prize from either academy during their careers. About one-third of the membership obtained three or more awards.

Professorships

We do not have accurate figures about failed attempts to obtain a teaching chair (which are rarely mentioned in biographical material) but we do know that quite a few eminent academicians had unsuccessful candidacies under their belts. The most notable of these was Claude Bernard, who never made it to the Faculty of Medicine.[21] More characteristic, perhaps, were those who met with success on a third, fourth, or fifth attempt.[22] Some individuals had to wait a very long time until a chair in their specialty became free. Marcel Proust's father, Adrien, waited many years for the chair of hygiene generally conceded to be his due because the incumbent, Appollinaire Bouchardat, refused to retire though he was almost completely deaf. It is said that when they met, Bouchardat would taunt the younger man by boasting about his good health and virility.[23] The last laugh was Proust's, however: a cabinet change brought one of his friends to the Ministry of Public Instruction and Bouchardat was forced to retire.

On average, academician-professors in the first half of the nineteenth century obtained chairs at the Faculty of Medicine when they were in their early forties (see Table 10.3). The age of appointment was highly variable in the population of 1821 and more uniformly youthful among academicians of 1861, among whom 40 percent were less than forty years old on their appointment. In later years professorships came increasingly late as a result of stiffer competition. Among academician-professors in 1901, only two men were appointed to the Faculty of Medicine before

TABLE 10.3 Average Age at Appointment to Professorship

	1821	1861	1901	1935
Faculty of Medicine	43.3	42.7	47.6	51.2
School of Pharmacy	35.1	46.1	38.6	41.3
Science and research	42.0	45.6	40.9	50.6
Veterinary education[a]		33.6		28.5
Military[a]		36.8		36.7

[a] Populations are combined because of the small numbers involved.

the age of forty. Among those of 1935, over 60 percent were past the age of fifty on their appointment to a professorship.

Professors in the institutions of science and research were appointed at a roughly comparable age to colleagues in medicine. The one exception is the population of 1901 when science professors were considerably younger at appointment. This seems to have resulted directly from the creation of new institutions, which named some very young men to their staffs. Positions in the École Pratique de Hautes Études, Institut Agronomique, and École de Physique et Chimie had nowhere near the status of chairs of traditional institutions and did not require the same accumulation of posts and honors which had become a prerequisite at the schools of medicine and pharmacy. However, five out of six chairs at the very prestigious Collège de France were also obtained by academicians under the age of forty-five in this cohort. This suggests that the rapid expansion of posts in the small domain of Parisian science accelerated careers throughout the system. By 1935, however, the average age of appointment to scientific institutions had risen by ten years to almost exactly the same age as appointment to the Faculty of Medicine.

The few professors at other sorts of institutions were appointed at a considerably younger age. The average age on appointment for pharmacist-academicians in 1935 was only forty-one, a full ten years younger than appointment to the Faculty of Medicine. It may be that the unofficial requirement for a doctorate of science at the School of Pharmacy served to shrink the available pool of eligible candidates and thus reduce competitive pressures. The young age of appointment to military medical schools is not very significant because such teaching posts were not usually permanent and did not represent the highest career levels that could be reached in the military. In a unique category were the handful of academicians with professorships at the School of Veterinary Medicine at Alfort, whose age of appointment remained very low in all our samples. They were, moreover, being appointed only a few years after receiving veterinary diplomas, also at an exceptionally young age.[24] Clearly rising educational requirements throughout the system of higher education had very little impact on veterinary education. It was not until the interwar period that the educational administration attempted to raise standards in this domain by creating a doctorate of veterinary science granted officially by the medical faculties.[25]

Professors occasionally moved from one chair to another within the same institution. This was inevitable since individuals regularly applied for a vacant chair even if it was not in their main field of specialized interest. *Permutation* to a more appropriate chair when one became available was standard practice. In the Faculty of Medicine, there was also a tendency to move from theoretical chairs, in which lectures took place on faculty premises, to more prestigious clinical chairs, which centered all activities in a hospital service. Since most clinicians had to spend time in hospitals as part of their responsibilities outside the faculty, this concentration of effort in a single locale simplified busy careers.

There was, however, little movement of professors between the Faculty of Medicine and other institutions of medical education. Although Vauquelin served as professor of chemistry at the medical faculty while acting as director of the School of Pharmacy, no academician in any of our four samples held a chair at both this faculty and School of Pharmacy or at the faculty and the Veterinary School at Alfort. A number of faculty professors among the academicians of 1820 held important posts in the Napoleonic army. But the only professor at Val-de-Grâce in any of the four populations who obtained a chair at the Faculty of Medicine was Broussais, who was appointed by the new government of the July Monarchy after the Revolution of 1830.

There was, however, considerable career movement between the medical schools on one hand and the various scientific institutions on the other. The nature of scientific careers rewarded by membership in the Academy of Medicine changed over the course of the nineteenth century. In the first half of the century intimate links united the Faculty of Medicine and the institutions of science like the Collège de France, Muséum d'Histoire Naturelle, and Paris Faculty of Sciences. Of the ten academicians of 1820 who taught in the latter three institutions no less than seven also occupied chairs at the Faculty of Medicine and another was at the School of Pharmacy. Among those of 1861 four out of seven men in scientific institutions were also at the faculty and another taught at the Veterinary School at Alfort.

Among academicians of 1901, however, only three out of twenty men in scientific institutions also occupied chairs at the Faculty of Medicine. Four others were professors at the School of Pharmacy, confirming our previous data on the close links between this institution and the scientific domain at the turn of the century. Two other academicians of 1901 moved to scientific institutions from military medical schools and another migrated from Alfort. Still, nearly 50 percent of the academicians in scientific and research institutions did not hold posts in any of the institutions of medical education, suggesting that medical laboratory research was becoming an autonomous career. This became even more evident in the twentieth century. Among the twenty academicians in 1935 with posts in scientific institutions, thirteen (65 percent) did not hold posts in institutions of medical education.[26]

Although there were cases in which a professor of science like Jean-Baptiste Dumas was rewarded with a post in a medical school, the more normal movement was to start at a medical institution. From here, outstanding scientists went on to coveted chairs at the Sorbonne (Adolphe Wurtz), the Muséum d'Histoire Naturelle (Constant Duméril), or the Collège de France (Marcelin Berthelot). Successful clinicians might aspire to the chair of medicine at the Collège de France. The new scientific institutions created late in the nineteenth century were less prestigious than the Faculty of Medicine. But they nevertheless represented hierarchical advancement for professors at Alfort and Val-de-Grâce. Such movement, it should be emphasized, did not necessarily mean that medical posts were abandoned. In many though not all cases, actual teaching might be farmed out to an assistant, with the formal title remaining in the hands of the incumbent. This possibility of holding several different posts (*cumul*) was one of the few methods of financially rewarding outstanding professors within the system of bureaucratically rigid salaries.

Even after a chair in an institution of education or science had been obtained, competition and advancement continued. Some of those who achieved professorial status went on to administrative positions in their institutions or within the state education system. The proportion of academicians with such posts was remarkably stable: 16 percent among those in both 1821 and 1861, 17 percent in 1901, and 19 percent in 1935. In the early nineteenth century a significant number were inspectors of higher education (a post that was abolished in the 1880s) and in the early twentieth many sat on the various administrative commissions that now proliferated. But in all of our populations, a majority were deans or directors of faculties or schools.

One does not get the feeling that such positions, particularly the direction of the Faculty of Medicine, were particularly desirable and certainly not for clinicians. It may be significant that with the exception of the founding deans of the Faculty of Medicine, Michel-Augustin Thouret and Jean-Jacques Leroux, the most successful and longest serving deans were outside the mainstream of clinical medicine. Orfila (seventeen years) was a chemist and toxicologist, Wurtz (eleven years) was a chemist, Paul Brouardel (thirteen years) was an expert in forensic medicine and public health, and Henri Roger (thirteen years) was a physiologist. This is not, upon reflection, surprising. Clinicians who had spent their professional lives in hospitals, becoming virtual dictators in their wards, would not have found it easy to cope with a rigid educational administration, an equally rigid hospital administration which ran the clinics on which faculty teaching depended, and huge numbers of chronically disgruntled and frequently disruptive medical students. Furthermore, the few thousand francs that supplemented the dean's professorial salary was insignificant when measured against potential earnings from private practice.[27] It may be that such positions represented real power in the autocratic regimes preceding the Third Republic. But this power was counterbalanced by the instability that went along with being a political appointee at a time when regimes changed frequently. And as institutions of higher education after 1870 become more collegially run (within the limits of administrative centralization), deans undoubtedly lost some of their influence.[28]

If moving into the administration had only limited appeal for many academicians, there remained rewards to compete for. Many professors were by now patrons. Their disciples had to be placed in the junior and intermediate posts available in faculty laboratories and clinics (and by the twentieth century in hospitals), as well as navigated through the most prestigious *concours* and elections. But they were not just competing on behalf of others. They too remained dependent on colleagues if they aspired to be elected to the honorific academic institutions. Membership in the Academy of Medicine was the norm for professors at the Faculty of Medicine, but those in other institutions had to work hard for this honor. And only from a fifth to a quarter of the academicians in any of our populations would go on to obtain the most coveted of prizes, admission to the Academy of Sciences.

The Academies

It was in the early nineteenth century possible to become a full member of the Academy of Medicine by passing through associate membership status. Among our sample of academicians in 1861, some 38 percent began in junior positions with the vast majority appointed resident (Parisian) associates during the 1820s. Once associate status was eliminated in 1835, movement through the ranks of the academy became uncommon. On rare occasions, someone living outside Paris and appointed a corresponding member of the academy might return to the capital and be appointed a titular member. This happened to only two individuals in any of our four populations.[29]

Nearly all academicians, therefore, were appointed directly to full membership. With the exception of those named by the government in 1820, academicians were elected by their peers. By the late nineteenth century the underlying mechanisms were similar to those determining entry to the Faculty of Medicine (and the Academy of Sciences). Patrons competed in placing their protégés; alliances and *combinaisons* were forged. As we saw in Chapter 2, academicians were on average appointed in their mid- to late forties throughout most of the nineteenth century (excepting the population of 1820). Members in 1935, however, had been appointed a good deal later in their lives (average 56.5 years of age), paralleling the rising age of medical professorships.[30]

Once elected, academicians could compete for some of the academy's own honorific posts. From one-quarter (population of 1901) to a little over one-third (that of 1861) of the academicians were elected to the post of honorary annual president. Election reflected longevity at least as often as it did real intellectual eminence. (Academicians liked to honor their *doyens*.) In any case, presidential contests did not arouse much passion. Election to the post of permanent secretary was more significant and could provoke considerable emotion, as did the very close contest in 1887 between Jaccoud and Bergeron. Even at this stage, old patronage ties could be significant. One of Georges Debove's last acts before retiring as permanent secretary of the Academy of Medicine in 1920 was to help his lifelong protégé, Charles Achard, win election to replace him.[31] But at this stage of academicians' careers, rivalry centered above all on the struggle to become a member of the Academy of Sciences.

The pinnacle of success in an elite medical career was election to the Academy of Sciences (AS). When a suitable vacancy opened up in that institution, the aspirant would visit the sitting members in order to line up support.[32] Henri Roger tells a wonderful, possibly apocryphal, tale of a botanist competing for a place in this academy. His strategy for winning over those he visited was to prepare cards listing the research of each academician. By carefully studying the relevant card before a visit, he was able to discuss and suitably praise his host's scientific accomplishments. After one such visit, the candidate left particularly pleased with his eloquence only to realize to his horror that he had during the last hour been praising not his host's research but that of another academician. He had mistakenly pulled out and studied the wrong card. According to this version of the story, the very elderly academician voted for him anyway, telling colleagues that it was useful to have a colleague in the academy to remind him of early research that he could no longer recall.

Throughout the nineteenth century the average age at election to the AS rose for members of the Academy of Medicine; it was around 53 for academicians in 1821 and 1861 and 55.6 for those in 1901 before it jumped to 66.3 for those in 1935. Many of those appointed to the Academy of Medicine in 1820–21 were already members of the AS. But from then on the standard pattern was for election to the Academy of Medicine to precede election to the AS by an average of from seven to ten years. Even by the standards of the elitist Academy of Sciences, medical members of the AS were recruited at an advanced age; the medical section of the AS was consistently among the two or three sections of that academy with the highest average age at election.[33] Elite medicine in Paris dwarfed all the other scientific sectors from which the AS recruited its members, creating enormous competitive pressures.

TABLE 10.4   Membership in the Academy of Sciences

	1821	1861	1901	1935
AM populations in AS (%)	26	23	20	21
AM in AS in specific year (%)	14	13	14	12
Full AS members in AM in				
specific year (%)	20	16	21	17
Faculty professors in AS (%)	46	52	19	21
Index	1.8	2.3	0.97	1.0
Science professors in AS (%)	100	100	57	63
Index	3.8	4.3	2.9	3.0
Professors in major science schools[a] (%)	100	10	89	91
Index	3.8	4.3	4.5	4.3
Professors of pharmacy in AS (%)	33	29	63	29
Index	1.3	1.3	3.2	1.4

Key: AM = Academy of Medicine; AS = Academy of Sciences; Index = percentage of AS members in a category divided by the percentage of AS members in the academy as a whole.
[a] Collège de France, Paris Faculty of Science, Muséum d'Histoire Naturelle.

Approximately one-quarter of the members of the Academy of Medicine in 1821 had been or were to be elected to the AS as full or associate members (see Table 10.4). To some extent, this rate of membership is inflated because of an unusually high turnover of academicians appointed in 1820–21. Even so, the proportion of members of the AS in later populations fell only slightly and remained quite steady throughout the nineteenth and twentieth centuries. Likewise the proportion of full AS members in our sample years who were members of the Academy of Medicine remained steady.

The reason for this stability was the continued existence of a section of medicine and surgery in the AS with six places out of a total membership of sixty-six. In addition, the section of anatomy and zoology in the AS usually held a handful of medical practitioners of anatomy and one finds members of the Academy of Medicine in such nonmedical sections as chemistry, zoology, and rural economy.[34] There was thus a very large medical presence in the AS throughout the nineteenth and early twentieth centuries. While no one minded that laboratory scientists working in medical institutions were well-represented, there was some resentment of the large place allotted clinical medicine, too practical to be considered a "real" science.[35] In 1825 the zoologist Geoffroy Saint-Hillaire campaigned to have the section of medicine and surgery eliminated altogether.[36] As the century progressed, such feelings intensified and infiltrated the medical section itself. In 1872 two members of the section, Claude Bernard and Gabriel Andral, in supporting their candidate for a contested vacancy, proposed that doctors and surgeons be limited to four places with the remaining two reserved explicitly for physiologists. They were unsuccessful and a surgeon was elected.[37] It nevertheless seems to have become accepted that two of the six places in the section be reserved for physiologists.[38] More generally, the place of clinical medicine in the Academy of Sciences decreased in the following years.

Throughout the nineteenth century, those members of the Academy of Medicine who were or would become professors in a Parisian institution of science had the best chance of reaching the AS (see Table 10.4). Both types of appointment were forms of recognition granted by the scientific elite and decisions in both were often made by the same individuals. Among academicians of 1821 and 1861, every one of the handful of academicians with an appointment in a scientific institution was elected to the AS. Such men were approximately four times as likely to be appointed to the AS as members of the Academy of Medicine generally. The much larger contingent of individuals in these institutions in the samples of 1901 and 1935 was no longer certain of election to the AS but remained in a favored position. About 60 percent of those in scientific institutions in the populations of 1901 and 1935 were elected to the AS, making them about three times as likely to obtain this honor as members of the Academy of Medicine generally.

Even this figure is misleading since it lumps together individuals in traditional institutions like the Collège de France with those in newer and less prestigious institutions like the Institut Pasteur. Of the twenty men in the populations of 1901 and 1935 with chairs at the Collège de France, Faculty of Sciences, or Muséum d'Histoire Naturelle, no fewer than eighteen were also members of the AS.

Unlike the major institutions of science, the Paris Faculty of Medicine lost much of its special link with the Academy of Sciences. In the samples of 1821 and 1861, about half of all professors at the Faculty of Medicine were also members of the AS. In some cases, of course, they also taught in scientific institutions. But even those who did not had a good chance of entering the AS. Professors in that institution were about twice as likely as the average academician to be elected to the AS. Among academicians of 1901 and 1935, only about 20 percent of the admittedly larger contingent of professors of medicine made it to the AS, their chances being pretty much equal to those of other academicians. If one excludes the small number of professors at the Faculty of Medicine who also held a post in a scientific institution, faculty professors in fact had somewhat lower chance of reaching the AS than did academicians generally.

Like the growing separation between professorships at the Faculty of Medicine and those in scientific institutions, the declining place of the Faculty of Medicine in the AS suggests a growing rift between the worlds of clinical medicine and scientific research. In filling medical spots in the AS early in the nineteenth century, that institution had chosen predominantly from the staff of the faculty, especially those individuals who also held posts in scientific institutions. As the personnel in scientific institutions expanded and separated from the world of the medical faculty, members of the AS were increasingly elected from within its ranks at the expense of medical professors. The latter were not of course excluded completely from the AS since the section of medicine continued to be predominantly clinical. But their numbers were reduced by half from the population of 1861 to that of 1901 (from fourteen to seven). The total rose slightly in the population of 1935 (to nine). But since the total contingent of professors grew as well, an individual professor's chance of election improved little.

The small School of Pharmacy had a rather different relationship historically with the AS. In the samples of 1821 and 1861, about 30 percent of the professors were appointed to the AS, giving them a slightly higher than average chance of election. In the late nineteenth century, however, the school of pharmacy became closely associated with scientific institutions because, one surmises, of the presence on its staff of

Marcelin Berthelot, one of the two permanent secretaries of the AS during this period. One consequence, we saw, was the growing presence of its professors in scientific institutions. (An alternative perspective would see this as an example of the colonization of pharmacy by academic chemists.) Another consequence was the election to the AS of about two-thirds of its professors, giving professors of pharmacy a chance at election more than three times better than that of academicians generally. This favorable situation did not persist, and among academicians in 1935 professors of pharmacy had about the same chance of election to the AS they had during most of the nineteenth century.

Once elected to the AS, medical members could aspire to the various honorific posts that were available. Members of the Academy of Medicine had a reasonably good chance, for instance, of being elected officers of the AS providing that they were members of the latter institution for a significant length of time before they died. The presidency of the AS, which was an annual and nonrenewable appointment, was the most likely honor to be obtained. Close to half of all medical academicians in the AS in all four of our populations were elected to such posts, only slightly less than the proportion for nonmedical members.

If we examine the one post that clearly reflected intellectual stature rather than longevity or amiability, that of permanent secretary, we get a somewhat different impression of the role of medical men in the AS. Seventeen men were named to this key post between 1803 and 1914.[39] Of these, eleven individuals were responsible for "physical sciences," which included medicine. (The other six served as secretaries for the "mathematical" sciences.) Within the former group, the Academy of Medicine was well represented: we find two associate members (Cuvier and Pasteur) and three full members (Dumas, Vulpian, and Berthelot) of that institution. But only one of these, Vulpian, was a clinician and a member of the medical section of the AS. And he served in this post for only two years. Out of 212 worker-years served by the seventeen permanent secretaries (1803–1914 x 2 secretaries), only two years were served by a representative of the Parisian medical elite. This suggests that the stature of medical science in the AS was somewhat more complex and problematic than the simple calculation of honorific positions would suggest.

An indication that this was indeed the case is provided by a close examination of the academic eulogies and necrological notices read in the AS.[40] Unlike honorific positions, necrological notices in the AS reflected real intellectual stature within the scientific community. Among members of the AS in 1821, members of the Academy of Medicine did almost as well as nonmembers in attracting necrological notices. But only one of the ten members of the Academy of Medicine appointed to the AS after 1821 was so honored. And this relative neglect of members of the Academy of Medicine continued among the members of the AS in 1861. Things improved slightly for members in 1901 and 1935: but members of the Academy of Medicine in the AS were still honored with necrologies in the latter institution about half as often as nonmedical colleagues. The section of medicine and surgery was the least likely of all the sections of the AS to see its members honored by necrologies.

It is not easy to interpret this relative neglect. It may be that successive permanent secretaries felt free to ignore medical members because these were likely to be the subjects of *éloges* in the Academy of Medicine. Cuvier certainly gave this impression in the last years of his tenure.[41] Later Claude Bernard and Jean Vincent were the subjects of necrological notices but Nobel Prize winner Charles Richet was not. At the very least, the lack of such posthumous acknowledgments suggests considerable distance separating the medical from the scientific elite, despite their coexistence in various academies. This parallels a similar process of distancing seen in Chapter 2, where we examined the representation of the scientific community within the Academy of Medicine.

As the nineteenth century advanced, recruitment to the Academy of Medicine was increasingly governed by an ever more rigid ladder of posts and honors obtained through intense competition. Critics charged that the system was unfair and that it inhibited the development of medical science.[42] Whatever the truth of this charge, it is certain that competitive pressures increasingly delayed entry into the upper ranks of the elite. As a result, the academy's membership in the twentieth century, like that of the Faculty of Medicine and Academy of Sciences, became quite elderly. One wonders to what extent this aging process contributed to the perceived crisis of French medicine during the interwar years; it certainly must have had profound effects at the institutional level.

Within this system, those who made it to the summit came to wield awesome powers over the careers of younger men. Internship training, junior and intermediate level clinical and laboratory posts at the faculty, support in *concours*, and eventually elections to the faculty and academies were some of the plums which patrons could offer. Aspirants to the medical elite took over much of the day-to-day scut work of healing and research and became indispensable collaborators of patrons. Nonetheless, patronage had its limits since the Parisian medical world, unlike that of, say, philosophy or chemistry, was a large one in which there were many patrons to choose from and play off against one another. Furthermore, hierarchical patronage was not the only feature of the system. Horizontal links between members of the same generation could extend well beyond narrow coteries, especially if, as was the case in the 1850s and 1860s, members of a generation viewed themselves as exemplars of a radically new vision of medical science.[43]

A final consequence of the changes described in this chapter is the enormous expansion in the amount of effort that had to be invested in the struggle for posts. The time spent in a purely medical milieu, listening, teaching, observing, writing, and campaigning for posts and honors, was inordinate. This, as much as growing disciplinary specialization, may account for the apparent separation and differentiation of the medical elite from the scientific elite. One is tempted to ask whether, as might be expected, the social horizons of academicians narrowed accordingly. We shall take up this question among several others in Chapter 11.

NOTES

1. I have not here examined the various categories of corresponding and associate members discussed more briefly in Chapter 2.

2. The proportion decreased to 13 percent and 8 percent in the samples of 1901 and 1935 respectively.

3. The number appointed annually varied from about 30 early in the century to 60 or 65 late in the century. From 1802 to 1902, there were 3,300 individuals appointed Parisian hospital interns. Raymond Durand-Fardel, *L'Internat en médecine et en chirurgie des hôpitaux et hospices civils de Paris: centenaire de l'internat, 1802–1902* (1903), p. ix.

4. See, for instance, Jean Quénu, *Notre internat* (1971), and Alexandre Guéniot, *Souvenirs anecdotiques et médicaux, 1856–1871* (1927).

5. Jacques Fossard, *Histoire polymorphe de l'internat en médecine et chirurgie des hôpitaux et hospices civils de Paris*, 2 vols. (Grenoble, 1982), vol. 1, p. 9. For an illuminating study of this institution, see Leonard C. Groopman, "The *Internat des Hôpitaux de Paris*: The Shaping and Transformation of the French Medical Elite, 1802–1914," Ph.D. diss., Harvard University, 1986.

6. Ambitious but marginal physicians courted interns socially, invited them to observe experiments, or came by to teach them instrumental techniques they had developed. For examples, see Guéniot, *Souvenirs*, pp. 103, 124–28.

7. Quénu, *Notre internat*; Paul Le Gendre, *Du Quartier Latin à l'Académie (reminiscences)* (1930).

8. Less than 10 percent of the doctors and pharmacists in the population of 1821 had been interns.

9. The proportion of academicians with degrees in pharmacy ranged from a high of 14 percent in 1821 to a low of 11 percent in 1901.

10. On scientific pharmacy in the nineteenth century see Alex Berman, "Conflict and Anomaly in the Scientific Orientation of French Pharmacy, 1800–1873," *Bulletin of the History of Medicine* 37 (1963), 440–62.

11. The proportion of hospital staff without teaching or research appointments declined from 28 percent in the population of 1901 to 2 percent in that of 1935.

12. Among academicians in 1861, some 23 percent of faculty professors had never been *agrégés*; among those of 1901, the figure was 0 percent, and among those of 1935 it was 7 percent.

13. Henri Roger, *Entre deux siècles: souvenirs d'un vieux biologiste* (1947), p. 134.

14. Charles Achard, *La Confession d'un vieil homme du siècle: souvenirs du temps et de l'espace* (1943), p. 56.

15. This issue is discussed in George Weisz, "Reform and Conflict in French Medical Education, 1870–1914," in *The Organization of Science and Technology in France, 1808–1914*, ed. Robert Fox and George Weisz (Cambridge, 1980).

16. Achard, *La Confession*, p. 57.

17. See, for example, G. Debove, "Éloge de J.-M. Charcot," *MEM* 39 (1900), pp. 12–14, and especially Paul Le Gendre, *Un médecin philosophe: Charles Bouchard, son oeuvre et son temps (1837–1915)* (1924), pp. 42–45. Gratitude to patrons for such help became commonplace in the autobiographies that academicians began writing in the twentieth century. See, for example, Antonin Gosset, *Chirurgie, chirurgiens* (1941), pp. 156–58.

18. On the research ideal and its effects on medical faculties see George Weisz, *The Emergence of Modern Universities in France, 1863–1914* (Princeton, N.J., 1983), chap. 5.

19. For an amusing description of this process, see Roger, *Entre deux siècles*, pp. 155–75.

20. On the prizes of the Academy of Sciences see Maurice Crosland and Antonio Gálvez, "The Emergence of Research Grants within the Prize System of the Academy of Sciences, 1795–1914," *Social Studies of Science* 19 (1989), 71–100.

21. Among the academicians of 1861, six are known for certain to have failed in attempts to obtain a faculty chair. There were undoubtedly others.

22. The surgeon Velpeau was appointed on his fifth attempt at a chair while the physician Piorry was appointed on his sixth.

23. When he was seventy-nine, Bouchardat once mischievously told Proust that his career was coming to an end. He then dampened Proust's excitement by explaining that he knew he was getting old since for the last several months he had been forced to pay women to have sex with him. Roger, *Entre deux siècles*, pp. 157–58.

24. Veterinarian-academicians consistently obtained their professional diplomas in their very early twenties. They were at graduation from five to six years younger than graduating doctors and pharmacists.

25. Roger, *Entre deux siècles*, p. 241. The veterinary schools did not have the status of faculties and thus could not formally grant doctorates.

26. Of the remaining seven, three men were at the faculty, two at the School of Pharmacy, and two more at Val-de-Grâce.

27. In 1875 the editor of one medical journal, commenting on the recent decision of Wurtz to step down as dean of the medical faculty, suggested that the task had become so onerous that it either needed to be divided among several different people or should become a full-time job commanding a far higher salary. *Note sur le décanat des facultés de médecine. Extrait de la Gazette médicale de Paris* (1875).

28. For an account of how one individual was elected dean see Roger, *Entre deux siècles*, pp. 183–84.

29. The venereologist Philippe Ricord became a full member in 1850, fourteen years after his appointment as correspondent; the veterinarian Auguste Chauveau was appointed correspondent in 1864, national associate in 1876, and full member in 1891.

30. While the general trend applies to all academicians, members of the veterinary and basic science sections tended to be elected at a somewhat earlier age than other academicians, suggesting that competition was somewhat less intense in these areas.

31. Achard, *La Confession*, p. 79.

32. On "visits" see Maurice Crosland, *Science under Control: The French Academy of Sciences, 1795–1914* (Cambridge, 1992), pp. 221–24.

33. The section of medicine and surgery had the highest average age at entry among all sections of the AS in 1821, and the second highest in 1861, 1901, and 1935. Calculated from *Index biographique des membres et correspondants de l'Académie des Sciences* (1968).

34. There was, however, a decline in the number of academicians in the nonmedical sections of the AS; eight in 1861, seven in 1901, and five in 1935 (with four of these in the section of chemistry).

35. Members of the AS also resented the large amounts of money which the medical section controlled as a result of the Montyon legacy of the 1820s.

36. A. Latour, "Une révolution à l'Académie des Sciences," *Union médicale*, 3e sér. 13 (1872), 823–24.

37. Ibid., 825–29.

38. Crosland, *Science under Control*, p. 165.

39. Ibid., p. 121.

40. These are mentioned in the listing for each academician in *Index biographique des membres de l'Academie des Sciences*.

41. In a single *éloge* devoted to Hallé, Corvisart, and Pinel presented in 1827, Cuvier discussed the difficulty of evaluating medical men and stated explicitly that the presentation of *éloges* in the Academy of Medicine allowed his own tributes to these three men to be brief. Georges Cuvier, *Recueil des éloges historiques lus dans les séances publiques de l'Institut Royale de France*, 3 vols. (Strasbourg, 1819–27), vol. 3, p. 343. He presented no more *éloges* of medical men after that date.

42. Weisz, "Reform and Conflict"; Jean-François Picard, "Poussée scientifique ou demande de médecins? La recherche médicale en France de l'Institut national d'hygiène à l'INSERM," *Science Sociales et Santé* 10 (1992), 47–106.

43. For an illuminating examination of the rise of this reformist generation and its take-over of the Faculty of Medicine and the academy, see Bernard Brais, "The Making of a Famous Nineteenth-Century Neurologist: Jean-Martin Charcot," M. Phil. thesis, University College London, 1990.

11

The Medical Elite in French Society

In this chapter we shall attempt to situate the Parisian medical elite within larger social structures of family and class. The task is considerably more difficult than charting careers because social categories lack the concreteness of dates of a successful *concours* or appointment, and relevant data are more difficult to obtain. Before undertaking any analysis, moreover, we must first establish reliable indicators of social position and useful categories of social differentiation. We will consider a number of social characteristics about which (1) it is possible to find usable information and (2) there is a tradition of research that makes comparison possible.

One of our underlying questions, though by no means the only one, has to do with the relationship between changing social indicators and the evolving career structures described in the previous chapter. In a number of cases, data are sufficiently rich to justify strong arguments for links between the two domains. In most situations, however, our data permit only speculative suggestions.

Geographical Origins

Members of the academy were predominantly born in France. Only 3 percent of the four hundred or so academicians in our sample were born outside the national borders. Most came from neighboring European countries like Switzerland (three members) or the Netherlands (two); two other academicians were born in France's overseas colonies. The religious affiliation of families is not ordinarily included on public documents, but the vast majority of academicians seem to have been of Catholic origin. Only 4 percent have been identified as belonging however tenuously to a non-Catholic religious group. Half of these were Protestants and another half were of Jewish extraction. A Protestant (Pierre Boullay) was appointed to the academy in 1820, whereas the first Jew in our sample, Michel Lévy, was appointed in 1850. Thirteen of sixteen academicians of Protestant or Jewish origin were appointed

257

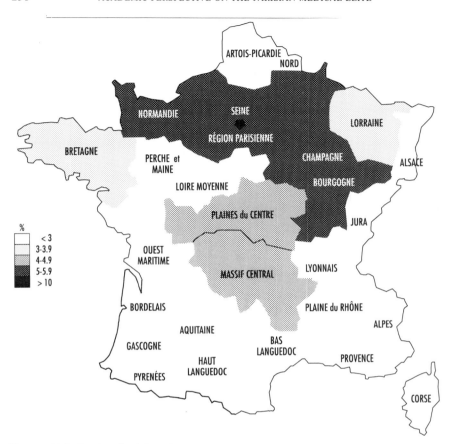

FIGURE 11.1. Regional origins of members of the Academy of Medicine (1820, 1861, 1901, 1935, combined).

during the Third Republic, as was one lone Greek of the Orthodox faith (Photinos Panas). Members of minority religious groups made up over 9 percent of the membership in 1901 and 5 percent in 1935.

The proportion of academicians born in Paris increased from 22 percent in 1821 to 33 percent in 1935.[1] Academicians born outside the capital were likely to be from neighboring regions: the Paris basin, Champagne, Normandy, and Burgundy and, at the outer limit, the Center Plain and the Massif Central. Together with the capital, these regions accounted for 62 percent of the academicians in our four samples combined.[2] Southern regions like Languedoc and Aquitaine, which had produced quite a few academicians earlier in the century, were no longer doing so by the end. Though most regions supplied at least some academicians, a few consistently did not: Corsica, Gascony, and, more surprisingly, the Rhone Plain, Lower Languedoc, and the Nord region.[3]

TABLE 11.1   Geographical Origins of Academicians, by percent

	1821	1861	1901	1935
Paris	22	30	29	33
Large cities	22	9	6	12
Chef-lieu	15	13	19	16
Rural	37	45	43	34
Unknown or born abroad	4	2	3	4
Number	110	97	98	93

Geographical proximity to Paris clearly played a key role in recruitment to the academy. But the cases of the Nord and the Lyonnais, both relatively close to Paris but producing few academicians suggest that the existence or lack of alternatives was also significant, for the regions of heavy recruitment to the academy do not include the biggest French cities, Lyon, Marseilles, Bordeaux, and Lille. In fact, the proportion of academicians born in large cities other than Paris declined fairly significantly during the nineteenth century (see Table 11.1).

The most plausible explanation has to do with a growing abundance of local elite medical careers in the large cities. Here hospitals, secondary schools of medicine, and, after 1870, new medical faculties offered ambitious young men relatively more certain opportunities for medical success than did the highly competitive careers of the capital where family and social connections often did not reach. The lack of such alternatives probably explains the relative stability of recruitment of academicians from smaller administrative cities (*chef-lieu de département*), small towns, and rural areas. Those born here had little choice but to migrate if they aspired to an elite medical career.[4] That something like this process of discrimination took place during medical studies is suggested by the regional origins of Parisian interns, strongly resembling those of our academicians.[5] Paris together with the six regions that produced large numbers of academicians also produced nearly 60 percent of the interns during the last decades of the nineteenth century.

Aside from proximity and lack of alternatives, regional traditions may also have been at work. For a number of individuals from a region to have "made it" in Parisian medicine would have certainly been a source of pride for the region and a career model for the most ambitious students. Such compatriots might also become important contacts and patrons. A common theme in academic eulogies of the early nineteenth century is that of the friendless medical student from the provinces who comes to Paris with nothing but a letter addressed to a professor or hospital physician originally from the same region.[6]

Social Backgrounds

The social backgrounds of academicians, as measured by fathers' occupations,[7] remained fairly stable and within a relatively narrow social range over the century being discussed (see Table 11.2). From 40 to 50 percent had fathers in liberal or intellectual occupations (including middle-level civil servants), a group making up less than 1 percent of the total French population in the 1870s. Less than 20 percent of the fathers were members of the wealthier propertied classes or the high-level administrative castes; and these were usually in the more modest strata of these categories and tended to live outside the Paris region. The sons of great landowners, bankers, industrialists, and the highest ranking civil servants are notable for their absence. Although there were few academicians from the working class per se, the modest sectors of the bourgeoisie and small agriculture were well represented. Overall, the backgrounds of academicians appear modest in comparison with those of most other Parisian elites; only professors in the faculties of science and letters came from more humble backgrounds.[8]

Looking more carefully at the chronological evolution of our populations, we see a number of small shifts. The most striking one had to do with a decline in the proportion of sons of doctors. Secondarily, there was a smaller decline in the representation of the offspring of the propertied classes that was largely compensated by increased recruitment among the sons of the educated professions. Sons of the popular classes increased their place in the academy between 1821 and 1861, with stabilization occurring thereafter, while the place of small business remained stable.

Sons of doctors, pharmacists, and veterinarians made up more than a third of the membership in 1821, but this was largely due to the older academicians who, in conformity with a pattern characteristic of the *ancien régime,* followed their fathers into the profession.[9] This pattern was somewhat less evident in our three later populations. Sons of medical practitioners were slightly less numerous in 1935 than children of the popular classes and offspring of the other educated professions. Fathers, of course, are not the only source of family medical traditions. But even if we include grandfathers and uncles in our definition of medical origins, the pattern of decline of medical origins remains substantially unchanged, though the rhythm is somewhat altered.[10]

TABLE 11.2   Professions of Academicians' Fathers, by percent

Father	1821	1861	1901	1935
Propertied classes[a]	19	23	16	14
Medicine[b]	35	28	28	22
Medical elite as % of Medicine[c]	12	43	28	16
Educated occupations[d]	17	14	21	25
Small business[e]	13	11	12	15
Popular classes[f]	17	24	23	24
Number	96	83	90	87

[a] *Proprietaires, rentiers,* high civil servants, magistrates, state engineering corps.

[b] Doctors, pharmacists, veterinarians, professors of medicine.

[c] Includes Parisian professors of medicine, pharmacy, or veterinary medicine; members of Academy of Medicine; medical staff of Parisian hospitals; *agrégés.*

[d] Legal professions, professors of secondary and higher education, artistic and intellectual professions, middle-level civil servants.

[e] *Marchands, commerçants,* innkeepers.

[f] Artisans, *employés,* farmers, domestics, workers, low-level legal workers, primary teachers, *petits fonctionnaires.*

If the place of medical families in the academy declined, familial medical credentials became more impressive. Most of the fathers in 1821 were modest medical practitioners. Only 12 percent of the medical fathers were members of the Parisian elite.[11] Of the fathers of members in 1861, no less than 43 percent of the medical professionals belonged to the Parisian elite, suggesting that being born into the elite sectors of medicine provided young men with the professional models and personal connections useful for career success. Such self-recruitment from within the medical elite declined, however, in the late nineteenth and early twentieth centuries. In the sample of 1901, the proportion of medical fathers who were in the medical elite was down to a still substantial 28 percent; by that of 1935, it had fallen to only 16 percent. Furthermore, the proportion of Parisians among all medical fathers, which was approximately 50 percent in the first three populations—and which would seem to confirm the significance of direct links to the medical elite for earlier academicians—declined to 22 percent in that of 1935. This suggests that direct family ties were somewhat less pertinent in the twentieth century than they had been in the nineteenth. One would imagine that the system of *concours* was at least partly responsible for this state of affairs.

There is ample evidence to suggest that *concours* did not do away with subjectivity and favoritism in recruitment, although they probably did eliminate the truly incompetent. But public competitions do seem to have neutralized to some extent the advantages of those born into the medical elite by giving outsiders an opportunity to become known to potential patrons. Put another way, in an essentially personal system of elite reproduction, the problem for aspirants was to come to the attention of those with power, something that was impossible in the overcrowded lecture halls of the Paris Faculty of Medicine. In the late eighteenth and early nineteenth century, contexts in which to gain recognition and support were not numerous. Pinel was discovered by Thouret, future dean of the Paris Faculty of Medicine, when he submitted a manuscript for one of the prize competitions of the Société Royale de Médecine. Nicholas Vauquelin was a lodger in the home of the pharmacist René Cheradame, where he was discovered by Fourcroy, who was a frequent visitor to the household. By the 1820s it was common for students to accompany hospital physicians on their rounds. But getting noticed in the crowd was more difficult. Sons and other relatives of elite physicians had the great advantage of being already known.[12]

The *internat* solved this problem to some extent because successful candidates spent four years in very close proximity to a number of different mentors. (Ordinarily one changed wards at least once each year.) By the time they were ready for the postgraduate *concours*, they were well known to several different patrons. Consequently, family connections became less pertinent than ties established between master and protégé.

Nonetheless, family connections could still be useful. Judgments in *concours* were notoriously subjective and might be influenced by personal factors. Furthermore, as competition for internship posts with the best or most appropriate patrons intensified, students had to make contact quite early in their studies while they were externs or clinical volunteers. (The decision to take on an intern was made exclusively by the chief of service.) A well-placed word from an influential relative could thus prove extremely useful.[13]

Parallel to the decreasing role of medical families was increased representation for the sons of the educated and liberal professions. This is hardly surprising in light of the growing dominance of *concours*. Members of this category were especially likely to have a family history of cultivating the intellectual skills necessary for success in *concours*. Since these occupations had a socioeconomic status relatively close to that of medicine, it is also likely that ambitious children were able to find models of successful medical careers close at hand. It is not clear whether the twentieth-century decline in the proportion of individuals from the propertied classes reflects the relative lack of cultural models among these social groups or the fact that less difficult routes to economic success were available to the sons of the wealthy.

The small rise in the representation of the popular classes in the academy that took place in the first half of the nineteenth century was maintained in subsequent populations but without further increases. Members from modest social backgrounds seldom came from the most deprived sector of society. In both the nineteenth and twentieth centuries, they were likely to be the sons of skilled artisans (whose workshops were sometimes difficult to distinguish from small factories). By the twentieth century one finds significant numbers of white-collar employees and small farmers among the fathers. The vast majority of academicians in this category were not raised in Paris but in provincial towns and villages. Overall there seems to have been some justification for the medical elite's image of itself as a group of self-made men. But one also sees little sign of that relative democratization of recruitment that seems to have occurred in other elite sectors during the early decades of the Third Republic.[14] One explanation may have to do with our decision to categorize shopkeepers in the small-business group. If we combine the popular and small-business groups, we do in fact see a very small rise in their combined representation in the twentieth century.

However one counts them, the largest increase in the representation of the popular classes occurred in the population of 1861, the first with large numbers of individuals who had gone through *concours* for internships and the *agrégation*. While not precluding patronage and nepotism, the system of *concours* favored objective skills of memory and rhetoric, which benefited the clever student, whatever his social background. We can test this hypothesis to some extent by comparing academicians who had been interns with those who had not in the population of 1861 (see Table 11.3). This was the last group of academicians for whom the *internat* was not indispensable for elite careers. A number of striking differences are apparent.

TABLE 11.3   Professions of Fathers of Academician Interns and Noninterns in 1861, by percent

Father	Interns	Non-interns	1821
Propertied	23	23	19
Medicine	20	35	35
Medical elite as % of medicine	13	40	12
Educated	23	7	17
Small business	5	16	13
Popular	30	19	17
Number	40	43	96

Among interns, the number with fathers in medicine is quite low while the proportion from modest backgrounds is rather high. The opposite is true of noninterns, whose social profile resembles that of the entire population of academicians in 1820–21. Interns were also more likely to come from one of the other educated professions and less likely to come from the small-business sector.

These figures suggest that the competition for the *internat* worked in the short run to alter recruitment patterns to the medical elite. They seemed to benefit particularly those from modest backgrounds or from families with members in the educated professions. It is likely that at this transitional stage, ambitious young men from medical families had less need to become interns because they continued to have other avenues to medical success. Of the sixteen academicians who were sons of medical men but who did not pass through the *internat*, six or nearly 40 percent, were sons of members of the medical elite. Three others (20 percent) married the daughters of men in the medical elite. In contrast, only one of eight interns from medical families was the son (and son-in-law) of a member of the Parisian medical elite. Alternative paths to the medical elite, however, were in the process of being closed. By 1901 the vast majority of academicians in civilian clinical medicine and pharmacy had passed through the *internat* as well as through a variety of other posts and *concours*. This may partly account for the decline in the proportion of sons of the medical elite among academicians in our later populations.

Our population is too small to compare different specialty groups, but we can say a few things about the major groups of medical professionals, doctors, surgeons, and pharmacists.[15] In the first half of the nineteenth century there were no dramatic differences among these groups but all reflected the corporate traditions of the ancien régime. The privileged classes were best represented in the medical section. Surgeons frequently came from families in the artisan crafts while pharmacists were particularly drawn from small commerce.

In the twentieth century pharmacy became a haven for more modest social groups. Nearly half the academician pharmacists came from fairly humble backgrounds and there was a striking absence of fathers in the liberal and educated professions. Few academic surgeons, on the other hand, were from modest origins; both the popular and small business classes were conspicuous by their absence.[16] Surgery was also the specialty of choice for the sons of medical families. Among academicians in this latter category, the proportion of those in surgery rose from 34 percent (1821 and 1861 combined) to 46 percent (1901 and 1935 combined). This suggests a significant improvement in the twentieth century in the professional status of elite surgical careers, a hypothesis that will be confirmed in our discussion of the wealth of academicians.

A comparison of the social origins of professors at the Paris Faculty of Medicine with those of other academicians helps us better understand the social conditions useful for achieving success in French medicine (see Table 11.4). In 1821 professors in the academy were considerably more likely than other academicians to come from the propertied and high civil service classes. The overrepresentation is due to a relatively large number of sons of magistrates, which probably reflected the social disruptions of the revolutionary period. The disappearance of this group in later populations meant that the representation of privileged groups was pretty much the same among professors and other academicians.

Table 11.4   Profession of Fathers of Faculty Professors and Other
Academicians, by percent

Father	1821		1861		1901		1935	
	FM	NonFM	FM	NonFM	FM	NonFM	FM	NonFM
Propertied	35	10	22	23	16	13	18	13
Medicine	24	42	22	30	24	29	20	23
Medical elite as %								
of medicine	13	15	0	29	53	25	25	9
Educated	18	16	26	9	26	22	38	15
Small business	3	15	0	13	9	3	15	13
Popular	21	18	30	25	26	24	10	36
Number	34	62	27	56	35	53	40	46

Key: FM=Faculty of Medicine professors.

In 1821 there was also a significant difference in the proportion of sons of doctors, with nearly twice as many among nonprofessors as among members of the Paris faculty. The simplest explanation is that being from a medical family was an important advantage in entering the medical elite at the beginning of the nineteenth century but this advantage did not extend to the top rungs of the hierarchy, where other types of advantage—brilliance, acquaintances, and family members among the professors of the faculty—assumed greater importance. This discrepancy between professors and other academicians disappeared gradually as the proportion of the latter group from medical families declined. Similarly, small business in 1821 and 1861 was less well represented among professors than among other academicians, with differences disappearing in the later populations.

However, one important difference between professors and nonprofessors persisted. In the population of 1861, nonprofessors were more likely than professors to have fathers in the medical elite, supporting the view that the introduction of *concours,* initially favored outsiders to the medical elite. In the twentieth century, however, the situation was reversed. Those academicians from medical families appointed to the Faculty of Medicine were considerably more likely than other academicians with medical roots to have had a father in the Parisian medical elite. Two other differences between these groups emerged at different times (Table 11.4).

From the 1861 sample on, a larger number of faculty professors had fathers in the educated and liberal professions. This would seem to be connected with the system of *concours* which assumed importance at roughly the same time. Groups with traditions of education and culture would have had an important advantage in confronting successfully the system of examinations stressing memory, rhetorical skills, and quickness of response. More complex is the situation of the popular classes. In our first three chronological groups, these were slightly better represented among professors than among other academicians. The increasing importance of *concours* was clearly not a disadvantage for members of this category, who were unlikely to have prior personal contacts within the medical elite. But in a major reversal, the representation of the popular classes among professors in 1935 declined to less than half that of other academicians. Taken together with the higher proportion of fathers in the medical elite among professors, this shift suggests that the

TABLE 11.5   Professions of Fathers of Professors of Medicine,
Professors of Science, and Medical Practitioners, 1935, by percent

Father	AM FM	AM SC	NonAM MDs
Propertied	18	10	24
Medicine	20	15	18
Medical elite as % of medicine	25	9	3
Educated	38	20	20
Small business	15	25	12
Popular	10	30	26
Number	40	20	164

Key: AM=academician; FM=Faculty of Medicine professors; SC=Institutions of Science professors; MDs=doctors.

Faculty of Medicine in the twentieth century recruited from relatively more privileged and better educated social strata than other medical institutions or than it had in the past.

One plausible explanation for this reversal is that the sacrifices required for faculty careers in the twentieth century had reached the point where they either discouraged or defeated many young men with only modest cultural resources. Elite medical careers were becoming most attractive and most accessible to those with family educational traditions and sufficient financial means to get through the long and grueling period of apprenticeship.[17]

This interpretation is supported and refined by comparing, within the 1935 sample, professors at the medical faculty with those in the institutions of science and research, whose careers depended more on records of publication than on the system of *concours*. The latter were less likely to be of propertied, medical, or educated origins than the former (see Table 11.5). Few, in fact, had fathers in the medical elite. Conversely, they were more likely to be from the small-business or popular class. It is difficult to escape the conclusion that the system of medical *concours* in the twentieth century discouraged those without family capital or educational traditions from more traditional elite careers centered in the Faculty of Medicine. This is largely confirmed by an examination of a random sample of 164 Parisian doctors who were never elected to the academy but who were at an advanced stage of their career in 1935 (Table 11.5).[18] While the proportion of fathers in the propertied classes is slightly larger for these doctors than for professors, the proportion with popular family origins is considerably greater while the percentage from the educated and professional classes is a good deal smaller. Although the proportion from medical families is similar for nonacademicians and academician-professors, few of the former are from the medical elite.

Marriage

The social resources provided by family background could be substantially increased by the judicious choice of a marriage partner. Most academicians eventually married. Our figures on this point are incomplete but the proportion of those known for certain

TABLE 11.6   Age of Academicians at Marriage

	1821	1861	1901	1935
Academicians				
Number known	39	51	57	53
Median age	32	30	33	33
% over 40	26	10	19	23
Academicians–Faculty of Medicine				
Number known	22	20	23	23
Median age	31	31.5	35	33
% over 40	23	10	26	24
Academicians–institutions of science				
Number known	NS	NS	12	12
Median age	NS	NS	29.5	32.5
% over 40	NS	NS	17	17

NS=not significant.

never to have married declined from 13 percent in the samples of 1821 and 1861 to 7 percent and 4 percent in those of 1901 and 1935. To some extent the decline in the number of lifelong bachelors meant only that men who might have chosen early in the nineteenth century not to marry were, later in the century, likely to marry at a fairly advanced age (see Table 11.6).[19]

In the sample of 1821 marriage age was extremely variable, reflecting perhaps the social dislocations of the late eighteenth century. Marriage age stabilized at a relatively youthful level among the younger academicians of 1821 and all those of 1861. But among the academicians of 1901 the median age at marriage rose by three years and stayed at that level among the academicians of 1935. The proportion of men who married after the age of forty also rose sharply from the 1861 sample to the ones that followed. General societal pressures certainly delayed marriage among many privileged groups in the second half of the nineteenth century. Christophe Charle suggests that deferred marriage was especially characteristic of upwardly mobile men from the more modest classes of society. This description would certainly characterize many academicians in 1901. But mobility alone cannot explain the fact that academicians seem to have delayed marriage even longer than other elites of the period.[20] One must look, therefore, to the changing nature of elite careers to account for increasingly deferred marriage.

The fact that academicians of 1901 both graduated from medical school and obtained their first hospital post about two years later on average than their predecessors would likely have meant that they took longer to attain the professional status that enabled them to marry. One indication that this was indeed the case is provided by academicians who were professors at the Paris Faculty of Medicine and who therefore experienced these pressures with special force. Professors in the 1821 sample were slightly younger when they married than other academicians. If the discrepancy means anything at all, it is that future professors had somewhat earlier career successes that encouraged them to marry.[21] In the 1861 population professors generally married slightly later than academicians generally (1.5 years) and the discrepancy became greater in the population of 1901 (2 years). Among academicians in 1935, however, professors no longer delayed marriage longer than other academicians.

What seems to have been occurring in the second half of the nineteenth century was that future professors were investing so heavily in their careers that they were putting off marriage longer than other academicians. In fact, over one-quarter of those professors in the 1901 sample who married waited until after their fortieth birthday. In the population of 1935 professors and other academicians were indistinguishable in this respect. Everyone seems to have adjusted in a similar way to the by-now well-established career structure. As we shall see, this adjustment may have had something to do with the social circles into which academicians married.

That professors at the Faculty of Medicine experienced exceptional strains in their personal lives is confirmed by examination of a group that was only partially subject to the demands of the system of *concours*: professors in the institutions of scientific and medical research. In the sample of 1901 professors or their equivalents in these institutions were about three years younger when they married than academicians generally and five to six years younger than professors in the Faculty of Medicine. In the population of 1935 the gap had almost disappeared, probably because professors in scientific institutions were no longer being appointed to posts at a significantly younger age than professors at the medical faculty.

Fathers-in-law

Into what sorts of social milieu did academicians marry?[22] Moving from the population of 1821 through to that of 1901, we see some consistent patterns (see Table 11.7). Between the populations of 1821 and 1861 there was a decline in the incidence of marriage to the daughters of doctors. There no change in this respect between 1861 and 1901 but we do see a drop in the proportion of men who married into the medical elite. Clearly, during this period the medical elite was becoming less inward-looking and seemingly more closely associated with other privileged social groups. This tendency, however, was reversed in our last sample when marriage within the medical milieu, and the elite medical milieu in particular, became common once again.

TABLE 11.7 Professions of Fathers-in-Law of Academicians, by percent

Father-in-Law	1821	1861	1901	1935
Propertied classes	30	49	48	21
Medicine	40	28	28	38
Medical elite as % of medicine	42	45	27	69
Educated occupations	17	18	25	24
Small business	7	5	0	6
Popular classes	7	0	0	12
Number	30	39	40	34

At the beginning of the nineteenth century, marriage to daughters of the medical elite was commonplace among academicians, and particularly future professors at the Paris Faculty of Medicine. Among professors in the 1821 sample whose fathers-in-law are known to us, one can cite Baron René Desgenettes, who married the daughter of Jean Colombier, inspector of Parisian hospitals in the late eighteenth century, and thus became the brother-in-law of Thouret, the first dean of the postrevolutionary Faculty of Medicine. Women relatives could consecrate professional ties in other ways that do not show up in our figures. The bachelor Vauquelin had as his house-keeper the sister of his collaborator and patron, Fourcroy.

There was nothing unusual about such endogamous patterns; they were character-istic of many social groups of the period.[23] The world of elite medicine was one of intense social relations. Education was dominated by a form of apprenticeship and the ties binding master to those he trained were strong. As members of a relatively new elite, moreover, many leading doctors probably had limited social contact with the privileged classes of society even when they provided them with medical care. Conse-quently, marriage within the medical milieu reflected real affinities that were a product of the closed, guildlike character of French medicine. Scattered data suggest that academicians from medical families were more likely than other academicians to marry into medical families (50 percent vs. 34 percent) and into the medical elite (44 percent vs. 30 percent). There was certainly an element of career self-interest mixed in as well. An ambitious young man could not have been unaware of the advantages of having a well-placed father-in-law. And established medical figures could select their brightest students as sons-in-law and groom them to be institutional allies and pro-fessional successors. Sons, in contrast, did not always possess the requisite qualities for success in elite medicine.[24] Family relations could operate so powerfully because, we saw, the system of *concours* did not yet govern recruitment to the medical elite.

The growing prevalence of *concours* did not do away with patronage or personal influence. The relationship between master and student remained as strong as ever but patronage ties became increasingly disassociated from marital links. Among academicians of 1861 the incidence of marriage to the daughters of members of the medical elite was still high (Table 11.7). However, the incidence among professors at the Faculty of Medicine was greatly reduced. And in the sample of 1901 there were relatively few marital ties of this sort for anyone.

In addition to the impact of *concours*, changing marital strategies reflected the increasing integration of the medical elite with the educated and even privileged seg-ments of society. In both 1861 and 1901 nearly half the academicians for whom we have such information had married the daughters of men from the propertied classes.[25] These unions, however, were rarely contracted with the offspring of the great families of industry and finance. It was rather those slightly at the margins of great wealth who seemed most attracted to the medical elite.[26] Daughters of the edu-cated professional classes also seem to have received increased marital attention from aspiring members of the medical elite. As one would expect, few future academicians were attracted to poor girls; the daughters of the popular classes were totally absent from the samples of 1861 and 1901.

It would seem as if the spreading system of *concours* made familial patronage within the medical elite less important to aspiring candidates. On the other hand, years of preparation for *concours* in poorly paid junior positions created a need for the economic security that marriage into the propertied classes could provide. Our data suggest that the status of the medical elite had risen enough so that marriage to a potential medical star was attractive to prosperous families outside the medical milieu. Furthermore, there now seems to have been sufficient social contact between ambitious young doctors and the more privileged classes of society to enable meeting and courting to occur. Sometime such contacts took place in the home of the patron.[27] The rising age of marriage for the academicians of 1901 also had a role to play since well-established elite doctors would have likely been more attractive to prospective bourgeois families than, those just starting out.

Certainly the medical elite was reflecting wider social trends. High-level civil servants of the turn of the century were also less likely to marry within the civil service and more likely to marry into the propertied classes than their predecessors of an earlier generation. Even those in business married increasingly outside their own social sphere.[28] A new national elite was emerging in the second half of the nineteenth century in which boundaries between different occupational spheres seem to have been more fluid. The medical elite, however, benefited especially from the new social openness. The academicians of 1901 show a considerably higher propensity to marry into the propertied classes than say, professors in most nonmedical institutions of higher education.

However one interprets these data, a major change seems to have occurred among the academicians of 1935. The proportion of marriages into the propertied classes declined sharply while marriage within the medical milieu returned to the levels of the early nineteenth century. Instances of marriage into the medical elite reached a new high. Most surprisingly, academicians were once again marrying into the popular and small-business classes. The professors of medicine about whom we possess information showed pretty much the same marital proclivities as other academicians, but they gravitated particularly toward the educated and liberal professions. These social patterns may well explain the tendency of the professor-academicians of 1935 to marry at a younger age than their immediate predecessors. Not aiming so high in the social hierarchy meant that less in the way of achieved professional accomplishments was demanded of prospective husbands. Medical families in particular would have been sensitive to early indicators of future medical success.

There are a number of possible explanations for this shift away from bourgeois marriage. One possibility is that family patronage once again became increasingly important as a marginal advantage in the increasingly competitive struggle to succeed. A more likely possibility is that the rising social status of medicine made it possible to find economic security in a medical marriage. Two other explanations, however, fit the data particularly well.

First, marriage for "love" almost certainly played an increasingly important role in marital decisions. This would explain the reappearance in small numbers of women of popular-class origins among the wives of academicians. If this was indeed the case, one would expect a growing tendency toward medical marriages since cultural affinities and common interests necessary to affective relations would be more likely if wives had some experience with the intense professional lifestyle (not to say workaholism) characteristic of the milieu. It is significant that several academicians of 1935 married pioneering women doctors, a surprising choice if social status was the primary consideration. A good example is the pediatrician Robert Debré, whose marriage is not classified as medical in our statistics because his father-in-law was not a doctor. Debré seems at first glance to have been an exemplary worldly physician, with an unusually wide circle of friends and acquaintances, including Charles Péguy and Paul Valéry. He married the daughter of a well-known artist who was herself a doctor and actually went through the *externat* and *internat* with her husband.[29]

Second, it may be that as more and more in the way of professional achievement was expected of future academicians—*concours*, publication, competition for academic prizes—there occurred a retreat from the larger social world as the medical elite became more insulated and inward-looking.[30] Later in this chapter we shall come across other indicators that tend to confirm this hypothesis.

We can personalize many of the themes raised in this discussion by turning to the autobiographical writing of Charles Achard,[31] permanent secretary of the academy from 1921 to 1944. Achard followed the by-now classic trajectory of *internat* (which he combined with laboratory work) and junior positions under the patronage of another future permanent secretary of the academy, Georges Debove. Throughout these apprenticeship years, Achard was supported financially by his parents. But soon after his nomination as a Paris hospital physician in 1893 (after four unsuccessful *concours*), a financial disaster struck his family and forced him to support his parents. He began a private medical practice with the aid of patrons who sent him patients. He also assumed a number of paid medical posts, becoming a physician of the customs administration, head of Odilon Lannelongue's laboratory at the Faculty of Medicine, and director of a weekly medical journal.

He managed through all this to find time for research (at the expense of "leisure," he tells us) but his continued progress through the medical hierarchy was clearly now at risk. It was proposed to him on several occasions that he marry an heiress so that he might devote himself exclusively to the research that would lead to a professorship. But he declined, he tells us, because he felt that instead of freeing him from practice such a marriage might bring in a society clientele that would eventually overwhelm his real work. Achard then goes on to express a much more profound unease at the idea of marrying into the "bourgeoisie."

In that epoch (the last two decades of the nineteenth century), he tells us, it was necessary to observe certain rites to marry into the bourgeoisie. Ordinarily a family friend or acquaintance, often a "veritable marriage specialist," initiated contact between two families. A first contact might be arranged at a ball or *soirée mondaine* where the young man might ask the young woman to dance. If things worked out, the families soon became involved. "The external appearance and education of the girl was balanced against the social situation and prospects of the future husband."[32] This led to a series of rituals—bewildering to Achard—including the daily sending of flowers by the husband-to-be to his future bride. "The astonishing thing is that there were young men willing to confront the series of such tests of protocol. It is true that one married less and less within the bourgeoisie."[33]

It is probable that Achard was uniquely unsuited for marriage. He did not marry until he was nearly sixty and his wife died six months after the wedding. But his account, whether it is ethnographically accurate or not, expresses the distance between the world of medical *concours* and the impossibly foreign and exotic world of high society. It would not be surprising if the same sense of strangeness kept more typical young academicians within the social confines of medicine.

We are in a position to further analyze the families into which academicians married through the funds which brides brought into the marriage.[34] These for the most part confirm the results of our examination of the professions of fathers-in-law. Like the latter data, information on the bride's wealth suggests that the late nineteenth century represented a period of unique social openness and wealth for the medical elite.

By and large, academicians improved their economic situation when they married. Although we have data about the money which academicians brought into their marriages (the *apport*) for only a small proportion of academicians, it is suggestive. The amount which academicians brought into the marriage was quite low for those in 1861 (median, 13,900 francs.) The median wealth of young husbands doubled (to 28,943 francs) in the 1901 sample, undoubtedly reflecting the trend to later marriage. Median wealth declined very slightly (to 27,000 francs) in the population of 1935. A point worth making about the *apports* of academicians is that few of our subjects were rich when they married. Only one brought more than 500,000 francs into his marriage.

The median wealth of academicians' brides at marriage was three times as great as the median wealth of the husband in all three of the samples for which we have information. (This ratio was also pretty much the norm for all the late-nineteenth-century elites examined by Charle.) However, the academicians of 1901 married far wealthier women; the median sum brought in by wives was double that for 1861. Nearly half of all wives delivered more than 100,000 francs to the marriage; one brought the princessly sum of over 3 million francs.[35] This was one of the rewards of later marriages and greater social openness. Among the academicians of 1935, the median wealth of wives declined by nearly 13,000 francs. This was the price paid for earlier marriage among professors and the tendency to remain within medicine and the liberal professions. But this decline should not obscure the fact that academicians of the twentieth century could remain within their own narrow social sphere because they were themselves relatively comfortable when they married.

The Next Generation

Information in Table 11.8 on the professions of children of academicians is congruent with the results of our examination of marriages. In the population of 1821 a large proportion of sons and sons-in-law went into medicine; about one-third entered the medical elite. Sons were especially likely to continue family medical traditions while sons-in-law were more likely to achieve elite status. Clearly, we are yet again witnessing guildlike tendencies toward self-reproduction characteristic of the early nineteenth century. In fact, 13 percent of the academicians could boast of three successive generations of medical men in their families.[36]

Among the offspring of the academicians of 1861 one sees a series of features already familiar from our examination of the fathers-in-law of 1901. The proportion of those in the propertied classes and the educated bourgeoisie doubled. The proportion

TABLE 11.8   Professions of Sons and Sons-in-Law of Academicians, by percent

Occupation	1820			1861			1901			1935		
	Son	SIL	Total	Son	SIL	Total	Son	SIL	Total	Son	SIL	Total
Propertied	14	26	19	37	39	38	23	27	25	27	32	29
Medicine	69	53	64	37	27	32	46	40	43	48	32	42
Medical elite as % of medicine	28	44	33	25	45	33	22	53	33	34	69	44
Educated	16	18	16	23	34	28	31	29	31	22	34	27
Small Business										1	2	2
Popular		3	1	2		1		2	2	1		1
Number	51	34	85	43	41	84	71	48	118	67	41	108

of those in medicine was halved. The percentage of academicians with three generations in medicine was also reduced by nearly half. Sons and sons-in-law were increasingly abandoning the difficult and competitive life of medicine in favor of the more leisurely lifestyles of landed proprietors and educated professionals. But those choosing medicine were as likely to enter the medical elite as their predecessors. Sons-in-law, in particular, could be carefully chosen for their intellectual qualities; nearly half of those in medicine ended up in the medical elite.

Among the offspring of the academicians of 1901 one gets a preview of the marriage patterns of the academicians of 1935. One also gets closer to the general pattern of self-reproduction characteristic of French elites as a whole.[37] There was a sharp decrease in the proportion of those in the propertied classes, while the place of the intellectual and bureaucratic professions was maintained. The proportion of those in medicine increased considerably, though it did not return to the levels of the early nineteenth century; the percentage of those in the medical elite remained stable. As in the earlier population, sons were more likely to be in medicine, whereas sons-in-law were more likely to make it into the medical elite; over half the sons-in-law in medicine did so.

There were few changes among the offspring of the academicians of 1935 in spite of the fact that our sample includes several daughters who went into medicine.[38] This suggests that elite medical culture stabilized considerably in the twentieth century. The main difference from the earlier sample is a rise in the proportion of both sons and sons-in-law in the medical elite.[39] There was also a slight rise in the proportion of academicians in three-generational medical families, partially accounted for by the new opportunities for daughters to enter medicine.[40] Without entering into details, we should also point out that the progeny of professors had in every one of our four samples a greater tendency, more or less pronounced, to be in the medical elite. It is hardly surprising that the career advantages derived from being born or marrying into the medical elite were magnified when one did so at the very highest levels.

We see then a consistent pattern. The occupational profiles of the sons and sons-in-law of one generation of academicians prefigured the occupational profile of fathers-in-law of the next generation of academicians. The offspring of 1861 foretell the great social openness of the academicians of 1901; the return to medicine of the children of 1901 announces the shift back toward medical marriage among the next generation of academicians.

Wealth

Data on the wealth of academicians at their death confirms many of the tendencies already described.[41] I have been unable to find wills for all academicians and it is not at all clear if those missing are due to an absence of wealth to transmit or to the filing of wills outside Paris. More significantly, extensive data for the 1935 population have proven impossible to use because of continuous and rapid inflation starting in the 1920s and currency changes later. This is compounded by the fact that the introduction of income taxes encouraged individuals to underreport their wealth. Still the data we can use clearly suggest a remarkable rise in the economic status of academicians during the nineteenth and early twentieth centuries, which parallels their eruption into the wider world of bourgeois elites.

I have found wills for only twenty-nine of the academicians of 1821 (see Table 11.9). Six of these, including several well-known medical figures, left less than 20,000 francs to descendants. Only two men, the surgeons Baron Guillaume Dupuytren and Jacques Lisfranc, could be considered rich, leaving estates worth over 1 million francs.[41] The average estate was 367,015 francs while the median was less than 90,000 francs, giving some idea of the great variations in the wealth of this generation.

Among the forty-eight academicians of 1861 whose wills were located, the average estate was about one-third higher than that of its predecessors and the median several times higher. Six individuals left estates worth over 1 million francs and only three had estates worth less than 20,000 francs. The huge discrepancy between average and median characteristic of the earlier population was substantially reduced in the 1861 cohort, indicating a somewhat less unequal distribution of wealth.

The academicians of 1901 were the best documented of our populations, having provided seventy-three (out of a possible total of ninety-eight) wills. They were also by far the richest. Both the average and median estates were more than twice as large as those of their predecessors. Twenty-six individuals (more than one-third of those with wills) left estates worth more than 1 million francs. Only two individuals left less than 20,000 francs. The figures would have been higher still had we not adjusted for inflation the estates of the eight academicians who died after 1928. Among all the

TABLE 11.9　Value of Estates at Death, in francs

	1821	*1861*	*1901*
All academicians			
Total Number	29	48	73
Average	367,015	478,745	1,191,507
Median	89,596	250,947	690,570
Number over 1 million	2	6	26
Faculty professors			
Average	533,312	590,483	1,483,511
Median	143,764	434,379	1,031,737
Number over 1 million	1	2	17
Surgeons			
Average	1,321,584	642,772	1,574,522
Median	348,070	496,686	842,612
Number over 1 million	2	2	8

elites of the period, only the heads of business enterprises left significantly larger fortunes than did academicians, whose estates were on a par or slightly larger than the estates of upper-level managers and the wealthiest civil servants.[42]

Two overlapping subgroups stand out as especially successful financially in all three of our populations: surgeons and professors at the Faculty of Medicine. Both consistently left estates that were of higher value than those of other academicians and positively dwarfed the estates of professors in other institutions, including, somewhat surprisingly, the Faculty of Law. (Professors of pharmacy had the next highest estates, which were on average over 500,000 francs less than those of medicine.)[43] Of the thirty-two professors (out of thirty-six) in the population of 1901 for whom we have data, seventeen, or more than half, left estates worth over 1 million francs, and five of these had estates worth more than 5 million francs. Only three academician-professors left estates worth less than 200,000 francs.

Since salaries even for faculty professors were modest,[44] the most likely explanation for wealth of this magnitude is that hospital and faculty posts attracted a clientele from the most affluent classes of society to the private practices of academicians; the value of such practices increased over the course of the century along with the increased status of medicine and of elite posts in particular. We can see why marrying off daughters to the young men of this elite became so much more attractive to the bourgeoisie during the second half of the century. Such marriages may also have opened doors to a more affluent clientele (as Charles Achard feared). At the very least, this wealth explains how academicians could afford to move among the Parisian upper classes of the Third Republic. It would be useful to know whether the growing tendency in the twentieth century to marry within the elite medical world affected the economic status of academicians to any significant degree. Unfortunately, inflation in the twentieth century makes direct comparisons unreliable.

An analysis of the domiciles of academicians strikingly confirms our data on estates. Doctors usually based their private practices in their homes, making a good address a professional investment. The economic status of the neighborhoods in which they lived was an expression of their social and professional aspirations.[46] As early as 1861 academicians rubbed shoulders with the rich. More than half lived in neighborhoods classified as rich or very rich by Jacques Bertillon, the premier French statistician of the late nineteenth century.[47] In 1901 four out of every five academicians lived in such an affluent neighborhood. Whereas only 6 percent of academicians in 1861 had lived in *quartiers* classified as "very rich," the comparable figure in 1901 was 33 percent.

There are, however, major differences in this respect between academicians who were professors at the medical faculty and those who were not. In 1861 professors were more likely to be in rich neighborhoods than their academician colleagues outside the faculty. But neither was likely to reside in the very richest *quartiers*. In 1901, however, half the professors in comparison to less than one-quarter of the non-professors lived in the very richest neighborhoods. The difference can be explained in part by the fact that some of the academicians not at the medical faculty were pharmacists or veterinarians, professions that were less prestigious and certainly less lucrative than medicine. A large group of academicians held full-time laboratory positions while others held military appointments. Both groups had smaller resources

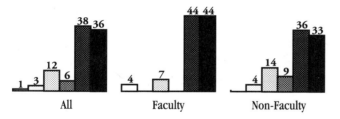

1861: 97 Academicians (27 Faculty, 70 non-Faculty)

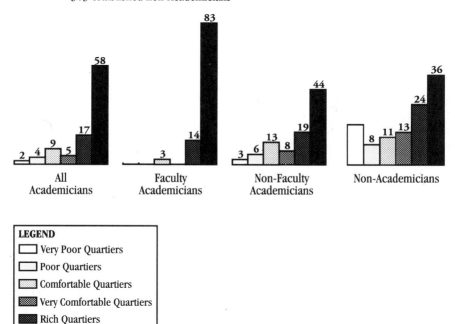

FIGURE 11.2. Domiciles by wealth of *quartier*. Classification of *quartiers* based on Bertillon.

and less need for a prestigious address than did those engaged in the private practice of medicine.

This becomes clearer when we compare the academicians of 1901 with a random sample of 294 Parisian physicians listed in a medical directory[48] of 1904 and who had been in practice at least twenty-five years, putting them at a career stage roughly comparable to that our academicians. They were less likely to end up in a rich neighborhood than were nonfaculty academicians but more likely to live in a very rich neighborhood. In fact, the main difference between the two groups had to do with

TABLE 11.10   Academicians Living in the Ten Most Expensive *Quartiers*, by percent

	1901			1935		
Level	*NonAM (1904)*	*All AM*	*Faculty AM*	*NonAM*	*All AM*	*Faculty AM*
1–5[a]	17	35	58	15	24	26
6–10[b]	12	21	31	17	22	23
Total %	29	56	89	32	46	49

Key: AM = academicians; NonAM = nonacademician practitioners.

[a] The four *quartiers* of the 8th arrondissement and the Porte-Dauphine area of the 16th.

[b] Saint-Thomas d'Aquin and Invalides (7th arrondissement), Chaussée d'Antin (9th), Chaillot (16th), and Plaine-Monceau (17th).

inequalities. Whereas it was rare for an academician to reside in medium to poor *quartiers*, nearly 41 percent of our nonacademician practitioners ended up in such surroundings.

Bertillon's classification does not enable us to analyze our 1935 sample because Paris changed significantly between the 1880s and the interwar years. We can, however, utilize another source, the *Livre Foncièr de Paris* of 1911, which enables us to calculate the average rent in each neighborhood,[49] in order to produce a classification of *quartiers* more appropriate to the early twentieth century. Since we already know that academicians did not live in poor neighborhoods, we will concentrate only on the ten most expensive ones.

Utilizing this categorization confirms the large-scale movement of the academicians of 1901 into the richest neighborhoods (see Table 11.10). Over half of all academicians and about 90 percent of the faculty professors lived in the ten richest *quartiers* as compared to 29 percent of nonacademician practitioners. Over one-third of academicians, and well over half of the faculty professors, lived in the five wealthiest *quartiers* in comparison to less than 20 percent of our nonacademician sample. In the population of 1935 there was a substantial retreat of academicians from the five wealthiest neighborhoods. In the case of faculty professors, the retreat from the wealthy *quartiers* (particularly the most expensive among them) was massive. Nonacademicians, in contrast, lived in these neighborhoods in about the same proportions as they had in 1904.[50]

These data do not necessarily mean that academicians of 1935 lived more modestly than their predecessors. It was possible to find magnificent lodgings in slightly less opulent neighborhoods. Nor was there a wholesale abandonment of the most affluent neighborhoods. Nearly one-half of academicians in 1935 lived in the ten most expensive *quartiers*. But in comparison with academicians of 1901 there was substantial movement out the neighborhoods of the very rich.

We can better understand what was going on if we remember that certain arrondissements are popularly considered to have a particular social character. The eighth was the home of the wealthy bourgeoisie while the fifth and sixth, where most Parisian institutions of higher education are located, were closely associated with university intellectuals.[51] If our data about the social openness of the medical elite in the late nineteenth century and its partial reintrenchment in the twentieth are correct, one would expect a movement out of the fifth and sixth arrondissements in the population of 1901 and some return there in 1935.

TABLE 11.11   Academicians Living in the Fifth and Sixth Arrondissements, by percent

Arrondissement	1861		1901		1935	
	All	*Faculty*	*All*	*Faculty*	*All*	*Faculty*
5th and 6th	28	30	22	8	25	28
Expanded[a]	40	48	41	25	42	45

[a]Saint-Thomas-d'Aquin and École Militaire in the 7th; La Salpêtrière and Croulebarbe in the 13th; Montparnasse in the 14th; and Necker in the 15th.

Overall, the proportion of academicians in the Latin Quarter diminished only slightly between 1861 and 1901 (see Table 11.11). But in the case of faculty professors, the wealthiest academicians in our sample, the change was dramatic. In 1861 nearly one-third of the faculty professors inhabited the fifth and sixth arrondissements; in 1901 less than 10 percent did; a larger proportion (14 percent) of nonacademician Parisian doctors in our random sample lived in these two arrondissements. Half the faculty professors, in fact, lived in the very bourgeois eighth arrondissement. In 1935 the proportion of all academicians in the Latin Quarter rose only slightly. But in the case of professors at the Faculty of Medicine, the proportion living in these arrondissements returned pretty much to the levels of 1861 while the proportion living in the eighth declined by about half. This return to the Latin Quarter is particularly striking in view of the fact that distances were far less daunting in 1935 than they had been in 1901 thanks to motorized transportation. Even if we expand the boundaries of the Latin Quarter to include *quartiers* bordering on the fifth and sixth arrondissements, our results remain substantially unchanged (Table 11.11).

One does not want to make too much of such data. They do, however, lend support to earlier data suggesting that the most successful members of the medical elite associated themselves in a variety of ways with the nonmedical bourgeoisie in the late nineteenth century and retrenched somewhat within the world of elite medicine in the twentieth. If this interpretation is correct, one would expect to find similar patterns of change among other indicators of social openness and isolation.

Political Office

The seeking of political office is a particularly telling marker of social openness because the desire for such office is already a sign of interests and concerns which transcend narrow professionalism and because success in the endeavor ordinarily requires considerable social resources. The evolution of political activity among our four samples strikingly parallels the data on marriage and children. There was little participation in national legislative bodies or in municipal and departmental assemblies among the academicians of 1821. Only one of the three men serving in a legislative body did so for more than a single term. Parisian professors in other disciplines, particularly the sciences, played a highly visible political role in the early nineteenth century. If the medical elite did not follow this example, it was, I have suggested elsewhere, due to the recentness of its emergence and its lack of political traditions.[52]

There was, however, a sharp increase in the incidence of political activity among the academicians of 1861 and 1901. About a dozen individuals in each population held political office of some sort. The figures in the former case are slightly misleading since, despite the large numbers involved, most academicians held local rather than national office and only briefly. In two cases a senate seat was essentially a symbolic reward which the government granted Claude Bernard and the surgeon Auguste Nélaton for achievement in other domains (and which they held only fleetingly until the fall of the empire).

Politicians at the national level in the academy of 1901 had all been elected to fairly lengthy terms in the Chamber of Deputies or the Senate and combined these positions with elected office at the local and regional levels. Furthermore, while the proportion of politically active professors in most other institutions of higher education declined substantially between 1861 and 1901, it remained stable in the case of the Faculty of Medicine. That faculty, in fact, now had the highest proportion of political activists among all the major Parisian institutions of higher education.[53]

These data reflect changing political conditions in nineteenth century France. Those for the population of 1861 suggest strong political aspirations and limited opportunities, until the Third Republic, at least; those for 1901 reveal the opening up of political life to the middle classes under the Third Republic. But if opportunities were available to many groups, the medical elite seems to have benefited particularly. Electoral activity required at least moderate wealth and extensive social contacts, both of which the academicians of 1901 possessed in abundance. To be sure, only one of our academician-legislators achieved ministerial rank and this was Marcelin Berthelot, a chemist and scientific mandarin who was in no way a typical member of the medical elite. This suggests that the political success of academicians did not go very deep.[54]

It is nonetheless surprising to note that only one academician of 1935, the obstetrician Amédée Doléris, was elected to the national legislature and only for a single term. He was, moreover, not very typical of academicians in that cohort. He did not hold a professorship and though he occupied a hospital post, he was not an *agrégé* and had won no prizes from either the Academy of Medicine or Sciences. It is true that had we chosen a slightly earlier date for our sample of academicians, we would have found another politically active member, Adolphe Pinard, who died in 1934. But this would not substantially change our figures or their interpretation.[55]

The retreat of academicians from politics was clearly not due to the disappearance of medical men generally from the national political stage.[56] It may, however, have something to do with the relative isolation of university intellectuals from political power, which Christophe Charle has observed among the Parisian elites of 1901 and which is linked to parallel but distinct processes of professionalization in the political and academic domains.[57] Since well over one-half of our academicians in 1935 were professors of one sort or another, we may be witnessing the belated adaptation of the medical elite to wider institutional processes. However one explains this phenomenon, however, the data on political activity would appear to confirm the hypothesis of growing professional insularity and isolation of the Parisian medical elite in the twentieth century.[58]

The data in the last two chapters suggest a dramatic change in the social characteristics of the medical elite in the last decades of the nineteenth century. Just as academicians were likely to be associated with the Faculty of Medicine and/or hospitals and to have passed through a long series of *concours*, they were likely to be relatively wealthy, to live in the same neighborhoods as other elites, and, frequently, to marry among them. Though rarely at the highest echelons of power, they were also well-represented in national politics.

It is this social ascent which gave resonance and grounding to Léon Daudet's delirious Swiftian novel *Les Morticoles*,[59] published in 1894, in which a traveler is stranded in a land ruled by doctors. Anyone who is not a doctor is sick. In fact, it is the medical elite which is dominant among the *Morticoles* and which is the true target of Daudet's satirical pen. Recruited through competitive examinations in "footlicking" (literally), engaged constantly in intrigues to obtain posts and honors, members of this elite cynically seek out wealth by exploiting rich patients even as they experiment cruelly on the poor and propagate materialistic atheism. Daudet, the son of the novelist Alphonse Daudet, had abandoned medical studies after, it is said, suffering an injustice in a *concours*. In the process of becoming a prominent polemicist of the extreme right, Daudet was hardly offering an objective account of the Parisian medical elite. But the entire satirical thrust of *Les Morticoles*, indeed its central conceit of a ruling class of doctors, depends for its effect on the new wealth and sociopolitical status of the Parisian medical elite that has been documented in this chapter.

In the twentieth century more subtle changes took place. Data on origins suggest that professorships in the Faculty of Medicine were becoming somewhat more socially exclusive, whereas more modest social origins were characteristic of the marginal professional groups in the academy. A range of indicators suggest a notable tendency toward social retrenchment and increased professional insularity. The nature of elite medical careers can only partially explain this phenomenon since these were already well established among the academicians of 1901, who exhibited a considerable degree of social openness. I should therefore like to present a somewhat more complex interpretation which is speculative but which accounts for our findings.

The medical elite in the nineteenth century found itself confronted by two different imperatives. On the one hand, there was a widespread desire to take what was regarded as its proper place in French society. This entailed participation in the political and administrative bodies which governed society[60] as well as maintaining regular social relations and even contracting marital alliances with members of the privileged classes. On the other hand, the medical elite was subjected to an increasingly rigid career structure that demanded an enormous investment of time and energy and that tended to segregate potential members within a narrow range of medical institutions.

The two imperatives were not completely contradictory. The rigorous system of recruitment helped raise the social and economic status of the medical elite and thereby facilitated the process of social integration. Conversely, marriage to daughters of wealthy families could provide the economic basis for the long period of study, publishing, and *concours* that was demanded. In the long run, however, the two imperatives were not compatible, and in the twentieth century the pendulum swung in the direction of the second. What is perhaps most astonishing is that the academicians of 1901 succeeded so well in combining social with professional success. This was, I suspect, a function of the unique conditions of the early Third Republic. Long thwarted social and political aspirations could now be given free rein. A new and uniquely open national elite was in the process of being formed and members of the medical elite rushed to take their places, despite their heavy professional obligations. That one-quarter of the academicians of 1901 never had children suggests that they achieved their dual aspirations only at the cost of considerable personal sacrifice.

Academicians in the twentieth century tended increasingly to function within the confines of the medical milieu. It was not just the rigorous system of competitions which isolated future academicians. Political life became less congenial as the certainties of early republicanism, based on the belief in laicism, science, education, and public health, disintegrated during the interwar period. As for marriage, a new emphasis on affective relations rather than social convenience encouraged the preference for shared culture and social background; the improved economic standing of medicine, moreover, ensured that medical marriages did not entail major economic sacrifices. It may also be the case that once the medical elite succeeded in becoming firmly ensconced within the national elite, academicians could allow themselves the luxury of turning inward.

NOTES

1. The proportion of Parisians among all French doctors increased even more quickly during this period, from 11 percent in 1847 to 20 percent in 1890.

2. Paris contributed 30 percent while the other six regions contributed 32 percent.

3. The five regions together produced only 2.5 percent of our entire sample of academicians.

4. The extent of rural recruitment is especially surprising considering that the rural population in France declined from 75 percent of the total population in 1851 to 49 percent in 1931.

5. My data on interns are calculated from Raymond Durand-Fardel, *L'Internat en médecine et en chirurgie des hôpitaux et hospices civils de Paris: centenaire de l'internat, 1802–1902* (1903).

6. This is a frequent motif in the eulogies of E. Pariset. See the funeral oration for Ollivier in Etienne Pariset, *Histoire des membres de l'Académie Royale de Médecine*, 2 vols. (1850), vol. 2, p. 598. Paul Le Gendre, *Un médecin philosophe: Charles Bouchard, son oeuvre et son temps (1837–1915)* (1924), p. 291, mentions that Bouchard, who grew up in Lyon, became mentor to several students of Lyonnais origin who were the sons of old friends or relatives. Charles Achard mentions utilizing letters from Alsatian relatives in order to get permission to work in the lab of Adolphe Wurtz, who was originally from Alsace. Charles Achard, *La Confession d'un vieil homme du siècle: souvenirs du temps et de l'espace* (1943), p. 42.

7. The professions of fathers come mainly from the birth certificates of academicians. The procedure used was to determine the exact date and place of birth of each academician, listed in *Index biographique des membres, des associés, et des correspondants de l'Académie de Médecine, 1820–1990* (1990). With this information, I wrote to the municipal authorities in the place of birth, who provided the information recorded on the certificate. Supplementary infor-

mation was provided by Christophe Charle, who generously made available to me his research data on professors at the Faculty of Medicine. At a later stage of research, I was able to find supplementary material in Françoise Huguet, *Les Professeurs de la Faculté de Médecine de Paris: dictionnaire biographique, 1794–1939* (1991); Christophe Charle and Eva Telkes, *Les Professeurs de la Faculté des Sciences de Paris: dictionnaire biographique, 1901–1939* (1989) and *Les Professeurs du Collège de France: dictionnaire biographique, 1901–1939* (1988).

8. The large historical literature on the various elites is nicely summarized in Christophe Charle, *Les Élites de la République, 1880–1900* (1987), esp. chap. 1.

9. Well over half the academicians of 1821 who had been born before 1750 were the sons of medical men. Among those born after 1750 the figure was 32 percent. On prerevolutionary patterns see Catherine Maille-Virole, "La Naissance d'un personnage: le médecin parisien à la fin de l'Ancien régime," *Historical Reflections* 9 (1982), and Adeline Daumard and François Furet, *Structures et relations sociales à Paris au milieu de XVIIIe siècle* (1961).

10. The proportion of medical families defined in this broader way is 44 percent in 1821, 35 percent in 1861, 28 percent in 1901, and 29 percent in 1935.

11. For the definition of the term "medical elite" as it is used in this discussion see the notes to Table 11.2.

12. However, they might inherit enemies as well as supporters. Much of the autobiography of J. Quénu is taken up with the difficulties created for him by his father's old enemy Henri Hartmann. Jean Quénu, *Notre internat* (1971).

13. Charles Richet claimed to have chosen medicine as a profession because "the *grande situation* of my father, professor at the faculty, eminent surgeon, could be of great use to me in the noble profession of medicine." Charles Richet, *Souvenirs d'un physiologiste* (1933), p. 9. During his studies, he tells us, he was able to work in Wurtz's laboratory,"thanks to paternal protection."

14. Charle, *Les Élites*, pp. 64–65.

15. The number of veterinarians is too small to be included in this discussion.

16. While 61 percent of the pharmacists and 42 percent of physicians in the combined populations of 1901 and 1935 had origins in either the popular or small business classes, the figure for surgeons was 20 percent.

17. In a recent survey of retired doctors in France, a great many elderly doctors attribute their decisions to abandon further training and *concours* to financial constraints. Claudine Herzlich et al., *Cinquante ans d'exercice de la médecine en France: carrières et pratiques des médecins français, 1930–1980* (1993), p. 60.

18. A random list of doctors in practice for at least thirty years was compiled from the *Guide Rosenwald* of 1935. Doctors' student files were then consulted in the AJ16 series at the AN. In some cases a copy of the birth certificate was in the file. In most cases, however, the date and place of birth in the file enabled me to write to local authorities for information. Information was received about fathers' professions for about half the individuals on the original random sample.

19. Dates of marriage were initially discovered in succession registers at the AP, Series DQ7 and DQ8. These were supplemented by a variety of published biographical sources. This and later discussions of marriage include only data about *first* marriages. Remarriages have not been considered.

20. Charle, *Les Élites*, p. 260.

21. For instance, professors in this sample were on average nearly two years younger than other academicians when they obtained their medical degrees.

22. Succession registers often provide information about the marriages of academicians and about the wife. Thus some marriage contracts and, above all, wives' birth certificates containing information about academicians' fathers-in-law could be located.

23. See the examples in Adeline Daumard, *La Bourgeoisie parisienne de 1815 à 1848* (1962), p. 342. J.-P. Royer, R. Martinage, and P. Lecocq, *Juges et notables au XIXe siècle* (1982) also stress the role of nepotism in recruitment of magistrates; André-Jean Tudesq, *Les Conseillers généraux en France au temps de Guizot* (1967), pp. 458–59, emphasizes the importance of family connections among scientists.

24. Erwin Ackerknecht, "From Barber Surgeon to Modern Doctor," *Bulletin of the History of Medicine* 58 (1985), 545–53.

25. Many are identified on public documents as *propriétaires*. The term is a vague one; at least some of the fathers-in-law were probably defined in this way because they were retired from a profession or business. The term, however, does seem to have been associated with wealth in nineteenth-century France. The women who brought the most wealth into their marriage with an academician were often daughters of men described as *propriétaires*.

26. For instance, Charles Bouchard married Hélène Ruffer, daughter of the director of the London branch of the Lyon-based Banque Aynard. Mme. Bouchard's sister married into the provincial medical elite when she wed a student of Charcot, Antoine Peirret, who was to become professor of psychiatry at the Lyon Faculty of Medicine. (Paul Le Gendre, *Du Quartier Latin à l'Academie [reminiscences] [1930]*, p. 108.) O. Lannelongue, however, got closer to the social summit when he married the widow of the son of Count de Remussat (who was herself from a wealthy family with a fortune originating in the Rouen cotton trade). See Claude Vanderpooten, *Le Bistouri et la fortune: Odilon et Marie Lannelongue* (Condé-sur-Noireau, 1986).

27. At the height of his fame, for instance, Charcot held a regular weekly Tuesday evening soirée in which his interns mixed with the cream of Parisian literary and political society. Georges Guillan, *J.-M. Charcot, 1825–1893: sa vie—son oeuvre* (1955), pp. 30–37. Another figure of the period with wide social contacts was the urologist Félix Guyon. One of his interns, Théodore Tuffier, who was a member of the academy from 1918 to 1928, met his future wife, the daughter of a well-known currency exchanger, at the home of his mentor. See *Le Docteur Tuffier, 1857–1929: sa vie, ses travaux, ses enseignements* (n.d.), p. 16.

28. These figure are from Charle, *Les Élites*, pp. 272–75.

29. Robert Debré, *L'Honneur de vivre: témoignages* (1972).

30. The worldly and well-read Robert Debré writes that living the exhausting life of a young elite physician put an end to much of his cultural and social activity. Ibid., p. 152.

31. Achard, *La Confession*, pp. 57–60.

32. Ibid., p. 60.

33. Ibid.

34. My sources for this information are the succession registers at the AP, DQ7, DQ8; and the registers of marriage contracts at the Archives de l'Enregistrement.

35. The median sum among the fifteen wives of 1861 for which I have figures was 43,190 francs; for the forty-two wives of 1901, 88,497 francs; for the twenty of 1935, 74,900 francs.

36. This number refers only to the three generations examined: academicians, the generation immediately preceding (fathers and fathers-in-law), and the one following (sons, sons-in-law). The figures would be higher if grandfathers and grandsons were included.

37. Charle, *Les Élites*, p. 327, shows that about two-thirds of the offspring of businessmen were in business while 40 percent of the offspring of *fonctionnaires* followed careers in the civil service.

38. For a fascinating fictionalized account of the problems faced by daughters of the medical elite who chose to enter medicine see Colette Yver (Antoinette Huzard), *Princesse de science* (1907). I read the fifty-first edition of this book, indicating the extent of its popularity.

39. Some indication of the large number of sons of mandarins going into medicine during this period is the anecdote told by J.-P. Escande, who did his first hospital practicum (*stage*)

while a medical student with Pasteur-Vallery Radot. There were apparently enough sons of *patrons* in the group, for Pasteur-Vallery Radot to convoke them in his office and deliver the message that they should be worthy of their fathers. The story is recounted in Jacques Fossard, *Histoire polymorphe de l'internat en médecine et chirurgie des hôpitaux et hospices civils de Paris*, 2 vols. (Grenoble, 1982), vol. 2, p. 104.

40. The figures for three-generation families in the academy are very similar to the 9.75 percent found by Hertzlich et al., *Cinquante ans d'exercice*, p. 42, for retired doctors throughout France born before 1909.

41. The main sources for these data are the succession registers in the AP DQ7 and DQ8. These have been supplemented with data provided by Christophe Charle.

42. With the exception of these two individuals whose wealth has already been documented by other historians, specific individuals cannot be discussed in this context according to regulations governing the use of such administrative sources.

43. Charle, *Les Élites*, p. 365. His figures for professors at the medical faculty vary slightly from mine because he limits himself to those active in 1901 while my sample includes some academicians in 1901 who were later appointed professors.

44. Ibid.

45. A senior Parisian professor earned 15,000 francs annually during this period. On university salaries more generally see George Weisz, *The Emergence of Modern Universities in France, 1863–1914* (Princeton, N.J., 1983).

46. Addresses of all academicians are at the front of the volumes of the *Annuaire de l'Académie de Médecine*. Volumes for the years under consideration were used.

47. Jacques Bertillon, *Cartogrammes et diagrammes relatifs à la population parisienne* (1889).

48. *Annuaire médicale et pharmaceutique du docteur Roubaud*, published from 1848 to 1913.

49. *Livre Foncièr de Paris* (1911), pp. 12–19, Tableau II.

50. A random sample of 195 practitioners who were in practice at least thirty years but were never elected to the academy was selected from the major annual medical directory of the period, the *Guide Rosenwald* of 1935.

51. Crosland, *Science under Control*, p. 428. Maurice de Fleury, *Le Médecin* (1927), p. 43.

52. George Weisz, "The Medical Elite in France in the Early Nineteenth Century," *Minerva* 25 (1987), 163–64.

53. Charle, *Les Élites*, p. 411, gives a figure of 11.4 percent for the Faculty of Medicine as opposed to 9.3 percent for the Faculty of Law and 8 percent for the Faculty of Letters.

54. The lack of success at the cabinet level applied to physician-legislators more generally. See Jack D. Ellis, *The Physician-Legislators of France: Medicine and Politics in the Early Third Republic* (Cambridge, 1990).

55. Pinard was, like Doléris, an obstetrician. It is possible that practitioners of this specialty had an affinity for politics connected with concern for public health and eugenics. Nadine Lefaucher has argued that the separation of hospital obstetrics from gynecological surgery (which remained in the hands of hospital surgeons) stimulated elite obstetricians to view their field in broader sociopolitical terms. Nadine Lefaucheur, "La Résistible création des accoucheurs des hôpitaux," *Sociologie de travail*, 30 (1988), 353.

56. Matei Dogan, "Les Filières de la carrière politique en France," *Revue française de sociologie*, 8 (1967), 472, shows that there was only a slight decline in the proportion of doctors among legislators during the interwar period.

57. Charle, *Les Élites*, pp. 405–12.

58. A less conclusive confirmation of this interpretation is the fact that in each of our first three populations there were two academicians who had been elected to either the Académie

Française or the Académie des Sciences Morales et Politiques, suggesting some connection with the literary and intellectual elites. There were none among the academicians of 1935.

59. Léon Daudet, *Les Morticoles* (1984). For an illuminating reading of this work see Toby Gelfand, "Medical Nemesis in Paris, 1894: Léon Daudet's *Les Morticoles,*" *Bulletin of the History of Medicine* 60 (1986), 155–76.

60. For a good example of such demands in the name of the academy see J.-B. Barth, "Compte rendu des actes de l'Académie," *BAM* 2 (1873), xxvi–xxix.

Conclusion

I have covered considerable ground in the preceding pages. There is at the center of things the institutional history of the Academy of Medicine. The academy began in the early nineteenth century as an organization balancing scientific and public health roles. Because the operations of the state in public health remained restricted, because academicians showed deferential reluctance to offer unsolicited advice to the government, and because medical knowledge was in some ways highly inadequate, it was the evaluative scientific function which dominated academic life. The academy was a central intellectual institution of French medicine; its deliberations were closely monitored and frequently criticized by the medical press. It propagated and evaluated recent medical knowledge without, for the most part, seeking to impose institutional or professional consensus. Some of its debates loom very large indeed in the history of medicine.

By the twentieth century the academy was predominantly a public health institution. The rapid expansion of the state's role in prevention and health care and the expanding definition of public health to include various forms of private behavior provided many opportunities to apply medical expertise. At the same time, most of the evaluative scientific functions, with the exception of prize-granting, were quietly dropped. By the interwar period the main vestige of the academy's traditional role in medical science were the papers, usually not of the first rank, presented at its meetings and published in its *Bulletin*. Rather than providing detailed evaluations of deceased academicians, *éloges*, like the centenary celebrations that took place regularly, served chiefly to defend the international standing of French medicine. Traditional academic genres seem to have become increasingly incompatible with the extreme specialization taking over medical science.

The connection between medicine and science is a complex one. The popular view of this relationship is that medicine in the nineteenth century was largely unscientific as well as ineffective; that pathological anatomy and physiological experimentation brought intellectual advances without transforming medical practice very profoundly, until, in the twentieth century, medicine was revolutionized by experimental science. For those scientists and historians who see physics and chemistry as the paradigmatic sciences, medicine's scientific status, even today, remains doubtful. In France, it is frequently argued, the power of clinical medicine has seriously hampered the progress of experimental research.[1]

That nineteenth-century medicine (and frequently that of the twentieth century as well) does not fully conform to the criteria set by the exact sciences like physics and chemistry goes without saying. But this does not mean that it can be comfortably dismissed from the domain of science. The world of science in the early nineteenth century was heterogeneous and amazingly fluid. The organizers of the Academy of Sciences had no doubt that medicine belonged in that institution as it did in the Collège de France. Those members of the medical elite who followed anatomoclinical procedures were also graced with the certainty that they were doing "science." A physicist influenced by his own disciplinary norms might have disagreed (and probably did). But there is something profoundly ahistorical in the acceptance by historians of a single, normative definition of science; for the historical actors of the early nineteenth century, the precise nature of science was something to be worked out in the crucible of debate and practice.[2]

Members of the medical elite, of course, were not just scientists. A widely expressed cliché was that medicine was an "art" as well as a "science" and most doctors would have argued that exclusive concern with the advancement of knowledge at the expense of patient care was nothing short of unethical. The great majority of French doctors, certainly, had few pretensions to being scientists. But elite medicine in Paris was largely defined by its flourishing research sector.

It is at this point that the story begins to get complicated. I have suggested in several contexts that the research domain of medicine, closely associated initially with the larger scientific domain, became relatively more autonomous as medical science developed its own institutions and a distinctive professional culture. (It also became relatively autonomous from the medical profession, which was a source of considerable tension in the late nineteenth century.)[3] But at the same time, the evolving exact sciences were generating theories and research methodologies which introduced both strains and new possibilities to a medical science dominated by the evolving traditions of the anatomoclinical method.

If I have accomplished nothing else in this book, I hope to have at least convinced readers that the medical elite was not hostile to innovations in medical science. There were arguments, to be sure, about the validity of some innovations, and certain individuals were opposed in principle to changes of any sort. But at the summit of the professional hierarchy, the chief issue was how new methods of science could be integrated and combined with more traditional procedures. It was above all necessary to determine what constituted valid use of such methods. Some new procedures did not address medical concerns directly. The problem was how to move from, say, chemical analysis of waters or the blood to practical diagnosis or therapy; often the process depended on leaps in logic or highly speculative accounts of disease processes which might or might not be convincing. Even when a procedure more directly addressed medical questions, the weight to be given the results was not necessarily evident. And what was one to do if results contradicted clinical experience? Academicians did not usually oppose new procedures borrowed from the laboratory or elsewhere, but they were understandably inhospitable to claims that results derived from such procedures superseded clinical experience.

I do not mean to suggest that there were no serious tensions. The growing contingent of laboratory scientists in the medical elite, although increasingly well represented in the academy, certainly felt that its versions of science were underrepresented and underfunded in medical institutions. Their relative lack of participation in academic activities is surely expressive of some degree of alienation. The absence of support for introducing research grants, as the Academy of Sciences did, undoubtedly reflects the distance between clinical and laboratory elites. Recruitment into the medical elite was complicated by the need to reconcile research ability with those capacities capable of being judged by *concours*.[4]

As complex in its own way as the relationship between the medical elite and science is that between the medical elite and political power linked, as it so frequently is, to "fortune." By creating such institutions as the Faculty of Medicine and the Academy of Medicine, the central government, abetted by local authorities who administered the Parisian hospital system, created a national medical elite of an entirely new sort. Pariset's *éloges* express wonderfully the novel sense of power, prestige, and wealth which academicians now felt. Nonetheless, however elevated the status of the medical elite appeared to be, it was recognized to be low in comparison to that of the scientific elite. It was not just a matter of the relative lack of political and administrative appointments documented here; the conditions under which the academy operated—lack of facilities, tiny budgets—proclaimed its inferior status and energized periodic attempts at institutional reform. Even its role in public health, the fundamental rationale for the academy's existence, was surprisingly restricted and limited for the most part to low-level technical-administrative functions.

To some extent, this situation reflected the recent and rather circumscribed interest of the French state in medicine and public health. The public role of science was long-standing and, by the nineteenth century, institutionalized in the Academy of Sciences, the Sorbonne, the very prestigious *grandes écoles*, and the various state engineering corps. Apart from its utility and prestige value for governments seeking to be perceived as favorable to progress, scientific knowledge—more specifically mathematical knowledge—was a key symbolic component in the formation and definition of elite bourgeois status in France.[5] As the new kid on the block, medicine had none of these advantages. And one suspects that the limitations of the medical science of the era gave administrators little incentive to substantially extend the state's public health role and the academy's duties.

The relatively low status of medicine began to rise, we saw, in the second half of the nineteenth century. By the beginning of the twentieth century academicians were by any standards wealthy and politically well-connected. If there was some retreat from bourgeois "fortune" and especially political power as the century advanced, one can be fairly certain that this expressed the intense specialization of elite medical functions rather than any loss of status. The Academy of Medicine never achieved the funding levels of the Academy of Sciences. But its new premises—which it did not have to share with other academies—placed it on a status plane close if not exactly equal to the older institution. Perhaps most significantly, while the government pretty much abandoned the Academy of Sciences as an agency of its practical scientific activities, the Academy of Medicine took on more and more practical technical tasks. One could not say of the Academy of Medicine, as one could easily say of the Academy of Sciences, that its primary role in the twentieth century has been to provide honor to productive scientists. While the former institution has certainly performed this function for the medical elite, it has continued to serve the state in very direct ways as well.

It would be fairly easy at this point to frame the political rise of the academy in Foucauldian terms as yet another expression of the development of the "technologies" and "disciplines" that support and depend on "power." Such a framework would certainly have some explanatory power. It was the rise in medical "knowledge-power" which made pertinent and provided the satirical thrust of Léon Daudet's *Les Morticoles*, which treats the medical elite as a new kind of ruling class. However, I am doubtful whether the academy provides a particularly salient focus for any analysis of power that extends beyond the narrow medical domain.[6]

Insofar as its routine duties were concerned, the academy performed essentially gatekeeping functions. It determined which of many possible candidates could become approved secret remedies, spas, producers of serums and organic extracts. Academicians themselves were well aware of the distance between such tasks and "higher" scientific research. Efforts to develop public knowledge of relevance to administrative concerns seemed to many to be a futile undertaking because of the difficulties of collecting and utilizing the information provided by state agents. The academy was more successful when responding to specific questions from a ministry. But as we have seen, governments in the nineteenth century made an effort to restrict the academy to narrow technical issues. The scope of academic concerns broadened considerably in the twentieth century; however, the academy now functioned within a highly contentious system of pressure group politics where scientific prestige could not easily be translated into real influence. Its evaluative scientific practices were, I have argued, influential in the nineteenth century, but they were neither coercive nor especially constraining; in any case, they declined substantially in the twentieth century.

To be sure, the academy did on a regular basis call for the extension of state and medical power in such matters as compulsory vaccination, alcoholism prevention, and protection of infants. But whether such efforts were particularly successful is a matter for debate. After all, historians have determined that France lagged well behind Germany and Britain in the early twentieth century in introducing public health measures.[7] Some of the delays involved can be attributed to a political system that made institutional reform of any kind a tortuous obstacle course. Others can be ascribed to the crisis in public finances that stemmed from long resistance to the introduction of an income tax. But a close look at some of the academy's debates also suggests that many academicians shared the concern for privacy, fear of administrative intervention, and desire to protect individuals from state power that was characteristic of the medical profession and the French bourgeoisie generally. Thus while I do not dispute the growth of "medical power" in the nineteenth and twentieth centuries, it is not clear to me that institutions like the academy were necessarily central to this process. In more than a few cases, I suspect, medical knowledge was little more than an alibi for the extension of state power.[8]

Let me complete the circle of these concluding remarks by touching on the link between the rise of medical power in the second half of the nineteenth century and the development of medical science. It is absolutely clear to me that, like the creation of new medical institutions in the late eighteenth and early nineteenth centuries, the expansion of medical power and wealth in the late nineteenth and early twentieth centuries reflected political imperatives. Just as governments of the earlier period needed expertise independently of medicine's quite limited capacity to provide it, the expansion of state power in the later era required increasingly elaborate forms of expertise. It would, however, be foolish to deny either the significance of scientific developments in this later period or the increased capacity of medical science to provide more reliable forms of expertise than those available in the past. Likewise, the increased stature and affluence of the medical elite reflected in some measure the new prestige and recent successes of medical science.

It has become commonplace for historians to suggest that the main links between medicine and science at the end of the nineteenth century were rhetorical. It is argued that science added little of practical value to healing because it did not much increase the number of effective therapies available. It did, however, enable doctors to identify themselves with the cultural prestige and authority of laboratory science.[9] There is certainly truth to such claims. Medical associations did unquestionably identify themselves with science in polemical and highly opportunistic ways. But focusing exclusively on such efforts blinds us to the very profound ways in which the commitment to science constrained and shaped medicine.[10]

Furthermore, such arguments reduce medicine to practical therapeutics. Medicine, however, is (and has always been) also about understanding and explaining disease. This ability to understand and explain in ways congruent with the most up-to-date scientific knowledge constituted a major element in the appeal of "scientific medicine" at the turn of the century. Bacteriology in particular (but not uniquely) offered a powerful explanatory framework for disease causation that had immediate repercussions for public health and that offered realistic hope of eventual therapeutic breakthroughs, even as it subverted traditional medical certainties.

Medicine, moreover, was not a monolithic entity. Then as now, it encompassed many different groups and institutions. There is absolutely no question that for some, perhaps many doctors, identification with science was an occasional rhetorical and polemical strategy. But medicine also had its own elaborate research sectors exemplified in France by the Academy of Medicine. Within these sectors, the varieties of scientific activity were at the center of institutional life. Different models of science might be in conflict. The fundamental nature of medical science and its relationship to various paradigms and procedures borrowed from the physical and life sciences might provoke contentious debate. But science, as academicians understood it, provided the very cornerstone for the activities of the Academy of Medicine and the self-images of the medical elite.

NOTES

1. This extremely common view was propounded by Abraham Flexner, *Medical Education in Europe: A Report to the Carnegie Foundation for the Advancement of Teaching* (New York, 1912) and has been repeated regularly ever since, particularly by French medical reformers.

2. A similar argument is made by John Harley Warner, "Science in Medicine," *Osiris*, 2nd ser. 1 (1985), 37–58.

3. On this tension see George Weisz, "Reform and Conflict in French Medical Education, 1870–1914," in *The Organization of Science and Technology in France, 1808–1914,* ed. Robert Fox and George Weisz (Cambridge, 1980), pp. 283–307; and Martha L. Hildreth, *Doctors, Bureaucrats, and Public Health, 1888–1902* (New York, 1987).

4. Weisz, "Reform and Conflict."

5. On the social role of mathematical knowledge in France, see Terry Shinn, "Science, Tocqueville, and the State: The Organization of Knowledge in Modern France," *Social Research,* 59 (1992), 533–66.

6. The academy's power to reinforce medical hierarchies has been discussed at length in this book. I refer in what follows to medical power exercised in the wider social and political spheres.

7. See especially Allan Mitchell, *The Divided Path: The German Influence on Social Reform in France after 1870* (Chapel Hill, N.C., 1991); and Matthew Ramsey, "France," in *The History of Health and the Modern State,* ed. Dorothy Porter (Amsterdam, 1994).

8. I do not, of course, mean to suggest that no doctors were involved in these processes of "medicalization." I do suggest, however, that those most involved frequently constituted marginal minorities within institutional medicine. I also do not mean to suggest that the academy never tried to advance state power. But such initiatives were more rare than one might suppose and frequently sparked considerable opposition within the institution.

9. Versions of this argument can be found in Gerald L. Geison, "'Divided We Stand': Physiologists and Clinicians in the American Context," in *The Therapeutic Revolution: Essays in the Social History of American Medicine,* ed. Morris J. Vogel and Charles E. Rosenberg (Philadelphia, 1979), pp. 135–57; and S. E. D. Short, "Physicians, Science, and Status: Issues in the Professionalization of Anglo-American Medicine in the Nineteenth Century," *Medical History* 27 (1983), 51–68.

10. This argument is made by Barbara G. Rosenkrantz, "The Search for Professional Order in Nineteenth Century American Medicine," *Proceedings of the International Congress of the History of Science* (Tokyo, 1975), no. 4, pp. 113–24, and is developed by Warner, "Science in Medicine." Also see Nicholas Jardine, "The Laboratory Revolution in Medicine as Rhetorical and Aesthetic Accomplishment," in *The Laboratory Revolution in Medicine,* ed. A. Cunningham and P. Williams (Cambridge, 1992), pp. 304–23.

Select Bibliography

Abir-Am, Pnina. "A Historical Ethnography of a Scientific Anniversary in Molecular Biology: The First Protein X-Ray Photograph." *Social Epistemology* 6 (1992), 323–54.

Académie de Médecine. *Index biographique des membres, des associés et des correspondants de l'Académie de Médecine, 1820–1990.* 1991.

———. *Exposition sur l'histoire de l'Académie de Médecine, 1829–1970.* 1972.

———. *Centenaire de l'Académie de Médecine, 1820–1920.* Masson, 1921.

Académie des Sciences. *Index biographique des membres de l'Académie des Science.* Gauthier-Villars, 1968.

Achard, Charles. *La Confession d'un vieil homme du siècle: souvenirs du temps et de l'espace.* Mercure de France, 1943.

Ackerknecht, Erwin H. *Medicine at the Paris Hospital, 1794–1848.* Baltimore: Johns Hopkins University Press, 1967.

———. "Broussais, or a Forgotten Medical Revolution." *Bulletin of the History of Medicine* 27(1953), 320–43.

Adams, Thomas M. *Bureaucrats and Beggars: French Social Policy in the Age of the Enlightenment.* New York: Oxford University Press, 1990.

Baillière, J.-B., and son. *Histoire de nos relations avec l'Académie de Médecine, 1827–1871: lettre adressée à MM. les membres de l'Académie.* Baillière, 1872.

Bertillon, Jacques, Préfecture de la Seine. *Cartogrammes et diagrammes relatifs à la population parisienne.* Masson, 1889.

Borell, Merriley. "Origins of the Hormone Concept: Internal Secretions and Physiological Research." Ph.D. diss., Yale University, 1976.

Bourdelais, Patrice, and Raulot, Jean-Yves. *Une peur bleue: histoire du choléra en France, 1832–1854.* Payot, 1987.

Brais, Bernard. "The Making of a Famous Nineteenth-Century Neurologist: Jean-Martin Charcot." M.Phil. thesis, University College London, 1990.

Brockliss, Laurence W. B. "The Development of the Spa in Seventeenth-Century France." In *The Medical History of Waters and Spas,* ed. Roy Porter, *Medical History,* Supplement No. 10. London: Wellcome Institute for the History of Medicine, 1990, pp. 23–47.

———. "L'Enseignement médical et la Révolution: essai de réévaluation." *Histoire de l'éducation* 42 (1989), 79–110.

———. *French Higher Education in the Seventeenth and Eighteenth Centuries: A Cultural History.* Oxford: Clarendon Press, 1987.

Bulletin de l'Académie (Royale, Impériale, Nationale) de Médecine.

Cabanès, Dr. Augustin. "Notice historique sur l'Académie de Médecine." *Gazette des Hôpitaux* 66 (1893), 23–26.

Charle, Cristophe. *Les Élites de la République, 1880–1900*. Fayard, 1987.

Charle, Christophe, and Telkes, Eva. *Les Professeurs de la Faculté des Sciences de Paris: dictionnaire biographique, 1901–1939*. Institut National de la Recherche Pédagogique–Éditions du CNRS, 1989.

———. *Les Professeurs du Collége de France: dictionnaire biographique, 1901–1939*. Institut National de la Recherche Pédagogique–Éditions du CNRS, 1988.

Claus, Alisa. *Every Child a Lion: The Origins of Maternal and Infant Health Policy in the United States and France, 1890–1920*. Ithaca, N.Y.: Cornell University Press, 1993.

Coleman, William. *Yellow Fever in the North: The Methods of Early Epidemiology*. Madison: University of Wisconsin Press, 1987.

———. "The Cognitive Basis of the Discipline: Claude Bernard on Physiology." *Isis* 76 (1985), 49–70.

———. *Death Is a Social Disease: Public Health and Political Economy in Early Industrial France*. Madison: University of Wisconsin Press, 1982.

Cosma-Muller, Pascale. "Entre science et commerce: les eaux en France à la fin de l'Ancien Régime." *Historical Reflections* 9 (1982), 249–63.

Crawford, Elisabeth. "The Prize System of the Academy of Sciences, 1850–1914." In *The Organization of Science and Technology in France, 1808–1914*, ed. Robert Fox and George Weisz. Cambridge: Cambridge University Press, and Paris: Éditions de la Maison des Sciences de l'Homme, 1980), pp. 283–307.

Crosland, Maurice. *Science under Control: The French Academy of Sciences, 1795–1914*. Cambridge: Cambridge University Press, 1992.

Crosland, Maurice, and Gálvez, Antonio. "The Emergence of Research Grants within the Prize System of the Academy of Sciences, 1795–1914." *Social Studies of Science* 19 (1989), 71–100.

Cuvier, Georges. *Recueil des éloges historiques lus dans les séances publiques de l'Institut Royale de France*. 3 vols. Strasbourg: Levrault, 1819–27.

Darmon, Pierre. *La Longue Traque de la variole: les pionniers de la médecine préventive*. Perrin, 1986.

Daudet, Léon. *Les Morticoles*. Bernard Grasset, 1984.

Daumard, Adeline. *Les Bourgeois et la bourgeoisie en France depuis 1815*. Aubier, 1987.

———. *La Bourgeoisie parisienne de 1815 à 1848*. Éditions S.E.V.P.E.N., 1962).

Daumard, Adeline, and Furet, François. *Structures et relations sociales à Paris au milieu de XVIIIe siècle*. A. Colin, 1961.

Debré, Robert. *L'Honneur de vivre: témoignages*. Herman et Stock, 1972.

Delaunay, Paul. *La Vie médicale aux XVIe, XVIIe et XVIIIe siècles*. Hippocrate, 1935.

———. *Les Médecins, la Restauration et la révolution de 1830*. Extrait de la Médecine Internationale Illustrée, 1931.

———. *Le Monde médical parisien au dix–huitième siècle*. Rousset, 1906.

Desaive J. P., et al., eds. *Médecins, climat et épidémies à la fin du XVIIIe siècle*. Mouton, 1972.

Dictionnaire de médecine, 1st ed. 21 vols. Béchet Jeune, 1822–28.

Dictionnaire de médecine, 2nd ed. 30 vols. Béchet Jeune, 1832–46.

Dictionnaire des sciences médicales. 60 vols. Panckouke, 1812–22.

Dictionnaire des sciences médicales: biographie médicale, 7 vols. Panckoucke, 1820–25.

Duffin, Jacalyn. "Vitalism and Organicism in the Philosophy of R.-T.-H. Laënnec." *Bulletin of the History of Medicine* 62 (1988), 525–45.

———. "Laënnec: entre la pathologie et la clinique." Thèse 3e cycle, Université de Paris I, 1985.

Duhot, Émile, and Fontan, M. *Que sais-je? le thermalisme*. 2nd ed. Presses Universitaires de France, 1972.

Durand-Fardel, Raymond. *L'Internat en médecine et en chirurgie des hôpitaux et hospices civils de Paris: centenaire de l'internat, 1802–1902.* G. Steinheil, 1903.

Dureau, Dr. A. "Les Vicissitudes du logement de l'Académie de Médecine." *Chronique médicale* 2 (1895), 157–203.

Ebrard, Guy. *Le Thermalisme en France: situation actuelle et perspectives d'avenir. Rapport au Président de la République.* La Documentation Française, 1981.

Ellis, Jack D. *The Physician-Legislators of France: Medicine and Politics in the Early Third Republic.* Cambridge: Cambridge University Press, 1990.

English, Peter C. "Emergence of Rheumatic Fever in the Nineteenth Century." *Milbank Quarterly* 67 (1989), suppl. 1, 33–49.

Fabre, Dr., ed. *Dictionnaire des dictionnaires de médecine français et étrangers.* Baillière, 1850.

Fay-Sallois, Fanny. *Les Nourrices à Paris au XIXe siècle.* Payot, 1980.

Fleury, Maurice de. *Le Médecin.* Hachette, 1927.

Forgan, Sophie. "Context, Image and Function: A Preliminary Enquiry into the Architecture of Scientific Societies." *British Journal of the History of Science* 19 (1986), 89–113.

Fossard, Jacques. *Histoire polymorphe de l'internat en médecine et chirurgie des hôpitaux et hospices civils de Paris.* 2 vols. Grenoble: C.P.B.F., 1982.

Ganière, Paul. *L'Académie de Médecine: ses origines et son histoire.* Maloine, 1964.

Gauja, Pierre. *Les Fondations de l'Académie des Sciences (1881–1915).* Gauthier-Villars, 1917.

Geison, Gerald L. "'Divided We Stand': Physiologists and Clinicians in the American Context." In *The Therapeutic Revolution: Essays in the Social History of American Medicine,* ed. Morris J. Vogel and Charles E. Rosenberg. Philadelphia: University of Pennsylvania Press, 1979, pp. 135–57.

Gelfand, Toby. "Medical Nemesis in Paris, 1894: Léon Daudet's *Les Morticoles.*" *Bulletin of the History of Medicine* 60 (1986), 155–76.

———. *Professionalizing Modern Medicine: Paris Surgeons and Medical Science and Institutions in the Eighteenth Century.* Westport, Conn.: Greenwood Press, 1980.

Genty, Maurice. *Les Biographies médicales,* 6 vols. Baillière, 1927–39.

Gerbod, Paul. "Les 'Fièvres thermales' en France au XIXe siècle." *Revue historique* 277 (1987), 309–34.

Geyer-Kordesch, Johanna. "Court Physicians and State Regulation in Eighteenth-Century Prussia: The Emergence of Medical Science and the Demystification of the Body." In *Medicine at the Courts of Europe, 1500–1837,* ed. Vivian Nutton. London: Routledge, 1990.

Gillispie, Charles C. *Science and Polity in France at the End of the Old Régime.* Princeton, N.J.: Princeton University Press, 1980.

Goldstein, Jan. *Console and Classify: The French Psychiatric Profession in the Nineteenth Century.* Cambridge: Cambridge University Press, 1987.

Gosset, Antonin. *Chirurgie, chirurgiens.* Gallimard, 1941.

Goubert, Jean-Pierre. *La Conquête de l'eau.* Robert Laffont, 1986.

Grenier, Lise, ed. *Villes d'eaux en France.* Édition Institut Français d'Architecture, 1985.

Groopman, Leonard C. "The *Internat des Hôpitaux de Paris*: The Shaping and Transformation of the French Medical Elite, 1802–1914." Ph.D. diss., Harvard University, 1986.

Guéniot, Alexandre. *Souvenirs anecdotiques et médicaux, 1856–1871.* Baillière, 1927.

Guitard, E. H. *Le Prestigieux Passé des eaux minérales.* Société d'histoire de la pharmacie, 1951.

Hacking, Ian. *The Taming of Chance.* Cambridge: Cambridge University Press, 1990.

Hahn, Roger. *The Anatomy of a Scientific Institution: The Paris Academy of Sciences, 1666–1803.* Berkeley: University of California Press, 1971.

Hannaway, Caroline. "From Private Hygiene to Public Health." In *Public Health*, ed. T. Ogawa. Osaka: Taniguchi Foundation, 1981.

————. "Medicine, Public Welfare and the State in Eighteenth-Century France: The Société Royale de Médecine of Paris (1776–1793)." Ph.D. diss., Johns Hopkins University, 1974.

Herzlich, Claudine, et al. *Cinquante ans d'exercice de la médecine en France: carrières et pratiques des médecins français. 1930–1980.* Éditions INSERM, 1993.

Hildreth, Martha L. *Doctors, Bureaucrats, and Public Health, 1888–1902.* New York: Garland, 1987.

Hillemand, P., and Gilbrin, E. "Le père Elisée (1753–1817): Premier Chirurgien de Louis XVIII." *Histoire des sciences médicales* 14 (1980), 233–40.

Hillemand, P., Gilbrin, E., and Segal, A. "Le père Elisée et la réforme des études médicales." *Histoire des sciences médicales* 15 (1981), 159–65.

Huard, Pierre. *Sciences, médecine, pharmacie de la Revolution à l'Empire, 1789–1815.* Édition Roger Dacosta, 1970.

Huard, Pierre, and Imbault-Huart, M.-J. "La Première Séance de l'Académie Royale de médecine." *Bulletin de l'Académie Nationale de Médecine* 155 (1971), 414–23.

Huguet, Françoise. *Les Professeurs de la Faculté de Médecine de Paris: dictionnaire biographique, 1794–1939.* Institut National de la Recherche Pédagogique-Éditions du CNRS, 1991.

Imbault-Huart, M.-J. *L'École Pratique de Dissection de Paris de 1750 à 1822, ou l'influence du concept de médecine pratique et de médecine d'observation dans l'enseignement médico-chirurgical au XVIIIe siècle et au début du XIXe siècle.* Lille: Service de réproduction des thèses Université de Lille, 1975.

Jamot, Christian. *Thermalisme et villes thermales en France.* Clermont-Ferrand: Institut d' Études du Massif Central, 1988.

Jardine, Nicholas. "The Laboratory Revolution in Medicine as Rhetorical and Aesthetic Accomplishment." In *The Laboratory Revolution in Medicine*, ed. A. Cunningham and P. Williams. Cambridge: Cambridge University Press, 1992, pp. 304–23.

Jones, Colin. "The *Médecins du Roi* at the End of the *Ancien Régime* and in the French Revolution." In *Medicine at the Courts of Europe, 1500–1837*, ed. Vivian Nutton. London: Routledge, 1990, pp. 209–61.

Keel, Othmar. "The Politics of Health and the Institutionalization of Clinical Practice in Europe in the Second Half of the Eighteenth Century." In *William Hunter and the Eighteenth-Century Medical World*, ed. W. F. Bynum and R. Porter. Cambridge: Cambridge University Press, 1985, pp. 207–56.

————. "Cabanis et la généalogie de la médecine clinique." Ph.D. diss., McGill University, 1977.

La Berge, Ann F. *Mission and Method: The Early-Nineteenth-Century Public Health Movement.* Cambridge: Cambridge University Press, 1992.

La Berge, Ann F., and Feingold, Mordechai, eds. *French Medical Culture in the Nineteenth Century.* Amsterdam: Rodopi, 1994.

Latour, Bruno. *The Pasteurization of France.* Cambridge, Mass.: Harvard University Press, 1987.

Le Gendre, Paul. *Du Quartier Latin à l'Académie (réminiscences).* Maloine, 1930.

————. *Un médecin philosophe: Charles Bouchard, son oeuvre et son temps (1837–1915).* Masson, 1924.

Léonard, Jacques. "La Restauration et la profession médicale." *Historical Reflections* 9 (1982), 69–84.

————. *Les Médecins de l'ouest au XIXe siècle.* Lyon: Honoré Champion, 1976.

Lesch, John E. "The Paris Academy of Medicine and Experimental Science, 1820–1848." In *The Investigative Enterprise: Experimental Physiology in Nineteenth-Century Medicine*, ed. William Coleman and Frederick L. Holmes. Berkeley: University of California Press, 1988, pp. 100–138.

———. *Science and Medicine in France: The Emergence of Experimental Physiology, 1790–1855*. Cambridge, Mass.: Harvard University Press, 1984.

Littré, Émile. *Dictionnaire de médecine, de chirurgie, de pharmacie de l'art vétérinaire et des sciences qui s'y rapportent*. 16th ed. Baillière, 1886.

Littré, Émile, and Robin, Charles. *Dictionnaire de médecine, de chirurgie, de pharmacie, des sciences accessoires et de l'art vétérinaire*. 12th ed. Baillière, 1865.

Louis, Antoine. *Éloges lus dans les séances publiques de l'Académie de Chirurgie, 1750–1792*, ed. F. Dubois d'Amiens. Baillière, 1859.

Maindron, Ernest. *Les Fondations des prix à l'Académie des Sciences; les lauréats de l'Académie, 1714–1880*. Gauthiers-Villars, 1881.

Maretzki, Thomas. "Cultural Variation in Biomedicine: The *Kur* in West Germany." *Medical Anthropology Quarterly* 3 (1989), 22–35.

Matthews, John Rosser III. "Mathematics and the Quest for Medical Certainty: The Emergence of Clinical Trials, 1800–1950." Ph.D. diss., Duke University, 1992.

Maulitz, Russell C. *Morbid Appearances: The Anatomy of Pathology in the Early Nineteenth Century*. Cambridge: Cambridge University Press, 1987.

———. "Channel Crossing: The Lure of French Pathology for English Medical Students, 1816–36." *Bulletin of the History of Medicine* 55 (1981), 475–96.

Mémoires de l'Académie (Royale, Impériale, Nationale) de Médecine.

Ministère de l'Instruction Publique. *Enquêtes et documents relatifs à l'enseignement supérieur*. 124 vols. 1883–1929.

Mitchell, Allan. *The Divided Path: The German Influence on Social Reform in France after 1870*. Chapel Hill: University of North Carolina Press, 1991.

Muller, Pascale. "Les Eaux minérales en France à la fin du 18e siècle." Mémoire de maîtrise, Université de Paris I, 1975.

Murphy, Terry D. "Medical Knowledge and Statistical Methods in Early Nineteenth-Century France." *Medical History* 25 (1981), 301–19.

Nora, Pierre, ed. *Les Lieux de mémoire*. 3 vols. Gallimard, 1984–93.

Nouveau Dictionnaire de médecine et de chirurgie pratique. 40 vols. Baillière, 1864–86.

Nye, Robert A. *Masculinity and Male Codes of Honor in Modern France*. Oxford: Oxford University Press, 1993.

Nye, Robert A. *Crime, Madness and Politics in Modern France: The Medical Concept of National Decline*. Princeton, N.J.: Princeton University Press, 1984.

Odic, Charles. "Les Événements du 18 novembre 1822." Thèse en médecine, Université de Paris, 1921.

Outram, Dorinda. "Before Objectivity: Women, Wives and Cultural Reproduction in Nineteenth-Century French Science." In *Uneasy Careers and Intimate Lives: Women in Science, 1789–1968*, ed. P. Abir-Am and D. Outram. New Brunswick, N.J.: Rutgers University Press, 1987.

———. *Georges Cuvier: Vocation, Science and Authority in Post-Revolutionary France*. Manchester: University of Manchester Press, 1984.

———. "The Language of Natural Power: The *Éloges* of Georges Cuvier and the Public Language of Nineteenth Century Science." *History of Science* 16 (1978), 153–78.

Pariset, Etienne. *Histoire des membres de l'Académie Royale de Médecine*. 2 vols. Ballière, 1850.

Paul, Charles B. *Science and Immortality: The Éloges of the Paris Academy of Sciences*

(1699–1791). Berkeley: University of California Press, 1980.

Payer, Lynn. *Medicine and Culture*. New York: Henry Holt, 1988.

Peisse, Louis. *La Médecine et les médecins; philosophie, doctrines, institutions, critiques, moeurs et biographies médicales*. 2 vols. Baillière, 1857.

Picard, Jean-François. "Poussée scientifique ou demande de médecins? La recherche médicale en France de l'Institut national d'hygiène à l'INSERM." *Science Sociales et Santé* 10 (1992), 47–106.

Pichevin, R. "La Première Académie de médecine de Paris." *Bulletin de la Société Française d'Histoire de la médecine* 12 (1913), 196–231.

Piquemal, Jacques. "Succès et décadence de la méthode numérique en France à l'époque de Pierre-Charles-Alexandre Louis." *France médicale* 250 (1974), 11–22.

Postel, Jacques. "Philippe Pinel et le mythe fondateur de la psychiatrie française." *Psychoanalyse à l'Univesité* 4 (1979), 197–244.

Quénu, Jean. *Notre internat*. Doin, 1971.

Ramsey, Matthew. "Academic Medicine and Medical Industrialism: The Regulation of Secret Remedies in France." In *French Medical Culture in the Nineteenth Century*, ed. Ann F. La Berge and Mordechai Feingold. Amsterdam: Rodopi, 1994.

———. *Professional and Popular Medicine in France, 1770–1830: The Social World of Medical Practice*. Cambridge: Cambridge University Press, 1988.

———. "Property Rights and the Rights to Health: The Regulation of Secret Remedies in France, 1789–1815." In *Medical Fringe and Medical Orthodoxy, 1750–1850*, ed. W. F. Bynum and Roy Porter. London: Croom Helm, 1987, pp. 79–105.

———. "Traditional Medicine and Medical Enlightenment: The Regulation of Secret Remedies in the Ancien Régime." *Historical Reflections* 9 (1982), 215–32.

Recueil de travaux du Comité Consultatif d'Hygiène Publique de la France.

Richet, Charles. *Souvenirs d'un physiologiste*. J. Peyronnet, 1933.

Riley, James C. *The Eighteenth-Century Campaign to Avoid Disease*. London: Macmillan, 1987.

Roche, Daniel. *Le Siècle des lumières en province: académies et académiciens provinciaux, 1680–1789*. Mouton, 1978.

———. "Talents, raison et sacrifice: les médecins vus par eux-mêmes." *Annales ESC* 32 (1977), 866–86.

Roger, Henri. *Entre deux siècles: souvenirs d'un vieux biologiste*. L'Expansion Scientifique Française, 1947.

Rosen, George. *From Medical Police to Social Medicine: Essays on the History of Health Care*. New York: Science History Publications, 1974.

Rosenberg, Charles. "The Therapeutic Revolution." *Perspectives in Biology and Medicine* 20 (1977), 485–506.

Rosenkrantz, Barbara G. "The Search for Professional Order in Nineteenth Century American Medicine." In *Proceedings of the International Congress of the History of Science*. Tokyo: Taniguchi Foundation, 1975, pp. 113–24.

Roubaud, Dr. Félix. *Histoire du statistique de l'Académie Nationale de Médecine depuis sa fondation jusqu'à ce jour*. Baillière, 1852.

Rouxeau, Alfred. *Laënnec après 1806*. Baillière, 1920.

Rusnock, Andrea A. "On the Quantification of Things Human: Medicine and Political Arithmetic in Enlightenment England and France." Ph.D. diss., Princeton University, 1990.

Salomon-Bayet, Claire, ed. *Pasteur et la révolution pastorienne*. Payot, 1986.

Shinn, Terry. "Science, Tocqueville, and the State: The Organization of Knowledge in Modern France." *Social Research* 59 (1992), 533–66.

Short, S. E. D. "Physicians, Science, and Status: Issues in the Professionalization of Anglo-American Medicine in the Nineteenth Century." *Medical History* 27 (1983), 51–68.

Sigerist, Henry E. "American Spas in Historical Perspective." *Bulletin of the History of Medicine* 11 (1942), 133–47.

Staum, Martin S. *Cabanis: Enlightenment and Medical Philosophy in France*. Princeton: N.J.: Princeton University Press, 1980.

Sussman, George D. "Étienne Pariset: A Medical Career in Government under the Restoration." *Journal of the History of Medicine* 26 (1971), 52–74.

———. "From Yellow Fever to Cholera: A Study of French Government Policy, Medical Professionalism and Popular Movements in the Epidemic Crises of the Restoration and July Monarchy." Ph.D. diss., Yale University, 1971.

Triaire, Paul, ed. *Bretonneau et ses correspondants*. 2 vols. Alcan, 1892.

Tröhler, Ulrich. "Quantification in British Medicine and Surgery 1750–1830 with Special References to Its Introduction into Therapeutics." Ph.D. diss., University College London, 1978.

Vicq d'Azyr, F. *Oeuvres de Vicq d'Azyr, recueillis et publiés avec des notes et un discours sur sa vie et ses ouvrages*, ed. J. L. Moreau de la Sarthe. 6 vols. Duprat-Duverger, 1805.

Violet, Isabelle. "Le Mythe de la libération des aliénés de Bicêtre par Philippe Pinel pendant la Révolution Française." Travail d'Étude et de Recherches, Université de Paris IV–Sorbonne, U.E.R. d'Histoire.

Wallon, Armand. *La Vie quotidienne dans les villes d'eaux, 1850–1914*. Hachette, 1981.

Warner, John Harley *The Therapeutic Perspective: Medical Practice, Knowledge and Identity in America, 1820–1885*. Cambridge, Mass.: Harvard University Press, 1986.

———. "Science in Medicine." *Osiris*, 2nd ser. 1 (1985), 37–58.

Weiner, Dora B. *The Citizen Patient in Revolutionary and Imperial Paris*. Baltimore: Johns Hopkins University Press, 1993.

Weisz, George. *The Emergence of Modern Universities in France, 1863–1914*. Princeton: N.J.: Princeton University Press, 1983.

———. "Reform and Conflict in French Medical Education, 1870–1914." In *The Organization of Science and Technology in France, 1808–1914*, ed. Robert Fox and George Weisz. Cambridge: Cambridge University Press, 1980.

———. "The Politics of Medical Professionalization in France, 1845–1848." *Journal of Social History* 12 (1978), 3–30.

Yver, Colette (Antoinette Huzard). *Princesse de science*. Calmann-Lévy, 1907.

Zweibel-Muller, Pascale." *La Société de l'École de médecine et la santé publique en France de 1801 à 1821*." Thèse 3e cycle, École des Hautes Études en Sciences Sociales, no. 1663.

Index